Congenital Heart Disease in Adults

The publication of this monograph was supported by a research project of the Ministry of Health of the Czech Republic No 00000064203 – 6306.

Congenital Heart ♦ Disease in Adults

Jana Popelová MD PhD
Associate Professor of Medicine
Director, Program of Congenital Heart Disease in Adults
Department of Cardiac Surgery
Hospital Na Homolce
Prague
Czech Republic

Erwin Oechslin MD FRCPC FESC
Director, Adult Congenital Heart Disease
Peter Munk Cardiac Centre
University Health Network/Toronto General Hospital
Toronto, ON
USA

Harald Kaemmerer MD VMD FESC
Professor of Internal Medicine
Deutsches Herzzentrum München
Klinik für Kinderkardiologie und Angeborene Herzfehler
München
Germany

Martin G St John Sutton FRCP FAHA FACC FESC FASE
John W Bryfogle Professor of Cardiac Imaging
University of Pennsylvania Medical Center
Division of Cardiology
Philadelphia, PA
USA

With illustrations by

Pavel Žáček MD PhD
Department of Cardiac Surgery
Charles University Hospital
Hradec Králové
Czech Republic

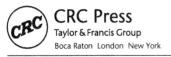

CRC Press
Taylor & Francis Group
Boca Raton London New York

CRC Press is an imprint of the
Taylor & Francis Group, an **informa** business

First edition: © Grada Publishing as, 2003, Praha, Czech Republic (in Czech)

First published 2008 by Informa UK Ltd

Published 2019 by CRC Press
Taylor & Francis Group
6000 Broken Sound Parkway NW, Suite 300
Boca Raton, FL 33487-2742

© 2008 by Taylor & Francis Group, LLC
CRC Press is an imprint of Taylor & Francis Group, an Informa business

First issued in paperback 2019

No claim to original U.S. Government works

ISBN 13: 978-0-367-45257-5 (pbk)
ISBN 13: 978-1-84184-584-5 (hbk)

References

Deanfield J, Thaulow E, Warnes C, et al. Management of grown up congenital heart disease. The task force on the management of grown up congenital heart disease of the European Society of Cardiology. European Heart J 2003; 24: 1035–84.
Therrien J, Dore A, Gersonz W, et al. Canadian Cardiovascular Society Consensus Conference 2001 update: recommendations for the management of adults with congenital heart disease. Part I. Can J Cardiol 2001; 17(9): 940–59.
Therrien J, Gatzoulis M, Graham T, et al. Canadian Cardiovascular Society Consensus Conference 2001 update: recommendations for the management of adults with congenital heart disease. Part II. Can J Cardiol 2001; 17(10): 1029–50.
Therrien J, Warnes C, Daliento L, et al. Canadian Cardiovascular Society Consensus Conference 2001 update: recommendations for the management of adults with congenital heart disease. Part III. Can J Cardiol 2001; 17(11): 1135–58.

Contents

Foreword

In the latter part of the 19th century, congenital heart disease (CHD) was of little clinical interest because diagnoses were almost exclusively made at necropsy, and treatment was wholly lacking. In 1936, Maude Abbott's *Atlas of Congenital Heart Disease* appeared,[1] and just over a decade later, Helen Taussig's *Congenital Malformations of the Heart* followed.[2] Even so, CHD in adults was not even a theoretical consideration. However, after the 1940s, advances in surgery and in diagnostic techniques resulted in what the authors aptly characterize as 'one of the biggest success stories in medicine.'

In 1973, 'the changing population of congenital heart disease' was recognized in the literature,[3] and CHD in adults began to evolve as a new subspecialty. In 1983, *Congenital Heart Disease After Surgery*[4] highlighted the impressive benefits of operation, but recognized that benefits were qualified by postoperative residua and sequelae that required medical care well into adulthood if not for a lifetime. In the United States, the first book to carry the title *Congenital Heart Disease in Adults*,[5] currently in its third edition, appeared in 1991. In 2003, *Diagnosis and Management of Adult Congenital Heart Disease* was published in the United Kingdom,[6] and, in 2005, the first Japanese text on Adult Congenital Heart Disease was published.[7] And now *Congenital Heart Disease in Adults* appears from Eastern Europe in a fine English translation (Informa Healthcare, London). Originally published in Czech in 2003, the book consists of 23 chapters, well constructed and well illustrated. The major congenital malformations – unoperated and postoperative – are featured, and are nicely supplemented by chapters on the historical background, the prevalence, the heterotaxies,

cyanosis in adulthood, postoperative residua and sequelae, psychosocial problems, and terminology. The literature is current.

The new English translation from the Czech Republic is a welcome geographical addition to the recent books on adult CHD from the United States, the United Kingdom, and Japan – all gratifying testimonies to the worldwide interest in this still growing cardiovascular subspecialty.

Joseph K Perloff MD
Streisand/American Heart Association Professor of Medicine and Pediatrics, Emeritus
Founding Director, Ahmanson/UCLA Adult Congenital Heart Disease Center

References

1. Abbott ME. Atlas of Congenital Cardiac Disease. New York: American Heart Association; 1936.
2. Taussig HB. Congenital Malformations of the Heart. New York: Commonwealth Fund; 1947.
3. Perloff JK. Pediatric congenital cardiac becomes a postoperative adult. The changing population of congenital heart disease. Circulation 1973; 47: 606–19.
4. Engle MA, Perloff K. Congenital Heart Disease After Surgery. Yorke Medical Books: New York; 1983.
5. Perloff JK, Child JS. Congenital Heart Disease in Adults. WB Saunders Co: Philadelphia; 1991.
6. Gatzoulis MA, Webb GD, Daubeney PEF. Diagnosis and Management of Adult Congenital Heart Disease. Churchill Livingstone: London; 2003.
7. Niwa K. New Illustrated Textbook of Cardiology. Adult Congenital Heart Disease. Medical View Co Ltd: Tokyo; 2005.

Preface

The outcome of surgical correction of congenital heart disease (CHD) has reached major advances over the past 30 years. New and more complex surgical and interventional procedures, applicable in infants, are emerging. As a result, some cardiologists have started to believe that CHDs in adulthood are of little importance, because they have been either surgically managed in childhood or they are of little hemodynamic significance. They also believed that severe, inoperable CHD cannot reach adulthood. Because of this misconception, but also because of its inherent complexity, until recently CHD was outside the main focus of interest in adult cardiologists.

However, the numbers of adults with CHD are today growing rapidly. Patients undergoing surgery as children in the 1950s–1970s have now become middle-aged individuals. The 1980s saw the advent of new surgical procedures and catheter-based interventions, the long-term outcomes of which we are now learning of. In addition, patients undergoing palliative surgical procedures in childhood also survive and, if provided reasonable conservative therapy, some patients with inoperable CHD may also live to reach adulthood. Some types of CHD, considered of little importance in childhood, may require surgery in adulthood. CHDs which are first operated on in adulthood may have a worse prognosis and more residual findings than if corrected in childhood.

Residual findings and arrhythmias may not manifest themselves clinically until some time after surgery. Even hemodynamically significant residual defects may be tolerated well for some time; however, they result in structural changes in the myocardium. These do not manifest themselves by clinical problems until several decades after surgery. The problem is, by that time, the myocardial changes may have already become irreversible. This explains why all these patients must be on constant follow-up and in time indicated for intervention or reoperation.

CHDs in adulthood show a low prevalence and huge heterogeneity. No controlled randomized studies in adults with CHD which furnish data to use in our decision-making have been conducted to date. Current guidelines are based on empirical observations and on data provided by studies involving small numbers of patients, and often date several decades back when the range of diagnostic and therapeutic options was much smaller compared with the arsenal available today. Criteria for indication and management applicable to children cannot be automatically applied to CHD in adulthood. In adulthood, CHD are joined by other conditions and complications such as coronary artery disease, hypertension, arrhythmia, acquired heart disease, diabetes mellitus, chronic obstructive lung disease, renal and hepatic dysfunction, impaired coagulation, and so on, appreciably increasing the risk associated with surgery. Making decisions about future strategy in adults is often very difficult. A decision has to be made between surgery carrying a risk and a life limited by CHD, even though these patients may have become accustomed to, and have come to terms with, their condition. Even today, the outcome of operation and reoperation for CHD in adulthood depends primarily on the body of experience that the department of cardiac surgery has with surgery for CHD and subsequent postoperative care.

The issue of CHD is becoming an integral part of adult cardiology and is receiving increased attention worldwide.

Jana Popelová

1

History

Until the early 20th century, it was difficult, if not impossible, to establish the diagnosis of congenital heart disease (CHD) during a patient's lifetime. As a result, CHD drew mostly the attention of pathological anatomists.[1–3] Remarkably, as late as 1934, only one of 62 cases of atrial septal defects demonstrated by autopsy was diagnosed during a patient's lifetime.[4]

The first to describe an open arterial duct was the Greek physician Galenos in the 2nd century AD.[5] In the 15th century, Leonardo da Vinci recognized a patent foramen ovale. Tetralogy of Fallot, while actually described by the Danish anatomist and theologian Nicolas Steno as early as 1673, was not diagnosed in vivo until 1888, by Arthur Fallot, hence the term.[6] In 1879, Henri Roger not only described the morphology but also the clinical features of a minor ventricular septal defect, consequently sometimes referred to as Roger's disease.[7]

The 20th century witnessed a remarkable development of diagnostic methods followed, after World War II, by a turbulent development of cardiac surgery.

Diagnosis of congenital heart disease

Several imaging modalities are used to confirm CHD when it is suggested by the symptoms and physical examination. In previous years, diagnosis and treatment of congenital cardiac disease often depended on cardiac catheterization. In the past decades, however, the number of diagnostic catheterization procedures has steadily declined in favor of interventional procedures, and imaging methods have shifted toward the use of less invasive and noninvasive techniques. Echocardiography, magnetic resonance imaging (MRI) and computerized tomography (CT) have gained a well-established role in the morphological and functional assessment of the heart and the great vessels.[8]

Noninvasive echocardiography started in the 1970s–1980s. In the late 1980s, 80% of children were referred for surgery exclusively on the basis of noninvasive diagnosis, without catheterization. As adults are much more difficult to examine by ultrasound than children, transesophageal echocardiography, affording accurate diagnosis of CHD in

adults, was another major step forward. Three-dimensional (3D) reconstruction, intravascular ultrasound and tissue velocity imaging may yield new insights into the anatomy and function of the heart.

MRI is extremely useful for delineation of the anatomy of the heart and great vessels, as well as for nonquantifiable assessment of blood-flow characteristics. The high resolution of this technique provides excellent spatial separation without limitations in the orientation of views. The development of specific techniques (fast gradient-echo, velocity mapping, echo planar imaging, myocardial tagging, and spectroscopy) allows quantification of physiological and pathological hemodynamic conditions. In particular, 3D-MRI reconstruction clearly demonstrates complex arrangements and clarifies morphology of complex CHD. Using MRI-fluoroscopy techniques, some centers have started to carry out balloon angioplasty of stenotic lesions, as well as radiofrequency ablation under MRI guidance.[9] The late gadolinium enhancement technique provides assesment of the fibrosis and scarring of the myocard of the left or right ventricle. The clinical indications for MRI in adults with congenital cardiac disease are well established for the evaluation of anatomy and/or function. It is considered a gold standard for the evaluation of the systolic function of the right ventricle.

Several newer CT technologies (e.g. spiral and multislice CT, dual-source CT) are in use as minimally invasive procedures: the high resolution of the images provide excellent spatial separation. A CT angiography is an important examination before reoperation.

Unfortunately, neither MRI, nor CT, nor ultrasound can accurately define intraluminal pressures and pulmonary vascular resistance. Therefore, catheterization is currently the only way to measure systemic or pulmonary pressure and resistance.[10]

However, today, catheter-based methods are no longer used for diagnostic purposes only, and may replace certain cardiac surgical procedures in CHD.[11,12] Balloon atrioseptostomy in the critically ill newborn with uncorrected transposition of the great arteries was reported as early as 1966;[13] balloon percutaneous valvuloplasty of pulmonary artery stenosis in 1982;[14] and balloon valvuloplasty of aortic stenosis in 1984.[15] Balloon angioplasty, possibly combined with stenting, can be used to manage aortic recoarctation, or even native aortic coarctation.[16–20]

Table 1.1   *First transcatheter procedures in congenital heart disease (CHD)*

Procedure	Year	Reference
Balloon atrioseptostomy	1966	Rashkind, Miller[13]
Balloon valvuloplasty of pulmonary stenosis	1982	Kan, White, Mitchell et al[14]
Balloon valvuloplasty of aortic stenosis	1984	Lababidi, Wu, Walls[15]
Balloon dilatation of aortic coarctation	1983	Lock, Bass, Amplatz et al[16]
Transcatheter closure of patent arterial duct	1966	Porstmann, Wierny, Warnke[21]
Transcatheter closure of atrial septal defect	1974	King, Mills[22]
	1997	Mašura, Gavora, Formanek, Hijazi[23]
Transcatheter closure of ventricular septal defect	1987	Lock, Block, McKay, Baim, Keane[24]

Table 1.2   *Milestones in the history of surgery for congenital heart disease (CHD)*

Anomaly	First surgical treatment	Surgeon
Patent ductus arteriosus	1938	R Gross, Boston[25]
		EK Frey, Düsseldorf
Aortic coarctation	1944	C Crafoord, G Nylin, Stockholm[27]
	1945	RE Gross, CA Hufnagel, Boston
Aortopulmonary shunt in a cyanotic patient (Blalock–Taussig anastomosis)	1944	A Blalock, Baltimore[28]
Fallot's tetralogy	1954	CW Lillehei, Minneapolis
Atrial switch for transposition of the great arteries	1958	A Senning, Stockholm[30]
	1963	WT Mustard, Toronto[31]
Arterial switch for transposition of the great arteries	1975	AD Jatene, Brasilien[32]
	1976	MH Yacoub, London[33]
Univentricular heart total cavo-pulmonary connection (TCPC)	1968	F Fontan, Bordeau[34]
	1988	M de Leval, London[37]

Closing a patent arterial duct was the first catheter-based closing procedure in CHD, performed by Porstmann in 1966.[21] After the advent of technically more sophisticated devices, and detachable spirals in particular, interventional closure of patent arterial ducts has found even broader acceptance. It is not only adult patients with CHD who have benefited from the development of the interventional closure of an atrial septal defect or a patent foramen ovale. While the possibility of catheter-based closure of atrial septal defects was initially reported in 1974,[22] the method has found a wide acceptance since the 1990s, when technically sophisticated occluders such as the Amplatzer septal occluder became available.[23] The transcatheter closure of ventricular septal defect is used for muscular defects, and for some perimembranous ventricular septal adefects.[24]

Cardiac surgery

The first successful ligation of an open arterial duct was undertaken in 1938 in the USA by Robert E Gross in Boston,[25] and independently by Emil Karl Frey in Germany.[26] The first surgery of coarctation of the aorta was performed by Clarence Crafoord from Stockholm, using Gross's technique, in 1944.[27] Palliative subclavian and pulmonary anastomosis in tetralogy of Fallot was first created by Alfred Blalock, as suggested by the pediatric cardiologist Helen Taussig, in 1944.[28] While the first to operate on an atrial septal defect on the closed heart was Sondergaard in 1950, an atrial septal defect was closed in the open heart using direct suture by Gross in 1952. Closure of a ventricular septal defect and correction of tetralogy of Fallot in the open heart and 'on pump' was pioneered by Lillehei in 1954 and Kirklin (in the USA) in 1955.[29] Techniques of managing transposition of the great arteries by redirecting venous return at atrial level were proposed by Ake Senning from Stockholm[30] and by William Mustard from Toronto.[31] Anatomical correction of transposition ('arterial switch') was devised by Adibo Jatene in Sao Paulo[32] and Magdi Yacoub in London.[33]

Until the late 1960s, patients with univentricular circulation were significantly impaired. In 1968, the concept of total right heart bypass became reality, when Fontan performed his first atriopulmonary connection in order to place the pulmonary and systemic circulation in series in a patient with tricuspid atresia with pulmonary stenosis. Since the initial report, published in 1971 by Fontan and Baudet,[34] the original technique of Fontan has undergone several modifications. Total cavo-pulmonary connection (TCPC) was introduced in 1988 by M de Leval. Meanwhile, the Fontan operation has been extensively applied not only for patients with tricuspid atresia but also for palliation of a wide variety of complex cyanotic congenital heart defects with only one ventricle, precluding biventricular repair.[35,36]

References

1. Rokitansky C. Die Defecte der Scheidewande des Herzens. Vienne, 1875.
2. Ebstein W. Uber einen sehr seltenen Fall von Insufficienz der Valvula tricuspidalis, bedingt durch eine angeborene hochgradige Missbildung derselben. Arch Anat Physiol 1866; 33: 238.
3. Baillie M. Morbid Anatomy of Some of the Most Important Parts of the Human Body, 2nd edn. London: Johnson and Nicol, 1797.
4. Roesler H. Interatrial septal defect. Arch Intern Med 1934; 54: 339.
5. McManus BM. Patent ductus arteriosus. In: Roberts WC, ed. Adult Congenital Heart Disease. Philadelphia, PA: FA Davis, 1987: 455–76.
6. Fallot A. Contribution á l'anatomie pathologique de la maladie bleue (cyanose cardiaque). Marseille Medical 1888; 25: 418.
7. Roger H. Clinical researches on the congenital communication of the two sides of the heart by failure of occlusion of the interventricular septum. Bull de l'Acad de Méd 1897; 8: 1074.
8. Kaemmerer H, Stern H, Fratz S et al. Imaging in adults with congenital cardiac disease (ACCD). Thorac Cardiovasc Surg 2000; 48: 328–35.
9. Moore P. MRI-guided congenital cardiac catheterization and intervention: The future? Catheter Cardiovasc Interv 2005; 66: 1–8.
10. Fox JM, Bjornsen KD, Mahoney LT, Fagan TE, Skorton DJ. Congenital heart disease in adults: catheterization laboratory considerations. Catheter Cardiovasc Interv 2003; 58: 219–31.
11. Andrews RE, Tulloh RM. Interventional cardiac catheterisation in congenital heart disease. Arch Dis Child 2004; 89: 1168–73.
12. Holzer R, Cao QL, Hijazi ZM. State of the art catheter interventions in adults with congenital heart disease. Expert Rev Cardiovasc Ther 2004; 2: 699–711.
13. Rashkind WJ, Miller WW. Creation of an atrial septal defect without thoracotomy. JAMA 1966; 196: 991–2.
14. Kan JS, White RI, Mitchell SE et al. Percutaneous balloon valvuloplasty: A new method for treating congenital pulmonary valve stenosis. N Engl J Med 1982; 307: 540–2.
15. Lababidi Z, Wu RJ, Walls TJ. Percutaneous balloon aortic valvuloplasty: results in 23 patients. Am J Cardiol 1984; 53: 194–7.
16. Lock JE, Bass JL, Amplatz K et al. Balloon dilatation angioplasty of aortic coarctation in infants and children. Circulation 1983; 68: 109–16.
17. Sohn S, Rothman A, Shiota T et al. Acute and follow-up intravascular ultrasound findings after balloon dilatation of coarctation of the aorta. Circulation 1994; 90: 340–7.
18. Yetman AT, Nykanen D, McCrindle BW et al. Balloon angioplasty of recurrent coarctation: a 12-year review. J Am Coll Cardiol 1997; 30: 811–16.
19. Rao PS. Coarctation of the aorta. Curr Cardiol Rep 2005; 7: 425–34.
20. Shah L, Hijazi Z, Sandhu S, Joseph A, Cao QL. Use of endovascular stents for the treatment of coarctation of the aorta in children and adults: Immediate and midterm results. J Invasive Cardiol 2005; 17: 614–18.
21. Porstsmann W, Wierny L, Warnke H. Der verschluss des D.a.p. ohne thorakotomie (1. Mitteiliung). Thoraxchirurgie 1967; 15: 199–203.
22. King TD, Mills NL. Nonoperative closure of atrial septal defects. Surgery 1974; 75: 383–8.
23. Mašura J, Gavora P, Formanek A, Hijazi ZM. Transcatheter closure of secundum atrial septal defects using the new self-centering Amplatzer septal occluder: Initial human experience. Cathet Cardiovasc Diagn 1997; 42: 388–93.
24. Lock JE, Block PC, McKay RG, Baim DS, Keane JF. Trancatheter closure of ventricular septal defects. Circulation 1988; 78: 361–8.
25. Gross RE, Hubbard JP. Surgical ligation of a patent ductus arteriosus. Report of first successful case. JAMA 1939; 112: 729.
26. Kaemmerer H, Meisner H, Hess J, Perloff JK. Surgical treatment of patent ductus arteriosus: A new historical perspective. Am J Cardiol 2004; 94: 1153–4.
27. Crafoord C, Nylin G. Congenital coarctation of aorta and its surgical treatment. J Thor Surg 1945; 14: 347–61.
28. Blalock A, Taussig HB. The surgical treatment of malformations of the heart in which there is pulmonary stenosis or pulmonary atresia. JAMA 1945; 128: 189.
29. Stephenson LW, John W. Kirklin: Reminiscences of a surgical resident. J Card Surg 2004; 19: 367–74.
30. Senning A. Surgical correction of transposition of the great vessels. Surgery 1959; 45: 966.
31. Mustard WT. Successful two stage correction of transposition of the great vessels. Surgery 1964; 55: 469.
32. Jatene AD, Fontes VF, Paulista PP et al. Successful anatomic correction of transposition of the great vessels: A preliminary report. Arq Bras Cardiol 1975; 28: 461.
33. Yacoub MH, Radley-Smith R, Hilton CJ. Anatomical correction of complete transposition of the great arteries and ventricular septal defect in infancy. Br Med J 1976; 1: 1112–14.
34. Fontan F, Baudet E. Surgical repair of tricuspid atresia. Thorax 1971; 26: 240–8.
35. de Leval MR. The Fontan circulation: What have we learned? What to expect? Pediatr Cardiol 1998; 19: 316–20.
36. van Doorn CA, Marc R de Leval. The Fontan operation in clinical practice: Indications and controversies. Nature Clinical Practice Cardiovascular Medicine 2005; 2: 116–17.
37. de Leval MR, Kilner P, Gewillig M, Bull C. Total cavo-pulmonary connection: a logical alternative to atriopulmonary connection for complex Fontan operation. Experimental studies and early clinical experience. J Thorac Cardiovasc Surg 1988; 96: 682–95.

2

Prevalence of congenital heart disease in adulthood

Congenital heart disease (CHD) refers to all morphological anomalies of the heart and large blood vessels present at birth. A CHD may manifest itself clinically at any time during one's life. Cardiomyopathies and arrhythmias without structural changes are not classified as CHD.

The prevalence of CHD at birth varies between 6 and 10 per 1000 live births.[1–3] The fetal prevalence of CHD is higher. CHD is found in 20% of abortions, in 10% of stillborn and 1% of live-born children.[1]

CHD is one of the biggest success stories in medicine. However, the prevalence of CHD in adulthood is difficult to describe as the introduction of new diagnostic and therapeutic modalities has dramatically changed both survival and the survival pattern during the last five decades. In addition, mortality has to be taken into account. Whilst the highest mortality rates for CHD were originally reported for children below the age of 1, since 1986 death from CHD has been most common in the adult population over 20 years of age.[4] In the 1950s, only 20% of children with complex CHD reached adulthood: today, 90% or more of these children are surviving into adulthood due to great advances in medicine. As a consequence, the population of adults with CHD is larger than the pediatric population, and most deaths from CHD occur in adults.

Still, it is critical to know the number of adults with CHD in order to provide adequate human and structural resources and care for these patients. In the USA, the number of adults with CHD is estimated to be 800 000, with 15% having severe complex CHD, 38% moderate CHD, and 47% 'simple' CHD.[2] Empirical data on the changing epidemiology of CHD were first scant in the Canadian province of Quebec: in 2000, the prevalence was 4.09 per 1000 adults for all CHD and 0.38 per 1000 (9%) for those with severe lesions.[5] A tsunami is approaching the adult health care system: an increasing number of adolescents with complications are maturing into adulthood, so challenging the adult health care system.

There are congenital heart defects which go undetected in childhood and do not manifest themselves until adulthood. These are, primarily, bicuspid aortic valves, reported to occur in 1–2% of the population. Another common type of CHD, which may occasionally not be diagnosed until adulthood, is an atrial septal defect. Other types of CHD remaining undetected until adulthood occur more rarely.[6]

References

1. Hoffman JIE. Congenital heart disease: Incidence and inheritance. Pediatr Clin North Am 1990; 37: 25–43.
2. Warnes CA, Liberthson R, Danielson GK et al. Task Force 1: The changing profile of congenital heart disease in adult life. J Am Coll Cardiol 2001; 37(5): 1170–5.
3. Hoffman JI, Kaplan S. The incidence of congenital heart disease. J Am Coll Cardiol 2002; 39: 1890–900.
4. Somerville J. Grown-up congenital heart (GUCH) disease: Current needs and provisions of service for adolescents and adults with congenital heart disease in the UK. Report of the British Cardiac Society Working Party. Heart 2002; 88 (Suppl I): 1–14.
5. Marelli AJ, Mackie AS, Ionescu-Ittu R, Rahme E, Pilote L. Congenital heart disease in the general population: Changing prevalence and age distribution. Circulation 2007; 115: 163–72.
6. Popelová J, Kölbel F, Dostálová P, Voříšková M. Echocardiography in adults with congenital heart disease. Exp Clin Cardiol 1999; 4(2): 89–93.

3

Atrial septal defect

Anatomical notes

- *Secundum atrial septal defect* (ASD; Figure 3.1): This defect is the most common form of congenital malformations in adults, accounting for about 70% of all defects at the atrial level. It is located at the level of the oval fossa, or dorsally to it, and is called secundum defect, in spite of the fact that the oval fossa is primum septum. There may be multiple defects (fenestrated interatrial septum). It is caused by a deficit, perforation or absence of the thin flap valve of the oval fossa (septum ovale) derived from the septum primum and attached to the atrial septum from the side of the left atrium (Figure 3.2). In adulthood, in the presence of severe atrial dilatation, whatever the cause, the flap valve may become insufficient to overlap the rim, resulting in acquired ASD (Figure 3.3). In contrast, excessive tissue of the oval fossa valve results in the formation of an atrial septal aneurysm, bulging into the right atrium; it may present with multiple fenestrations. From

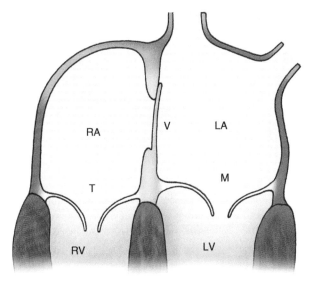

Figure 3.2
Anatomy of atrial septum: RA, right atrium; T, tricuspid valve; RV, right ventricle; V, valve of oval fossa; LA, left atrium; M, mitral valve; LV, left ventricle.

the side of the right atrium, the defect is limited by a protruding rim of the oval fossa, what is known as the limbic septum, with the upper and lower parts. The limbic septum separates the defect from the atrial walls, orifices of the venae cavae, and atrioventricular valves (Figure 3.3). In large defects, the limbic septum may be absent and the defect may extend to different distances, most commonly posterioinferiorly and -superiorly to the mouth of the caval veins.

- *Superior sinus venosus defect* (Figure 3.4): This defect is due to abnormal development of the sinus venosus in relation to the pulmonary veins, it is not a defect in the interatrial septum and accounts for about 5–10% of communications between the atria; it is localized below the entry of the superior caval vein. The superior sinus venosus defect is often localized within the mouth of the superior caval vein (the superior caval vein overrides the rim of the fossa ovalis – a characteristic anatomical feature), thus entering both atria (biatrial connection). This type of defect is frequently (in 80–90%) associated with partial anomalous return of the right upper pulmonary

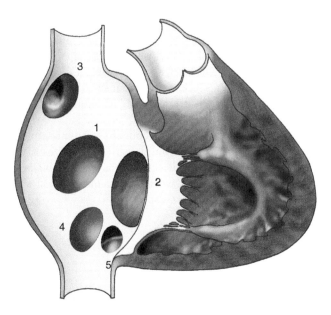

Figure 3.1
Atrial septal defects: 1, type secundum; 2, type primum (incomplete atrioventricular septal defect); 3, type sinus venosus superior; 4, type sinus venosus inferior; 5, unroofed coronary sinus defect.

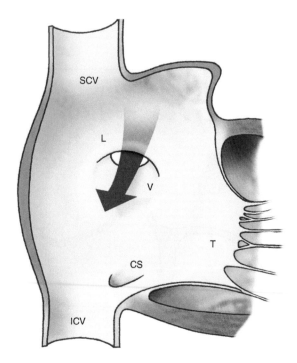

Figure 3.3
Anatomy of atrial septum, view from right atrium, acquired atrial septal defect: SCV, superior caval vein; ICV, inferior caval vein; CS, coronary sinus; T, tricuspid valve; L, valve of oval fossa.

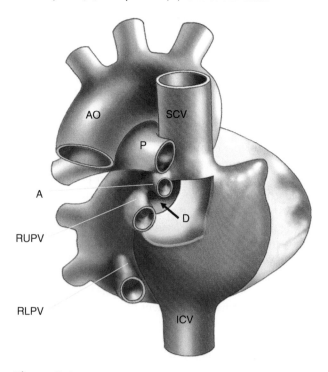

Figure 3.4
Sinus venosus superior atrial septal defect with partial anomalous pulmonary venous connection of right upper pulmonary vein (RUPV) and accessory pulmonary vein (A) into junction of superior caval vein (SCV) and right atrium. Superior caval vein overrides the defect. AO, Aorta; RLPV, right lower pulmonary vein; D, defect; ICV, inferior caval vein; P, right pulmonary artery branch.

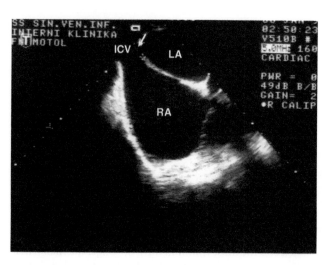

Figure 3.5
Sinus venosus inferior defect (arrow) with inferior caval vein (IVC) overriding the defect. Transesophageal echo, modified transversal view. LA, left atrium; RA, right atrium.

vein, which empties into the upper part of the right atrium or directly into the superior caval vein.

- *Inferior sinus venosus defect*: This defect is rare and accounts for about 2% of all defects at atrial levels; it is localized in the mouth of the inferior caval vein and is occasionally associated with partial anomalous return of the right lower pulmonary veins. A solid lower rim is absent with the defect. The Eustachian fold may constitute a false rim of the defect and detour blood from the vena cava inferior to the left atrium. This type of defect may thus be an undetected cause of cyanosis in adulthood (Figure 3.5).
- *Defect of the coronary sinus (unroofed coronary sinus)*: This is a very rare defect: the defect is in the wall separating the coronary sinus from the left atrium (Figure 3.1). It is usually associated with persistence of the left superior vena cava, emptying into the left atrium or into the coronary sinus.

ASD of the ostium primum type constitutes an incomplete form of atrioventricular septal defect (see Chapter 5). It accounts for 15–20% of all defects at atrial level. *Patent foramen ovale* is not considered a defect; it occurs in 25–30% of the population at large (see Chapter 4).

Prevalence

ASD is a frequent congenital heart disease (CHD), accounting for about 9–11% of all CHD in childhood. Given the good natural prognosis and the fact the defect is frequently not diagnosed until adulthood, ASD accounts for 22–30% of all CHD in series of adult patients. It is the most frequent CHD in adults (except bicuspid aortic valve). It can occur in isolation or in association with other cardiac defects.

Pathophysiology

An ASD allows shunt blood flow between the atria. The magnitude and direction of blood flow depends on the size of the defect and on the filling properties/pressures of both ventricles. Under normal circumstances, the difference between pressures in either atrium is low, and the left-to-right direction of the shunt is due to the higher compliance of the right ventricle and right atrium. A left-to-right shunt at the atrial level results in a volume overload and dilatation of the right ventricle and pulmonary artery; at a later stage, in the presence of tricuspid regurgitation, regurgitant volume through the tricuspid valve contributes further to dilatation of the right heart chambers (Figures 3.6 and 3.7). In conditions associated with a reduction in left ventricular compliance and an increase in left atrial pressure (systemic hypertension, left heart failure, mitral valve dysfunction), the magnitude of the left-to-right shunt increases. Simultaneous right-to-left shunt occurs in the presence of increased right atrial pressure, significant tricuspid regurgitation directed into the defect, or in cases where the vena cava superior or inferior is superimposed to the left atrium in sinus venosus type defects.

At younger ages, increased pulmonary blood flow does not result in severe pulmonary hypertension, as the pulmonary vascular bed may dilate considerably. The rise in pulmonary artery pressure in childhood and young age is therefore limited and is due to a high pulmonary blood flow rate (hyperkinetic pulmonary hypertension). However, a high pulmonary blood flow occurring for a number of years results in endothelial injury of the pulmonary vessels, depletion of the vasodilator reserve, and pulmonary vascular bed remodeling. Pulmonary vascular resistance is usually normal in youth, but may rise in elderly individuals. Pulmonary arterial pressure in the presence of ASD increases with age, particularly after 50 years of age, whilst the size of the shunt remains the same.[1] Factors contributing to the rise in pulmonary artery pressure include actual changes in the pulmonary vascular bed. In some cases, it may also be deteriorated by postcapillary pulmonary hypertension associated with left-heart disease, and hypoxic pulmonary hypertension in the presence of chronic lung disease. A severely dilated pulmonary artery in older age may be associated with formation of mural thrombi and distal embolism into the pulmonary vascular bed, which may also worsen the pulmonary hypertension (Figures 3.8–3.10). Underlying genetic factors can modify the phenotype and predispose the patient to the development of severe pulmonary vascular disease in the presence of a shunt at the atrial level: the high pulmonary blood flow can trigger the development of pulmonary vascular disease.

During exercise, pulmonary artery pressure tends to rise in healthy individuals too, and is proportionate to cardiac output. However, the rise in pulmonary artery pressure in individuals over 50 years of age is steeper. Older adults with ASD have been shown to have an abnormal rise in pulmonary artery pressure compared with controls.[2] Patients with ASD

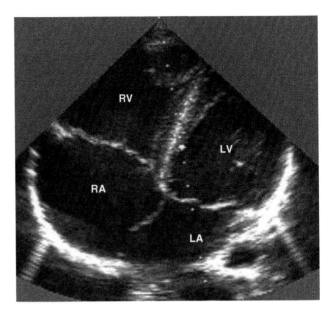

Figure 3.6
Transthoracic apical four-chamber view of atrial septal defect type secundum. Dilatation of the right ventricle (RV) and right atrium (RA) due to the left-to-right shunt through atrial septal defect, which may be seen as a drop-out in the atrial septum. LA, Left atrium; LV, left ventricle.

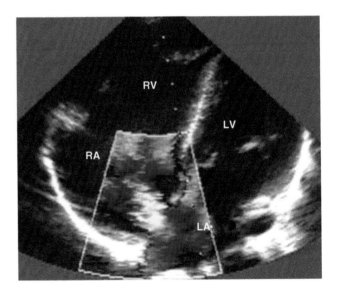

Figure 3.7
Transthoracic four-chamber view showing severe left-to-right shunt (red colour) due to atrial septal defect. RV, Right ventricle; RA, right atrium; LV, left ventricle; LA, left atrium.

and pulmonary hypertension have significantly reduced oxygen consumption during exertion; in patients without significant pulmonary hypertension, peak oxygen consumption correlates inversely with the size of the left-to-right shunt.[3]

Defect closure is followed by a fall in pulmonary artery pressure, even in older patients, unless there is irreversible, advanced disease in the pulmonary vascular bed

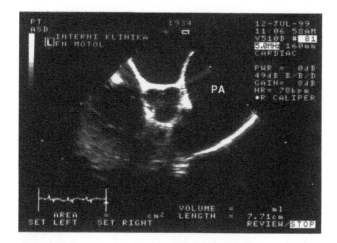

Figure 3.8
Transesophageal echo, severely dilated pulmonary artery (PA) to 77mm in 65-year-old lady with unoperated atrial septal defect.

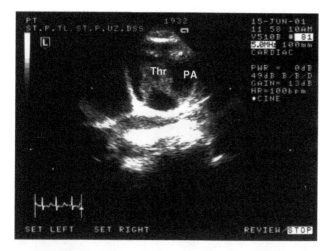

Figure 3.9
Transesophageal echo, another adult patient with thrombus (Thr) in dilated pulmonary artery (PA), persisting after atrial septal defect closure.

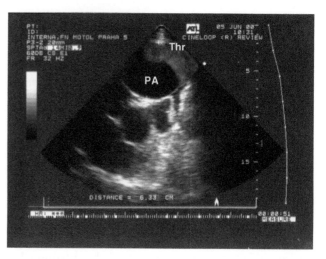

Figure 3.10
Parasternal transthoracic echo with severely dilated pulmonary artery (PA) up to 63mm with thrombus (Thr) in an adult patient with unoperated sinus venosus defect with pulmonary hypertension.

and the oppression of the left ventricle over a prolonged period of time result in its hypoplasia with a risk of left-heart failure following defect closure.

Clinical findings and diagnosis

A typical feature of ASD in adulthood is its prolonged asymptomatic course. In their youth, many patients with even a major ASD practiced sports experiencing no problems at all. Symptoms set in insidiously, most often after the age of 40 or 50. In women, the clinical status may deteriorate during pregnancy or after delivery. In adults with an ASD who are less than 40 years of age, there is no correlation between symptoms (NYHA class) and the size of a shunt. But, the development of symptoms does correlate with age.[5] Most patients with an ASD who are in their sixties experience problems; however, exertional dyspnea and reduced physical fitness are usually ascribed to physiological changes associated with aging, and lifestyle is modified accordingly. Major and limiting problems are often experienced after 65 years of age.

The clinical course of a nonoperated ASD in adulthood may be significantly affected by associated cardiovascular disease such as hypertension, coronary artery disease, and mitral regurgitation, as the compliance and the filling pressure of the ventricles change with subsequent impact on the size and direction of the shunt at the atrial level. Patients with unoperated ASD over 60 years of age very often develop atrial fibrillation. Atrial fibrillation or atrial flutter is an age-related reflection of the atrial stretch, which seldom occurs in those younger than 40 years of age.[6]

(Eisenmenger syndrome). Eisenmenger syndrome is defined as an extreme form of pulmonary vascular disease with pulmonary artery pressures at or near systemic level, and reversed or bidirectional shunting at atrial, ventricular or arterial level. It is rarely associated with ASD (1–6%). A study has demonstrated a higher incidence of pulmonary hypertension in young patients with defects of the sinus venosus type.[4]

In ASD, the left ventricle is oppressed by a dilated right ventricle and its diastolic function is abnormal. However, its systolic function is usually normal and does not diminish until there is an appreciably paradoxical movement of the interventricular septum. Diastolic function of the left ventricle is adversely affected by the volume-overloaded right ventricle (interventricular interaction). Inadequate filling

Symptoms

- Reduced exercise tolerance, tiredness.
- Exertional dyspnea.
- Palpitations (due to supraventricular arrhythmia, frequent atrial fibrillation/atrial flutter in older age).
- Atypical chest pain (right ventricular ischemia).
- Frequent respiratory tract infections.
- Signs of right-heart failure.

Clinical findings

- The patients are usually pink; cyanosis suggests severe pulmonary hypertension with reversed shunting in the presence of a secundum ASD or superior sinus venosus defect; cyanosis can also reflect associated pulmonary stenosis, a coronary sinus defect or an inferior sinus venosus defect (with a prominent Eustachian valve directing the blood to the left atrium).
- Right ventricular heave.
- Ejection systolic murmur with a maximum at the left sternal border (increased blood flow through the pulmonary artery orifice, relative pulmonary stenosis); sometimes, a pulmonary ejection click can be heard.
- Wide and fixed split of the second heart sound above the pulmonary artery (delayed pulmonary artery valve closure); a loud pulmonary component reflects severe pulmonary hypertension.
- Diastolic murmur at the lower left sternal border (increased blood flow through the tricuspid orifice – relative tricuspid stenosis).
- The clinical findings and auscultation may be completely discrete and unremarkable.
- A pansystolic murmur can be heard in the presence of mitral regurgitation on the apex.

Electrocardiogram (ECG)

The rhythm can be sinus, atrial flutter or atrial fibrillation (after the age of 40). Coronary sinus rhythm reflects the absence of a sinus node and is frequently seen in the presence of a superior sinus venosus defect. A grade 1 atrioventricular block can be found in the presence of a primum ASD, but it can also be found in older patients with a secundum ASD. Right atrial overload can be present. Right axis deviation and right ventricular hypertrophy reflects right ventricular volume overload/hypertrophy. Incomplete right bundle branch block (shape rSr' or rsR' in leads V1–V3) is a feature of delayed activation of the dilated right ventricle.

Chest X-ray

The cardiac silhouette is enlarged (right atrium and right ventricle). A prominent, dilated pulmonary artery, dilated hilar vessels can be present, and a lifted cardiac apex reflects the presence of right ventricular dilatation. Pulmonary plethora

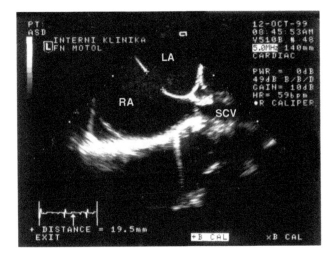

Figure 3.11
Atrial septal defect in transesophageal echocardiography. LA, Left atrium; RA, right atrium; SCV, superior caval vein.

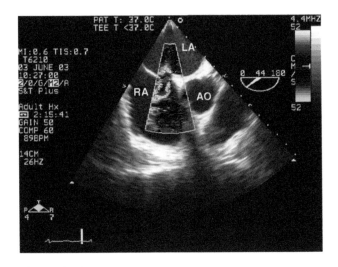

Figure 3.12
Transesophageal echocardiography, atrial septal defect with left-to-right shunt, color flow from the left atrium to the right atrium. Transesophageal echo, 44 degrees. LA, Left atrium; RA, right atrium; AO, aorta.

reflects increased pulmonary blood flow (left-to-right shunt). A small aortic knuckle reflects a chronic low systemic blood flow in the presence of an important left-to-right shunt.

Echocardiography

Exact assessment of the anatomy of the ASD often requires transesophageal echocardiography (TEE) in adults, in addition to transthoracic echocardiography. The following parameters are assessed:

- Presence and type of defect (Figures 3.11 and 3.12).
- Exact defect size is determined in at least two planes, the biggest measured size is of importance.

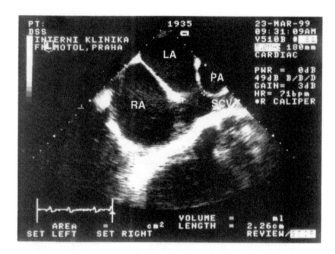

Figure 3.13
Transesophageal echocardiography, longitudinal view, sinus venosus superior defect (arrow). RA, Right atrium; LA, left atrium; PA, pulmonary artery; SCV, superior caval vein.

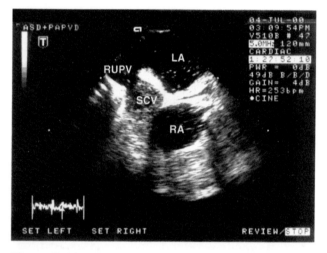

Figure 3.14
Transesophageal echocardiography, transversal view: Sinus venosus superior atrial septal defect with partial anomalous pulmonary venous connection of the right upper pulmonary vein (RUPV) entering superior caval vein (SCV) overriding the defect. Contrast agent enters left atrium (LA) from SCV.

- Distance of defect rims from other structures by TEE (atrioventricular valves, coronary sinus, superior and inferior caval veins, aorta).
- Quality of atrial septal margins around the defect (by TEE).
- Entry of pulmonary veins to rule out their anomalous return (Figures 3.13–3.15).
- Right ventricular size, its function and signs of volume overload (paradoxical movement of the interventricular septum).

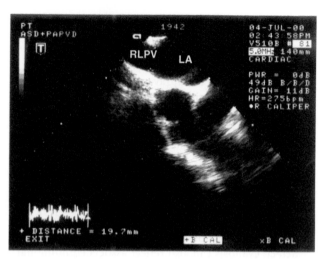

Figure 3.15
The same patient as in Figure 3.14. Transesophageal echo shows normal right lower pulmonary vein (RLPV) entering left atrium (LA).

- Magnitude of the left-to-right shunt using noninvasive calculation of the pulmonary to systemic blood flow ratio (Qp/Qs).
- Pulmonary artery pressure derived from noninvasive calculation of the right ventricular systolic pressure in the presence of tricuspid regurgitation (modified Bernoulli equation).
- Any other associated congenital anomalies, including another ASD, pulmonary stenosis, ventricular septal defect, etc.
- Size, and systolic and diastolic function of the left ventricle, which chronically fills inadequately.
- Mitral valve prolapse and magnitude of mitral regurgitation, if present (Figures 3.16 and 3.17).
- Width of the proximal segment of the main pulmonary artery with respect to the potential presence of pulmonary artery aneurysms and mural thrombi.

Catheterization

Catheterization is not required to establish the diagnosis of ASD. It is indicated:

- When there is a need to determine pulmonary vascular resistance and pulmonary vascular reactivity in the presence of pulmonary hypertension.
- In the presence of partial anomalous return of pulmonary veins, unless the course of all pulmonary veins is completely clear based on echocardiography, magnetic resonance imaging (MRI) or computerized tomographic (CT) angiography.
- To perform selective coronary arteriography in patients over 40 years of age, or in younger individuals with risk factors of coronary artery disease (CAD) or anginal

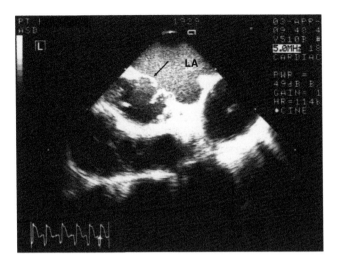

Figure 3.16
Transesophageal echo, longitudinal view: Mitral valve prolapse of the posterior cusp (arrow) with mitral valve degeneration and severe mitral regurgitation in large unoperated atrial septal defect in 70-year-old lady with severe congestive heart failure. Left atrium (LA) with spontaneous echocontrast.

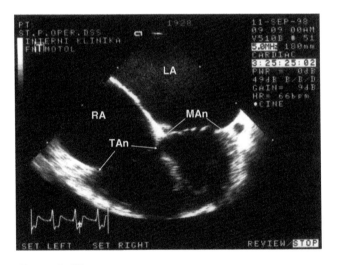

Figure 3.17
Transesophageal echo, transversal view: Atrial septal defect closed surgically at 67 years of age without annuloplasty of tricuspid and mitral valves. Persisting severe dilatation of tricuspid annulus (TAn) and mitral annulus (MAn) with mitral valve prolapse and severe residual tricuspid and mitral regurgitation. Severely dilated left atrium (LA) with spontaneous echocontrast and right atrium (RA).

pain, or if there is suspicion of congenital coronary artery anomaly or perioperative injury.
- Exceptionally to determine shunt size, only if the hemodynamic relevance of the defect is not clear from echocardiography.

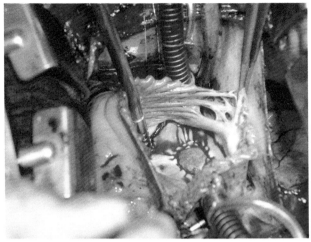

Figure 3.18
Surgical closure of atrial septal defect type secundum by pericardial patch. (Courtesy of J Spatenka, Prague, Czech Republic.)

Magnetic resonance imaging/ computerized tomographic scanning

Cardiac MRI is a very helpful diagnostic tool to assess pulmonary venous connection if there is any question about pulmonary venous connection by echocardiography. It is also the gold standard to calculate right ventricular volume and ejection fraction. CT scanning is an alternative if the patient is claustrophobic or if there is a contraindication of a cardiac MRI (e.g. a pacemaker).

Treatment

Management of ASD consists in its closure, which may be surgical with suture or a patch (Figure 3.18), or catheter based. Views over surgical treatment of asymptomatic ASD in adulthood were a debated issue. Indications for surgical and catheter-based closure of ASD may vary in future, especially if a long-term beneficial effect of catheter-based closure, without late complications, is confirmed. Another modern possibility is thoracoscopic robotic surgical closure (Figure 3.19).

ASD closure is indicated:

- In the presence of a significant left-to-right shunt (Qp/Qs >1.5:1) or a morphologically large defect (>10–15mm) with concomitant signs of right ventricular volume overload or with symptoms.
- If there is a history of paradoxical systemic embolism and contrast echocardiography documented right-to-left

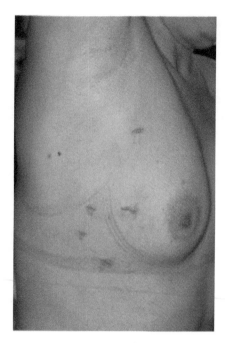

Figure 3.19
Small scars after surgical closure of large ASD by thoracoscopic robotic approach. (Courtesy of Dr Stepan Cerny, Department of Cardiac Surgery, Hospital Na Homolce, Prague, Czech Republic).

shunt, defect closure is indicated regardless of shunt magnitude, unless severe irreversible pulmonary hypertension is a contraindication to closure.

- Over 60 years of age and absence of symptoms do not rule out closure, especially if there is a significant shunt (Qp/Qs >2:1) and right ventricular volume overload.
- On atrial flutter or fibrillation, defect closure may be complemented with radiofrequency ablation, ablation of cavotricuspid isthmus or atrial surgery (Maze procedure).
- See 'pulmonary hypertension' (below) for contraindication. Relative contraindications for surgical closure may include a generally poor state of the patient with other serious conditions/comorbidities.

Surgical closure of atrial septal defect

All defects at the atrial level, with and without associated anomalies, can be closed surgically. All defects other than isolated secundum ASD, however, should be operated on by a CHD surgeon.[7–9] It is performed from midline sternotomy or, possibly, from a right-sided inframammary minithoracotomy ensuring a better cosmetic result. The best surgical cosmetic result is achieved by the thoracoscopic robotic approach (Figure 3.19). The defect is closed by direct suture or a pericardial or dacron patch.

Pulmonary hypertension in the presence of increased pulmonary vascular resistance (PVR ≥4 Wood units) poses a significantly increased operative risk and a poorer postoperative prognosis. The limit for contraindicating the procedure on grounds of a high PVR is not fully uniform, as factors such as the patient's biological age, and other comorbidities and conditions may also affect the postoperative course. A prerequisite for operability of patients with increased pulmonary artery pressure (>2/3 systemic arterial blood pressure) and increased PVR (2/3 systemic arteriolar resistance) is a net left-to-right shunt ≥1.5:1, or evidence of pulmonary artery reactivity when challenged with a pulmonary vasodilator (e.g. oxygen, nitric oxide and/or prostaglandins).[7,8,10]

Assessment of reversibility of pulmonary vascular disease using surgical pulmonary biopsy in adults is a matter of controversy given the risk involved with the procedure and the high likelihood of advanced changes. In addition, pathology expertise required in the assessment of these lung specimens may be an important limitation. Grades I and II of Heath-Edwards classification are considered reversible.

Catheter-based closure of secundum atrial septal defect

Because of the good outcome and low rates of complications, device closure has replaced surgical closure, and has become the method of choice to close morphologically suitable secundum ASD in the absence of any other associated defects.[10] Device closure cannot be performed in patients with a sinus venosus defect, ostium primum ASD, coronary sinus defects or in the presence of associated anomalies (e.g. anomalous pulmonary venous return). In the presence of pulmonary hypertension, it is appropriate to test the hemodynamic response to closure. There is no randomized trial and consensus on the appropriate anticoagulation or antiplatelet regimen after device closure; most operators prescribe aspirin alone or in combination with clopidogrel for 6 months (most trials used this regimen).[10] Infective endocarditis (IE) prophylaxis is indicated for at least 6 months (up to 12 months) following catheter-based closure.[11,12]

Catheter-based closure can only be performed in centers with adequate experience and adequate numbers of these procedures. Transesophageal echocardiography is an absolute must for proper assessment and suitability of the anatomy device closure. In addition to fluoroscopy, TEE or intracardiac ultrasound is used to monitor the procedure and deployment of the device. A closure can also be undertaken without X-ray control, only under control by transesophageal echocardiography,[13] or by intracardiac ultrasound.[14]

The size of the defect, as determined by transesophageal echocardiography, is not yet equivalent to occluder size. Occluder size is determined during catheterization according to maximum defect size, in which a balloon is inflated (what is known as 'stretched diameter') (Figures 3.20 and 3.21). A closure can only be performed if there is enough distance of defect margins from surrounding structures and the surrounding septum is of adequate quality.

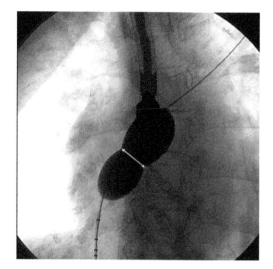

Figure 3.20
X-ray, measurement of stretched diameter ('waist') of atrial septal defect by inflated balloon during transcatheter closure.

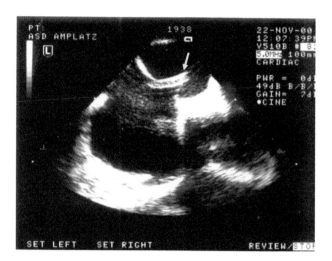

Figure 3.23
Transesophageal echo, longitudinal view: In the atrial septal defect (ASD) there is an introducer (arrow) of the Amplatzer system for ASD closure.

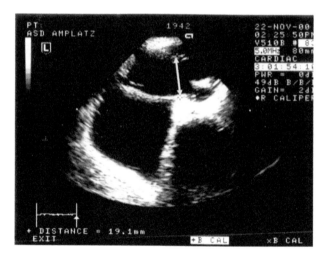

Figure 3.21
Transesophageal echo, longitudinal view: Measuring of the stretched diameter of the balloon during atrial septal defect closure by Amplatzer system.

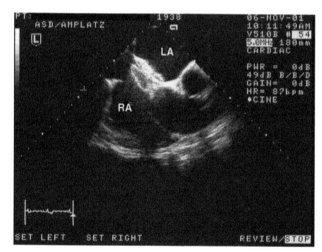

Figure 3.24
Transesophageal echo: Opening of both discs of the Amplatzer atrial septal occluder. Longitudinal view. LA, left atrium; RA, right atrium.

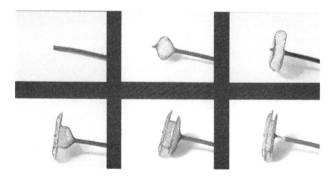

Figure 3.22
Amplatzer atrial septal defect (ASD) occluder for ASD closure. Two discs are connected by the neck, which is stenting the defect.

The most convenient and most frequently used device for closure of a secundum ASD in adults is currently the Amplatzer™ septal occluder (AGA Medical, Minnesota, USA).[15,16] This type of occluder features two discs connected with a neck closing (stenting) the defect and self-centering in the defect (Figures 3.22–3.25). The left atrial disc of the occluder designed for atrial defect closure is somewhat bigger than the right-side one. The occluder is made of elastic wire mesh and a thin nickel-titanium alloy wire, and is filled with a polyester material to help close the hole and provide a foundation for growth of tissue over the occluder after placement. Thrombus formation/growth of tissue inside the occluder results, within 3–6 months, in the disappearance of minor residual shunts which may be evident immediately after the

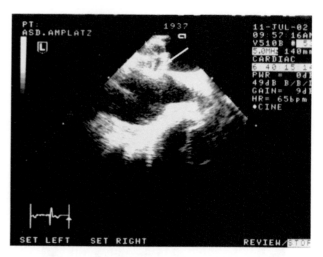

Figure 3.25
Right position of the Amplatzer atrial septal defect occluder (arrow), the rim from mitral valve is 10mm (crosses). Transesophageal echo, longitudinal view: LA, left atrium; RA, right atrium; RV, right ventricle.

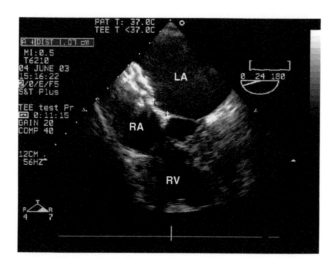

Figure 3.27
Transesophageal echo, longitudinal view: Wrong position of the left atrial disc of the atrial septal defect Amplatzer occluder (arrow), needing reposition.

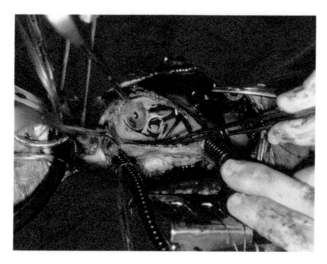

Figure 3.26
Amplatzer occluder completely endothelialized 5 months after implantation. View from right atrium. Another atrial septal defect close to the device. (Courtesy of Assistant Professor Jan Harrer, Hradec Králové, Czech Republic.)

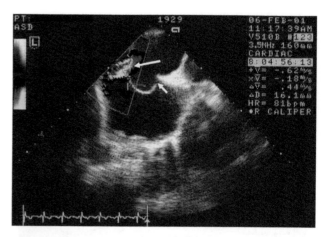

Figure 3.28
Transesophageal echo, color flow shows left-to-right shunt through one of two atrial spetal defects in aneurysmatic interatrial septum. Defects are marked with arrows.

procedure.[17,18] The occluder surface is completely endothelized after 3–6 months (Figure 3.26). Closure of a secundum ASD with the Amplatzer occluder device is possible, even in the case of an inadequate or absent anterosuperior septum (rim) in front of the aorta.[19] The Amplatzer occluder can be repositioned in the case of malpositioning (Figure 3.27). Of importance for adulthood is the fact that the Amplatzer occluder, unlike other types, can also be used with big defects measuring >20mm in diameter.[10,20–22] Currently, in the presence of appropriate morphology/anatomy, the Amplatzer occluder can be used to close defects with a stretched diameter measuring as much as 38–40mm. However, closure of larger defects (>20mm) and closure of defects with atrial septal aneurysm or those without an anterosuperior rim involve higher risk, are technically more demanding, and require greater experience and expertise. Two occluders may be used in multiple ASD (Figure 3.28), and the other defects should not be overlooked (Figure 3.26).

Efforts at reducing the content of metallic material in the occluder led to the development of new occluder types (e.g. Helex system[23]), and to complete elimination of metallic material, as with the newly tested, catheter-placed patch made of polyurethane foam.[24] Future research is directed at the development of a 'biodegradable' occluder whose body would resorb completely some time following full endothelization. Still, all newly introduced methods first warrant analysis of long-term results from a sufficiently large number of patients.

Complications of catheter-based artrial septal defect closure

In large series, using the Amplatzer occluder or the CardioSEAL/STARflex occluder, the complication rates were <10%, while serious complications occurred in the range of 0.3–1%.[17,18,20,25,26]

Complications of catheter-based ASD closure include:

- *Arrhythmia*, both during the procedure and within the first 3 months after the procedure; however, they are usually transient and their incidence is not high. They include atrial flutter or atrial fibrillation; and there have been rare reports of complete atrioventricular block.[27] The long-term risk of supraventricular arrhythmias is unknown.
- *Transient pericardial effusion.*
- *Thrombus of the left atrial disc*, possibly with peripheral embolism (Figure 3.29).
- *Occluder malpositioning* and its interference with surrounding structures, which may require surgical revision. If this complication is noted during the procedure, the Amplatzer occluder device can be repositioned or removed (Figure 3.27).
- *Occluder release and embolism* is one of the most serious complications, which may potentially require cardiac surgical revision. In large series, occluder embolism has been reported to occur in 1.4–3.5% of cases, and more frequently with bigger occluder models.[16,20,26] Embolism into the right ventricle and pulmonary artery is more frequent, while embolism to the left ventricle is rare. Because of the risk of device embolism, the Amplatzer septal occluder device is recommended to close defects measuring >18mm.[26]
- *Perforation of the right or left atrial wall or aorta* is a rare, but potentially lethal, complication; it requires acute cardiosurgical revision. Monitoring of patients during the first 24–48 hours after transcatheter closure is recommended (Figure 3.30).[28]
- *Occluder deformation* has been reported when using an oversize Amplatz occluder whose neck tends to bulge in smaller defects ('mushrooming'), with disc twisting, a rare complication.[29]
- *A rise in left atrial pressure* has been reported following catheter-based ASD closure in patients over 60 years of age, in as many as 39% of cases.[30]
- *Acute left-heart decompensation* is a potential risk in elderly patients with a small left ventricle or in patients with left ventricular diastolic dysfunction (e.g. a long history of hypertension). However, serious left-heart failure with pulmonary edema and the need for mechanical artificial ventilation after catheter-based ASD closure has only been described as a case report.[22,31] Pretreatment with an ACE inhibitor/angiotensin II inhibitor/calcium antagonists may be required to optimize hemodynamics/left ventricular filling pressures.
- *Air embolism* when using an improper technique of occluder insertion.
- Occluder insertion may interfere with right atrial structures such as *Eustachian valve and Chiari's network*.[29,32]

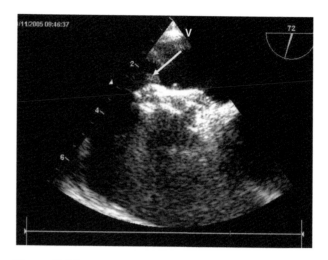

Figure 3.29
Thrombus on left atrial disc of the Amplatzer occluder (arrow), treated by anticoagulation without peripheral embolization. Transesophageal echo, 72 degrees. (Courtesy of Dr T Mráz, Cardiology, Hospital Na Homolce, Czech Republic.)

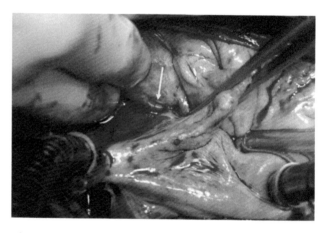

Figure 3.30
Perforation of the aorta (arrow) by Amplatzer occluder with tamponade, successfully treated by surgery. (Courtesy of Dr J Vojáček, Dept of Cardiac Surgery, FN Motol, Praha, Czech Republic.)

- *Hemolysis* has been reported very rarely.[33]
- *Local complications in the groin* after percutaneous puncture.

Complications of surgical atrial septal defect closure

- *Acute left-heart failure* after surgical ASD closure, leading to death or reoperation with a need for partial shunt restoration was reported in earlier series in about 2% of cases.[33a–33c]
- *Postpericardiotomy syndrome* with pericardial and pleural effusion.
- *Arrhythmia* is common after surgical ASD closure, especially in elderly patients; supraventricular arrhythmia is most often involved.[6]

- *Anomalous pulmonary vein orifice obstruction* by patch in sinus venosus type defect (redirection of the right pulmonary vein(s) through a baffle).
- *Cyanosis*, if the vena cava inferior has been inadvertently detoured to the left atrium.
- Local and systemic complications related to *cardiac surgical procedure*.

Residual findings after atrial septal defect closure

- *Residual shunts*: The criteria applicable to reoperation or reintervention in residual shunts are identical with those applying to primary defect closure.
  After surgical closure, residual shunts are seen more often in patients who underwent surgery when cardiac surgery was still in its infancy. In the very early series, residual shunts after surgery were relatively frequent, occurring in as many as 17% of cases.[34] The most frequent cause was cutting of suture through tissue or, possibly, unrecognized multiple defects. Currently, residual shunts occur in <2% of cases (Figure 3.31).
  After catheter-based closure, small residual shunts immediately after the procedure are present relatively often, particularly with a defect >20mm; however, their incidence declines substantially within 24 hours after the procedure. Depending on the occluder type, small, residual shunts tend to diminish or even disappear altogether over time. Use of the Amplatzer occluder device has been reported to be associated with an incidence of small, insignificant residual shunts of 0.8–2% at 3 months after the procedure, and a 0% incidence at 2–3 years after the procedure.[18,20,25,35]
- *Arrhythmia*: Atrial fibrillation is a frequent finding even after successful surgical ASD closure if the defect has not been operated on until adulthood. With ASD operated on in adulthood, the incidence of atrial fibrillation after 60 years of age is about 50%.
- *Unrecognized or residual-associated* CHD (anomalous pulmonary venous return, cor triatriatum, another defect, pulmonary artery stenosis, pulmonary artery regurgitation, etc.). Undetected CHD may occur in patients operated on before the advent of echocardiography. Their management depends on the hemodynamic relevance of these defects.

Risks associated with an unclosed atrial septal defect

- *Heart failure* is often seen in elderly patients (over 65 years of age) with a significant defect. It may be of a progressive nature with rapid deterioration of symptoms, especially in the presence of associated cardiovascular disease (hypertension, mitral valve regurgitation, CAD) and in the occurrence of atrial flutter/fibrillation. This complication may occur even in patients who have been asymptomatic throughout their lives and have tolerated their ASD well.

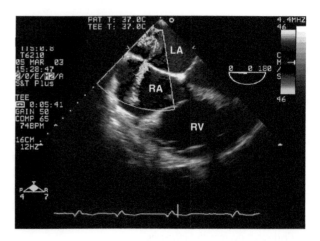

Figure 3.31
Small residual atrial septal defect with left-to-right shunt (color flow) persisting after surgical closure of the defect. Transesophageal echo, 0 degrees; LA, left atrium; RA, right atrium; RV, right ventricle – dilated.

- *Atrial fibrillation and atrial flutter* are frequent after 60 years of age in the presence of atrial dilatation on unclosed ASD, or even those that were closed late,[6] and pose a risk for systemic embolism. Chronic anticoagulation therapy is indicated in chronic atrial fibrillation.
- *Transvenous pacing* in the presence of an unclosed ASD carries the risk of paradoxical embolism into the systemic vascular bed. ASD closure before implantation of a transvenous system is required; implantation of an epicardial pacemaker system is an alternative.
- *Venous thrombosis* is associated with the risk of paradoxical embolism into the systemic vascular bed; the risk is increased during pregnancy, during delivery, and during hormonal contraception (in particular in smokers).

Pregnancy and delivery

Pregnancy and delivery are generally well tolerated, even by patients with an unclosed ASD with a significant left-to-right shunt. However, clinical symptoms may emerge or deteriorate during pregnancy or after childbirth. During pregnancy and delivery there is an increased risk of paradoxical embolization, regardless of the defect size. It is more appropriate to close the defect before planned pregnancy. Sudden major loss of blood, leading to hypovolemia, systemic vasoconstriction, reduced venous return, increase in the left-to-right shunt and a decrease in cardiac output, is poorly tolerated.[36] Pregnancy is contraindicated in patients with Eisenmenger syndrome.

Infective endocarditis

IE occurs rarely with any isolated defect at the atrial level, and endocarditis prophylaxis is not required. An increased risk for the development of IE is present immediately after surgical closure or catheter-based closure of an ASD. Measures for IE prevention must be adopted for 6–12 months after closure until the surgical patch/occluder surface have been covered with the endothelium; endocarditis prophylaxis is not required 6 (to 12) months after closure of an ASD.[11,12]

Follow-up

The cardiologist specialist in adult congenital heart disease (CHD) should follow: an unclosed ASD in adulthood, a surgically closed defect in adulthood, a defect after transcatheter closure in childhood or adulthood, ASD with pulmonary hypertension, with arrhythmia, with right or left ventricular dysfunction, with coexisting disease (CAD, hypertension, valve defects), or if residual findings after ASD closure during childhood are suspected.

The cardiologist without additional training in adult CHD may follow patients with a secundum ASD, closed in childhood or adulthood, and demonstrably free of residual findings, without residual shunt, pulmonary hypertension, arrhythmias and symptoms. Collaboration with a cardiologist with special training and expertise in adult CHD, or a center with an adult CHD program, is appropriate, and is required in the presence of residual defects or late complications or for septal defects other than the secundum type.[7–9]

Prognosis

ASD has a relatively good natural prognosis and patients with ASD may live into advanced age even without surgery.[37] In patients undergoing ASD closure before 24 years of age, the long-term survival does not differ from that seen in the general population at large.[38] Significantly shorter survival rates have been reported in patients with pulmonary hypertension (PAP $\geq$40mmHg) not having the ASD closed until after 24 years of age.[38] A closure in patients over 40 years of age, while reducing mortality, improving symptoms, reducing the incidence of functional deterioration and the incidence of heart failure compared with a conservatively managed control group, did not result in a reduced incidence of arrhythmia[6] or stroke on long-term follow-up. Independent mortality predictors were functional NYHA Class III–IV, PAP >40mmHg and Qp/Qs >3.5:1.[39]

The operative risk in young patients with ASD is minimal (<1%). However, with increasing age, the risk of surgery rises slightly, because of associated disease/comorbidity and pulmonary hypertension (3–6% mortality risk in elderly patients). ASD surgery is followed by a reduction in right ventricular size, even in patients operated on when over 40 years of age.[5] Still, sequelae of inadequate reversibility of hemodynamic changes, e.g. pulmonary artery dilatation with formation of in situ thrombi, and subsequent pulmonary embolism and pulmonary hypertension, tricuspid regurgitation, mitral regurgitation, and atrial fibrillation, may persist, even after successful ASD surgery, in adulthood.[6]

The issue of surgery in asymptomatic adults with ASD over 40 years of age was long debated. Exercise testing in fully asymptomatic patients of 40 years of age, with nonoperated ASD, revealed a significant reduction in functional exercise capacity and respiratory parameters compared with the population at large. Improvement of these parameters was not seen until after 10 years postoperatively, not during short-term postoperative follow-up.[40] In contrast, an increase in peak O_2 consumption, along with a reduction in right ventricular size, was noted as early as 6 months after catheter-based atrial septal closure in patients of 49 years of age, with few symptoms.[41]

An earlier, retrospective, nonrandomized study did not report any differences in mortality, and incidence of arrhythmia and heart failure between surgically and conservatively treated ASD.[42] However, even in this study, the group on conservative therapy showed a higher incidence of tricuspid regurgitation with a higher right ventricular systolic pressure; follow-up stopped when the patients reached 62–63 years of age. The point is, in our experience, it is just after 60 years of age that relatively rapid deterioration and complications occur in patients with unclosed ASD.

Conclusions from a large prospective randomized study supported the appropriateness of timely surgical ASD closure in adults over 40 years of age with few symptoms. A significant higher incidence of severe cardiovascular events was observed in a conservatively managed group.[43]

A convenient resolution of the dilemma whether or not to operate on adults with ASD with minimal symptoms is currently offered by the nonsurgical alternative of transcatheter defect closure. The latter approach does not require sternotomy or thoracotomy, the complication rate is low and the hospitalization time is shorter compared with surgical closure.[10,44–46] The success rate of transcatheter ASD closure is reported to be 89–100%, and depends on patient selection, occluder type, and experience at the center.

Catheter-based closure can also be used with advantage to manage defects in elderly, polymorbid patients and in those with pulmonary hypertension, who are at increased surgical risk.[47] Short- and medium-term outcomes of catheter-based ASD closure are very good – comparable with those reported for surgical defect closure. However, long-term outcome data of transcatheter ASD closure are not yet available.

References

1. Forfang K. Hemodynamic findings before and after surgery for atrial septal defect of the secundum type in middle-aged patients. Cardiology 1978; 63(1): 14–32.
2. Oelberg DA, Marcotte F, Kreisman H et al. Evaluation of right ventricular systolic pressure during incremental exercise by Doppler echocardiography in adults with atrial septal defect. Chest 1998; 113(6): 1459–65.
3. Kobayashi Y, Nakanishi N, Kosakai Y. Pre- and postoperative exercise capacity associated with hemodynamics in adult patients with atrial septal defect: A retrospective study. Eur J Cardiothorac Surg 1997; 11(6): 1062–6.
4. Vogel M, Berger F, Kramer A, Alexi-Meshkishvili V, Lange PE. Incidence of secondary pulmonary hypertension in adults with atrial septal or sinus venosus defects. Heart 1999; 82(1): 30–3.
5. Popelová J, Hlaváček K, Honěk T, Špatenka J, Kölbel F. Atrial septal defect in adults. Can J Cardiol 1996; 12(10): 983–8.
6. Gatzoulis MA, Freeman MA, Siu SC, Webb GD, Harris L. Atrial arrhythmias after surgical closure of atrial septal defects in adults. N Engl J Med 1999; 340: 839–46.

7. Therrien J, Dore A, Gersonz W et al. Canadian Cardiovascular Society Consensus Conference 2001 update: Recommendations for the management of adults with congenital heart disease. Part I. Can J Cardiol 2001; 17(9): 940–59.

8. Deandfield J, Thaulow E, Warnes CA et al. ESC Guidelines: Management of Grown-up Congnenital Heart Disease. Eur Heart J 2003; 24: 1034–84.

9. Landzberg MJ, Murphy JR DJ, Davidson Jr WR et al. Organization of delivery systems for adults with congenital heart disease. J Am Coll Cardiol 2001; 37: 1187–93.

10. Inglessis I, Landzberg MJ. Interventional catheterization in adult congenital heart disease. Circulation 2007; 115: 1622–33.

11. Wilson W, Taubert KA, Gewitz M et al. Prevention of infective endocarditis; guidelines from the American Heart Association. Circulation 2007; published ahead April 19, 2007.

12. Horstkotte D, Follath F, Gutschik E et al. ESC Guidelines on prevention, diagnosis and treatment of infective endocarditis. Eur Heart J 2004; 00: 1–37 (ESC website only: www.esc.org).

13. Ewert P, Daehnert I, Berger F et al. Transcatheter closure of atrial septal defects under echocardiographic guidance without X-ray: Initial experiences. Cardiol Young 1999; 9(2): 136–40.

14. Mullen MJ, Dias BF, Walker F et al. Intracardiac echocardiography guided device closure of atrial septal defects. J Am Coll Cardiol 2003; 41: 285–92.

15. Masura J, Gavora P, Formanek A, Hijazi ZM. Transcatheter closure of secundum atrial septal defects using the new self-centering Amplatzer septal occluder: initial human experience. Cathet Cardiovasc Diagn 1997; 42(4): 388–93.

16. Walsh KP, Tofeig M, Kitchiner DJ, Peart I, Arnold R. Comparison of the Sideris and Amplatzer septal occlusion devices. Am J Cardiol 1999; 83(6): 933–6.

17. Du ZD, Hijazi ZM, Kleinman CS, Silverman NH, Larntz K. Comparison between transcatheter and surgical closure of secundum atrial septal defect in children and adults: Results of a multicenter nonrandomized trial. J Am Coll Cardiol 2002; 39(11): 1836–44.

18. Chan KC, Godman MJ, Walsh K et al. Transcatheter closure of atrial septal defect and interatrial communications with a new self expanding nitinol double disc device (Amplatzer septal occluder): Multicentre UK experience. Heart 1999; 82(3): 300–6.

19. Arora R, Kalra GS, Singh S et al. Transcatheter closure of atrial septal defect using self-expandable septal occluder. Indian Heart J 1999; 51(3): 289–93.

20. Berger F, Ewert P, Dahnert I et al. Interventional occlusion of atrial septum defects larger than 20 mm in diameter. Z Kardiol 2000; 89(12): 1119–25.

21. Acar P, Saliba Z, Bonhoeffer P, Sidi D, Kachaner J. Assessment of the geometric profile of the Amplatzer and cardioseal septal occluders by three dimensional echocardiography. Heart 2001; 85(4): 451–3.

22. Losay J, Petit J, Lambert V et al. Pecutaneous closure with Amplatzer device is a safe and efficient alternative to surgery in adults with large atrial septal defects. Am Heart J 2001; 142(3): 544–8.

23. Zahn EM, Wilson N, Cutright W, Latson LA. Development and testing of the Helex septal occluder, a new expanded polytetrafluoroethylene atrial septal defect occlusion system. Circulation 2001; 104(6): 711–16.

24. Sideris EB, Toumanides S, Macuil B et al. Transcatheter patch correction of secundum atrial septal defects. Am J Cardiol 2002; 89: 1082–6.

25. Omeish A, Hijazi ZM. Transcatheter closure of atrial septal defects in children and adults using the Amplatzer Septal Occluder. J Interv Cardiol 2001; 14(1): 37–44.

26. Chessa M, Carminati M, Butera G. Early and late complications associated with transcatheter occlusion of secundum atrial septal defect. J Am Coll Cardiol 2002; 39: 1061–5.

27. Hill SL, Berul CI, Patel HT et al. Early ECG abnormalities associated with transcatheter closure of atrial septal defects using the Amplatzer septal occluder. J Interv Card Electrophysiol 2000; 4(3): 469–74.

28. Vojácek J, Mates M, Popelova J, Pavel P. Perforation of the right atrium and the ascending aorta following percutaneous transcatheter atrial septal closure. Interact CardioVasc Thorac Surg 2005; 4: 157–9.

29. Cooke JC, Gelman JS, Harper RW. Chiari network entanglement and herniation into the left atrium by an atrial septal defect occluder device. J Am Soc Echocardiogr 1999; 12(7): 601–3.

30. Ewert P, Berger F, Nagdyman N et al. Masked left-ventricular restriction in elderly patients with atrial septal defects: A contraindication for closure? Cathetr Cardiovasc Interv 2001; 52(2): 177–80.

31. Ewert P, Berger F, Nagdyman N et al. Acute left heart failure after interventional occlusion of an atrial septal defect. Z Kardiol 2001; 90(5): 362–6.

32. Onorato E, Pera IG, Melzi G, Rigatelli G. Persistent redundant Eustachian valve interfering with Amplatzer PFO occluder placement: Anatomico-clinical and technical implications. Catheter Cardiovasc Interv 2002; 55(4): 521–4.

33. Lambert V, Belli E, Piot JD, Planche C, Losay J. Hemolysis, a rare complication after percutaneous closure of an atrial septal defect. Arch Mal Coeur Vaiss 2000; 93(5): 623–5.

33a. Arciprete P, Vosa C, D'Angelo A, Pellegrino A, Cotrufo M. Ostium secundum atrial septal defect: is it a minor cardiac lesion? Ital J Surg Sci 1983; 13: 149–52.

33b. Bayer J, Brunner L, Hugel W et al. Acute left heart failure following repair of atrial spetal defects. Its treatment by reopening. Thoraachir Vask Chir 1975; 23: 346–49.

33c. Beyer J. Atrial septal defect: acute left heart failure after surgical closure. Ann Thorac Surg 1978; 25: 36–43.

34. Young D. Later results of closure of secundum atrial septal defects in children. Am J Cardiol 1973; 31: 16–22.

35. Berger F, Vogel M, Alexi-Meskishvili V et al. Comparison of results and complications of surgical and Amplatzer device closure of atrial septal defects. J Thorac Cardiovasc Surg 1999; 118: 674–80.

36. Oakley C. Heart Disease in Pregnancy, 1st edn. London: BMJ Publishing Group, 1997.

37. Webb GD, Gatzoulis MA. Atrial septal defects in the adults. Recent progress and overview. Circulation 2006; 114: 1645–53.

38. Murphy JG, Gersh BJ, McGoon MD et al. Long-term outcome after surgical repair of isolated atrial septa defect. N Engl J Med 1990; 323: 1645–50.

39. Konstantinides S, Geibel A, Olschewski M et al. A comparison of surgical and medical therapy for atrial septal defect in adults. N Engl J Med 1995; 333: 469–73.

40. Helber U, Baumann R, Seboldt H, Reinhard U, Hoffmeister HM. Atrial septal defect in adults: Cardiopulmonary exercise capacity before and 4 months and 10 years after defect closure. J Am Coll Cardiol 1997; 29(6): 1345–50.

41. Brochu MC, Baril JF, Dore A et al. Improvement in exercise capacity in asymptomatic and mildly symptomatic adults after atrial septal defect percutaneous closure. Circulation 2002; 106(14): 1821–6.

42. Shah D, Azhar M, Oakley CM, Cleland JGF, Nihoyannopoulos P. Natural history of secundum atrial septal defect in adults after medical or surgical treatment: A historical prospective study. Br Heart J 1994; 71: 224–8.

43. Attie F, Rosas M, Granados N et al. Surgical treatment for secundum atrial septal defects in patients >40 years old. J Am Coll Cardiol 2001; 38(7): 2035–42.

44. Thomson JDR, Aburawi EH, Watterson KG, Van Doorn C, Gibbs JL. Surgical and transcatheter (Amplatzer) closure of atrial septal defects: A prospective comparison of results and cost. Heart 2002; 87(5): 466–9.

45. Hughes ML, Maskell G, Goh TH, Wilkinson JL. Prospective comparison of costs and short term health outcomes of surgical versus device closure of atrial septal defects in children. Heart 2002; 88(1): 67–70.

46. Berger F, Ewert P, Bjornstad PG et al. Transcatheter closure as standard treatment for most interatrial defects: Experience in 200 patients with the Amplatzer Septal Occluder. Cardiol Young 1999; 9(5): 468–73.

47. Brauer VF, Gessner C, Hagendorff A, Pfeiffer D, Wirtz H. A hemodynamically active type II atrial septal defect in a 78-year-old patient. Indications for interventional catheter occlusion? Dtsch Med Wochenschr 2002; 127(1–2): 26–30.

4

Patent foramen ovale

Anatomical notes

Patent foramen ovale (PFO) is a relatively frequent variant of physiological state and a common finding in the general population; it is not classified as an atrial septal defect (ASD) or heart disease. It is an anatomically tunnel-like structure between the upper rim of the fossa ovalis limb and the fossa ovalis valve, and is the result of the lack of fusion of the septum primum and septum secundum (Figure 4.1). The length of the tunnel varies, ranging from 3 to 24mm, with a mean length of 9mm (Figures 4.2 and 4.3).[1-3]

Prevalence

In the first months of life, PFO is present in most children. In about 70% of cases, it later closes anatomically; in others it is closed functionally, since the pressure in the left atrium is somewhat higher compared with the right one.

In adulthood, anatomical patency of the foramen ovale persists in about 25–30% of the general population. In patients less than 55 years of age with a cerebrovascular

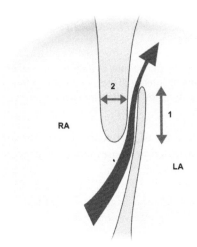

Figure 4.1
Patent foramen ovale. Red arrow shows right-to-left shunt, allowing the paradoxical embolization. 1, Lengths of the tunnel of foramen ovale; 2, width of the septum secundum; RA, right atrium; LA, left atrium.

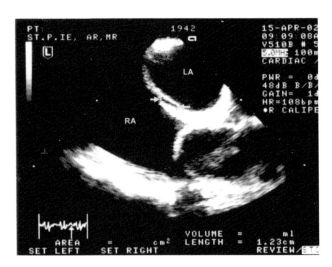

Figure 4.2
Measurement of the length of patent foramen ovale: transesophageal echo, longitudinal view (arrows).

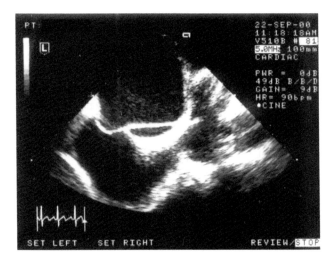

Figure 4.3
Large patent foramen ovale and small aneurysm of atrial septum.

event (CVE), and without risk factors of CVE, the incidence of PFO was higher at 40–54%.[4,5] In younger patients having a CVE, association has been shown with PFO and also atrial septal aneurysm.[6,7]

Pathophysiology

PFO plays an important role in fetal circulation, whereby oxygenated blood from umbilical veins and the vena cava inferior is preferentially directed through the Eustachian valve and PFO to the left atrium and into systemic circulation.

PFO in adults does not usually produce a significant shunt. Its potential risk is that it allows paradoxical embolism into the systemic vascular bed in the presence of venous thrombosis or right atrial thrombosis or thrombosis directly inside the PFO tunnel or atrial septal aneurysm, in hypercoagulation state or when using hormonal contraception.

A right-to-left shunt may be transient or intermittent: it is caused by increased right atrial pressure in pulmonary embolism or lung disease but, also, in cough, Valsalva maneuver or diving, and it may also be dependent on a change in position. The platypnea-orthodeoxia syndrome has been reported in elderly patients who are cyanotic and dyspneic when sitting – the problems resolve when lying. These complaints are explained by a right-to-left shunt in the presence of PFO and a prominent Eustachian valve, directing blood flow from the vena cava inferior to PFO.[8]

Diagnosis when suspecting paradoxical embolism

Transthoracic and transesophageal contrast echocardiography

In younger patients after a CVE or transient ischemic attack (TIA), transthoracic and transesophageal echocardiography is performed with concomitant administration of agitated saline contrast medium into a peripheral vein and using provocation maneuvers (cough, Valsalva maneuver). The risk for paradoxical embolism may depend on the potential size of the right-to-left shunt, as assessed by the appearance of microbubbles in the left atrium (Figures 4.4 and 4.5). PFO is judged to be present with the visualization of microbubbles in the left atrium within three cardiac cycles from the right atrial opacification.[7] Quantification of the number of bubbles appearing in the left atrium is not feasible because the number of bubbles depends on many factors. It was shown that in any PFO right-to-left shunting varies considerably, and that the magnitude of contrast shunting does not necessarily correlate with the true anatomical size of the PFO.[3] Transesophageal echocardiography is not superior to transthoracic echocardography to detect a right-to-left shunt by the use of agitated saline, as the use of sedation and the presence of the probe in the esophagus makes the performance of a Valsalva maneuver difficult. However, the transesophageal echocardiogram is superior to the transthoracic echocardiogram to delineate the structure of the interatrial septum and the PFO.

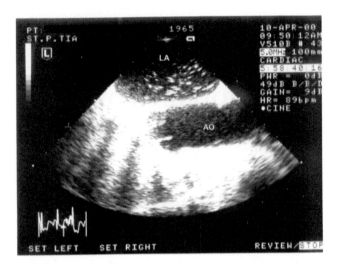

Figure 4.4
Right-to-left shunt in transesophageal echo, longitudinal view proved by contrast echocardiography: microbubbles in the left atrium (LA); AO, aorta.

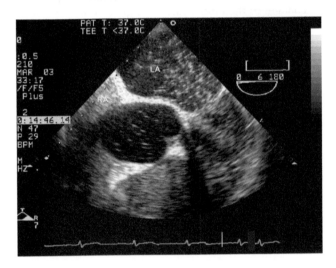

Figure 4.5
Positive contrast echocardiography in transesophageal echo microbubbles crossing interatrial septum via patent foramen ovale from right atrium (RA) to left atrium (LA).

In addition to the basic echocardiogram, the following information is assessed in transesophageal echocardiography in patients with CVE:

- Presence of PFO and right-to-left shunt by color Doppler or during intravenous echo-contrast medium administration.
- Presence of an atrial septal aneurysm (free 'floppy' septum with excursions to the right or the left atrium >10mm, or total excursion >15mm measured by M-mode through the redundant interatrial septum).
- Presence of thrombi in atria, particularly in the left atrial appendage.

- Spontaneous echo contrast in the left atrium.
- Function of the left atrial appendage, especially in supraventricular arrhythmia.
- Left ventricular thrombi in the presence of impaired kinetics.
- Atherosclerotic plaques in the ascending aorta, aortic arch and proximal descending aorta.

Transcranial Doppler examination

The potential for paradoxical microembolism into the cerebral arteries can also be assessed using transcranial Doppler with concomitant venous administration of an echo-contrast medium not passing through the pulmonary capillary bed. However, this technique detects microbubbles in the cerebral circulation not only in the presence of a PFO but also in the presence of any right-to-left shunt (e.g. VSD, intrapulmonary arteriovenous malformations, etc.).[9] Thus, the echocardiogram remains the gold standard to detect a PFO, as it provides both the presence and the location of the shunt.

Neurologic examination

Neurologic examination must identify the cause of CVE/TIA and rule out hemorrhage; it should be complemented by the carotid ultrasound and morphological visualization of the brain by computerized tomography (CT) or magnetic resonance imaging (MRI).

Examination by a cardiologist

Clinical examination, electrocardiogram (ECG), Holter monitoring, echocardiography.

Vascular examination

A source of thrombus is needed for paradoxical embolism. A Doppler ultrasound is performed to exclude deep vein thrombosis in the lower limbs and, alternatively, pelvic vein visualization by MRI/cardiac CT or venography.

Hematological examination

Hematological examination is designed to exclude thrombophilic states. The levels of protein C, S, antithrombin III, presence of anticardiolipin antibodies, activated protein C (APC) resistance, and homocystein levels are determined in addition to routine coagulation assays and D-dimer levels.

Genetic assay

Intended to search for evidence of factor V (Leiden) mutation (with APC resistance), prothrombin mutations, MTHFR mutation or their combination, etc.

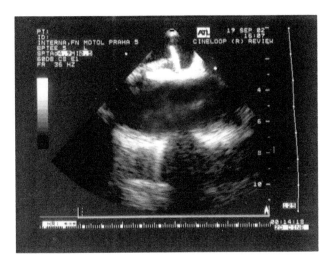

Figure 4.6
Amplatzer occluder closing patent foramen ovale; opened left atrial disc in the left atrium. Transesophageal echo.

Lung scan

Perfusion and ventilatory lung scan will reveal a previous lung embolism.

Treatment

Prevention strategies of recurrent CVE/TIA in the presence of a PFO may include: transcatheter or surgical PFO closure or, alternatively, anticoagulation or antiaggregation (antiplatelet) therapy.[10] However, there is no consensus about the best treatment to prevent cryptogenic stroke in the presence of a PFO because of the lack of a randomized studies evaluating the best treatment option.

A variety of occluders have been used for *catheter-based PFO closure*: Clamshell, Buttoned device, ASDOS, CardioSEAL/Starflex, PFO-Star, Amplatzer PFO, Helex. The Amplatzer device for PFO closure features a bigger right-atrium disc (Figures 4.6 and 4.7). Depending on the type of occluder to be used, the length of the PFO tunnel, septum secundum width, and PFO size on an inflated balloon are determined prior to the transcatheter closure. The completeness of the closure is tested by contrast echocardiography with provocation maneuvers after completion of the endothelialization of the device 6 months after the procedure (Figure 4.8).

Indication of catheter-based patent foramen ovale closure

- Cryptogenic CVE/TIA in younger age with documented paradoxical embolism via PFO after exclusion of any other factors (atherosclerosis, coagulopathy, vasculitis).

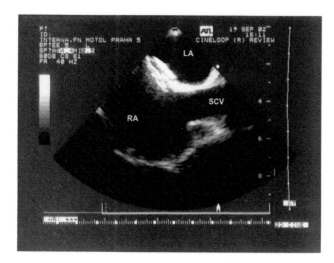

Figure 4.7
Patent foramen ovale closed by Amplatzer occluder.
RA, right atrium; LA, left atrium; SCV, superior caval vein.
Transesophageal echo, longitudinal view.

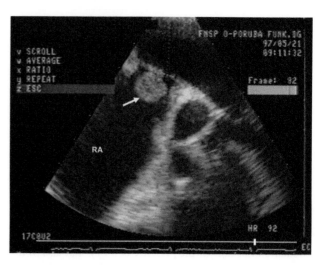

Figure 4.9
Transesophageal echo: Thrombus (arrow) in the
right atrium (RA). (Courtesy of Dr R Štipal, Faculty Hospital
Ostrava, Czech Republic.)

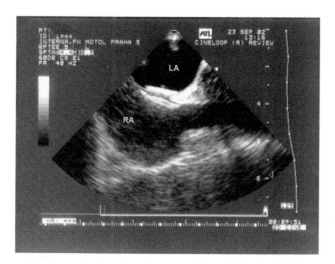

Figure 4.8
Patent foramen ovale closed by Amplatzer occluder with
no residual right-to-left shunt, proved by contrast
transesophageal echo.

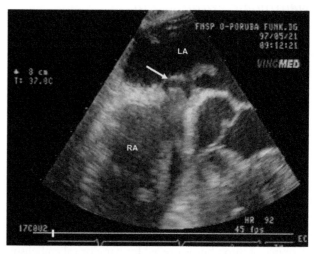

Figure 4.10
Thrombus (arrow) passing from right atrium (RA) to left atrium
(LA) via patent foramen ovale. Transesophageal echo. (Courtesy of
Dr R Štipal, Faculty Hospital Ostrava, Czech Republic.)

- A combination of PFO with atrial septal aneurysm and a
  history of CVE/TIA.
- Recurrent CVE/TIA on drug therapy with assumed
  paradoxical embolism via PFO (Figures 4.9 and 4.10).

Antiaggregation therapy is preferred in elderly patients, with
concomitant coronary artery disease, if a cause of CVE/TIA
other than paradoxical embolism is likely, and when anticoagulation therapy is contraindicated. *Anticoagulation therapy* is indicated in concomitant thrombophilic states,
deep vein thrombosis, pulmonary embolism, and atrial fibrillation. *Surgical management* of PFO is currently losing
ground. It is indicated in serious complications of catheter-
based closure if long-term anticoagulation and antiaggregation therapy is contraindicated; or if preferred by the
patient as an alternative to transcatheter closure following
drug therapy failure. It may be a method of choice for
patients with a metal allergy. Thoracoscopic surgical closure
is available in some centers.

In summary, the best method to prevent cryptogenic
stroke has still to be defined. There is no prospective study
demonstrating the superiority of one strategy over another
(antiplatelet therapy, anticoagulation, device/surgical PFO
closure). The threshold for device closure is declining

(simple technique, availability of the devices) and many PFO are closed, although there are no hard facts for a paradoxical emboli, in particular in patients with other risk factors such as a history of systemic hypertension, diabetes and plaques in the ascending aorta/aortic arch and nonobstructive plaques in the carotid arteries.

Pregnancy and delivery

Pregnancy and the period around delivery are associated with an increased risk for thromboembolic events. In patients with a history of paradoxical embolism, it is appropriate to perform transcatheter or surgical PFO closure before planned pregnancy to avoid anticoagulation and antiaggregation therapy during pregnancy, and a risk for recurrence.

Infectious endocarditis

Prevention of infectious endocarditis should be maintained for at least 6 months after transcatheter PFO closure.[11,12]

Follow-up

Patients with paradoxical embolism in the presence of PFO are examined and followed-up by a neurologist and a cardiologist/internist. Repeat follow-up by a cardiologist, including transthoracic echocardiography, is necessary following transcatheter PFO closure; a transesophageal echocardiogram may be required in the presence of a complication or residual shunt to describe the mechanism of/reason for the shunt.

Prognosis

No therapeutic approach will fully guarantee that neurological problems will never recur. The highest risk for ischemic CVE recurrence was associated with a combination of PFO with atrial septal aneurysm leading to CVE recurrence in 15.2% of cases at 4 years, even when salicylic acid (aspirin) was administered as a preventive measure. With PFO alone, the risk for CVE recurrence was lower when acetylsalicylic acid was administered.[13]

With *surgical closure*, TIA recurrence was seen in 7.5% of patients at 1 year and in 16.6% of patients at 4 years.[14] A risk factor for recurrence was multiple neurological events prior to closure. This emphasizes that factors other than the PFO may play a role in the pathomechanism of a TIA/stroke.

With *conservative treatment*, while prevention with warfarin was more effective compared with antithrombotic

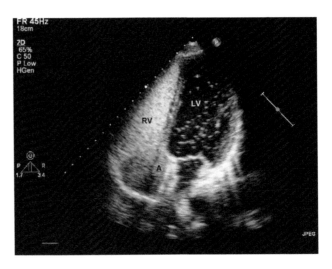

Figure 4.11
Residual right-to-left shunt after patent foramen ovale closure. Transthoracic echo, apical four champer view. RV, Right ventricle; LV, left ventricle; A, Amplatzer PFO occluder.

therapy in some studies, other studies reported no difference in efficacy.[15–17] The risk for CVE recurrence ranged between 2.3 and 17%. Anticoagulation and antiaggregation therapy is associated with a risk for bleeding complications.

After *catheter-based PFO closure*, the incidence of residual shunts is 4–11%, being lower when using newer occluder devices.[2,18,19] Residual shunts predispose to a higher incidence of recurrent neurological events (Figure 4.11).[20,21] The most common complications include occluder-related thrombosis (in 11–41% of cases depending on the extent of thrombosis), followed by occluder embolism and, rarely, tamponade.[22,23] While migraine can be experienced during the first weeks after closure, its incidence is lower in the long run compared with that prior to closure.

Recurrence of neurological events (TIA, CVE) and peripheral embolism after transcatheter PFO closure was 3.4–4.3% at 1 year and 5.9% at 3 years.[2,20] When using newer occluder devices, TIA/CVE recurrence was 0.9–1.5%/ year.[19,23]

Still, it has not been conclusively demonstrated whether or not transcatheter PFO closure in paradoxical embolism is superior to long-term anticoagulation or antiaggregation therapy. Data are affected by patient selection and different etiopathogenesis of CVE/TIA. Prospective randomized trials designed to compare transcatheter PFO closure with conservative treatment are ongoing.

References

1. Marshall AC, Lock JE. Structural and compliant anatomy of the patent foramen ovale in patients undergoing transcatheter closure. Am Heart J 2000; 140: 303–7.

2. Sievert H, Horvath K, Zadan E et al. Patent foramen ovale closure in patients with transient ischemic attack/stroke. J Interv Cardiol 2001; 14(2): 261–6.

3. Pinto FJ. When and how to diagnose patent foramen ovale. Heart 2005; 91: 438–40.

4. Lechat P, Mas JL, Lascault G et al. Prevalence of patent foramen ovale in patients with stroke. N Engl J Med 1988; 318: 1148–52.

5. Lamy C, Giannesini C, Zuber M et al. Clinical and imaging findings in cryptogenic stroke patients with and without patent foramen ovale. The PFO-ASA study. Stroke 2002; 33: 706–11.

6. Nighoghossian N, Perinetti M, Barthlet M, Adeleine P, Trouillas P. Potential cardioembolic sources of stroke in patients less than 60 years of age. Eur Heart J 1996; 17: 590–4.

7. Homma S, Sacco RL. Patent foramen ovale and stroke. Circulation 2005; 112(7): 1063–72.

8. Meier B, Lock JE. Contemporary management of patent foramen ovale. Circulation 2003; 107: 5–9.

9. Droste DW, Lakemeier S, Wichter T et al. Optimising the technique of contrast transcranial Doppler ultrasound in the detection of right-to-left shunts. Stroke 2002; 33: 2211–16.

10. Inglessis I, Landzberg MJ. Interventional catheterization in adult congenital heart disease. Circulation 2007; 115: 1622–33.

11. Horstkotte D, Follath F, Gutschik E et al. ESC Guidelines on prevention, diagnosis and treatment of infective endocarditis. Eur Heart J 2004; 00: 1–37 (ESC website only: www.esc.org).

12. Wilson W, Taubert KA, Gewitz M et al. Prevention of infective endocarditis; guidelines from the American Heart Association. Circulation 2007; published ahead April 19, 2007.

13. Mas JL, Arouizan C, Lamy C et al. Recurrent cerebrovascular events associated with patent foramen ovale, atrial septal aneurysm, or both. N Engl J Med 2001; 345(24): 1740–6.

14. Derani JA, Ugurlu BS, Danielson GK et al. Surgical patent foramen ovale closure for prevention of paradoxical embolism-related cerebrovascular ischemic events. Circulation 1999; 100 (19, Suppl II): 171–5.

15. Cujec B, Mainra R, Johnson DH. Prevention of recurrent cerebral ischemic events in patients with patent foramen ovale and cryptogenic strokes or transient ischemic attacks. Can J Cardiol 1999; 15(1): 57–64.

16. Bogousslavsky J, Garazi S, Jeanrenaud X, Aebischer N, Van Melle G. Stroke recurrence in patients with patent foramen ovale: The Laussane study. Neurology 1996; 46: 1301–5.

17. Mohr JP, Thompson JL, Lazar RM et al. Warfarin–aspirin recurrent stroke study group. A comparison of warfarin and aspirin for the prevention of recurrent ischemic stroke. N Engl J Med 2001; 34(20): 1444–51.

18. Hung J, Landzberg MJ, Jenkins KJ et al. Closure of patent foramen ovale for paradoxical emboli: Intermediate-term risk of reccurrent neurological events following transcatheter device placement. J Am Coll Cardiol 2000; 35(5): 1311–16.

19. Beitzke A, Schuchlenz H, Gamillscheg A, Stein JI, Wendelin G. Catheter closure of the persistent foramen ovale: Mid-term results in 162 patients. J Interv Cardiol 2001; 14(2): 223–9.

20. Windecker S, Wahl A, Chatterjee T et al. Percutaneous closure of patent foramen ovale in patients with paradoxical embolism: Long-term risk of recurrent thromboembolic events. Circulation 2000; 101(8): 893–8.

21. Wahl A, Meier B, Haxel B et al. Prognosis after percutaneous closure of patent foramen ovale for paradoxical embolism. Neurology 2001; 57: 1330–2.

22. La Rosee K, Krause D, Becker M et al. Transcatheter closure of atrial septal defects in adults. Practicality and safety of four different closure systems used in 102 patients. Dtsch Med Wochenschr 2001; 126(38): 1030–6.

23. Martin F, Sanchez P, Doherty E et al. Percutanneous transcatheter closure of patent foramen ovale in patients with paradoxical embolism. Circulation 2002; 106: 1121–6.

5

Atrioventricular septal defect

Division and anatomical notes

Atrioventricular septal defects (AVSD) constitute a spectrum of anomalies caused by abnormal development of endocardial cushions. AVSD is characterized by formation abnormalities of the atrioventricular valves (AV valves), the inferior part of the atrial septum, and the posterior part of the ventricular septum (Figure 5.1). Defects range from incomplete (partial) to intermediate to complete forms.

Incomplete (partial) atrioventricular septal defect

Incomplete (partial) AVSD, also referred to as 'ostium primum defect', is the most common form of AV canal defects. The interatrial communication is located between the inferior parts of the atrial septum (Figure 5.1b) and the bridging leaflets. An interventricular communication is lacking.

The AV valves insert at the same level. Within a common atrioventricular annulus lie two separate AV valve orifices. The anterior (= superior) and a posterior (= inferior) bridging leaflets are fused by leaflet tissue (connecting tongue) that lies in the ventricular septum. In the left-sided valve the

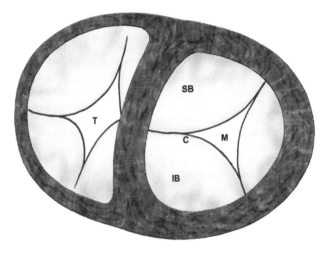

Figure 5.2
Incomplete atrioventricular septal defect: the cleft of the anterior 'mitral' valve cusp is in fact the commissure (C) between superior bridging leaflet (SB) and inferior bridging leaflet (IB). M, Mitral orifice; T, tricuspid orifice.

apposition line of the anterior (= superior) and a posterior (= inferior) bridging leaflet form what is called a 'cleft'. In fact, this 'cleft' is a commissure between the upper and lower bridging cusps on the left side of the atrioventricular valve (Figures 5.2 and 5.3). There may be a 'cleft' in the right-sided AV valve as well; the right-sided valve has four leaflets.

Moreover, the arrangement of the papillary muscles is different in the left ventricle. The aortic valve is displaced anteriorly and to the right ('unwedged'). In the left heart, there is a disproportion between the inflow and outflow tracts. The distance from the left ventricular apex to the aortic valve is considerably longer than that to the left AV valve, resulting in left ventricular outflow tract elongation ('gooseneck deformity').

Intermediate atrioventricular septal defect

Intermediate AVSD represents the least frequent type (Figure 5.4). It refers to a primum atrial septal defect (ASD), a common AV valve annulus and a restrictive interventricular communication. The ventricular septal defect (VSD) is located between the bridging leaflets and the crest of the ventricular septum. With a common AV valve, it resembles a complete AVSD. However, the

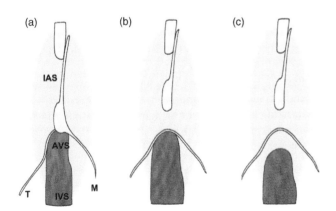

Figure 5.1
Atrioventricular septal defect (AVSD): (a) normal relation between interatrial septum (IAS), atrioventricular septum (AVS), interventricular septum (IVS), and septal cusps of tricuspid (T) and mitral (M) valves; (b) incomplete AVSD (atrial septal defect type primum); (c) complete AVSD (complete atrioventricular septal defect).

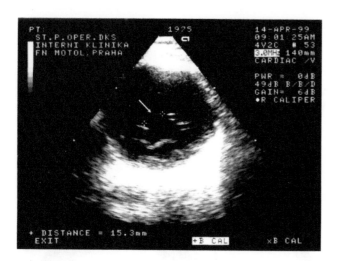

Figure 5.3
Cleft of the anterior mitral valve cusp (arrow) in incomplete atrioventricular septal defect. Transthoracic echo, short axis at the level of mitral valve.

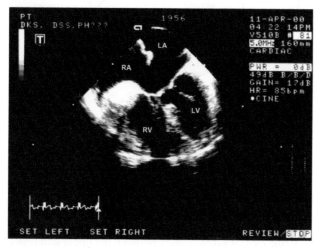

Figure 5.4
Intermediate type of atrioventricular septal defect: large ostium primum atrial septal defect, common atrioventricular valve, the chordal attachment covers the ventricular part of the defect with only minor shunt at the level of ventricles. Transesophageal echo, transversal four-chamber view. RA, Right atrium; RV, right ventricle; LA, left atrium; LV, left ventricle.

bridging cusps of the valve are attached to the top of the ventricular septum, thus dividing the common AV valve into a 'mitral' and a 'tricuspid' part: these attachments also diminish the ventricular component of the defect (Figure 5.5).

Complete atrioventricular septal defect

Complete AVSD involves unrestricted communication between both atria and both ventricles (Figure 5.1c). There

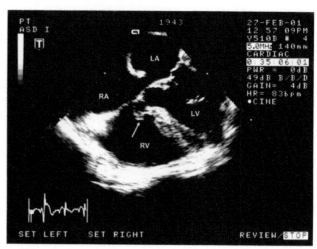

Figure 5.5
Intermediate atrioventricular septal defect in adulthood, small ostium primum atrial septal defect, attachment of the atrioventricular valve into ventricular septum completely covers the ventricular defect by pseudoaneurysm (arrow). Transesophageal echo. RA, Right atrium; RV, right ventricle; LA, left atrium; LV, left ventricle.

is an atrial septal (ostium primum) defect, a nonrestrictive ventricular septal inflow defect, and a single, common, usually five-cusp, AV valve, which is not attached to the ventricular septum. The valve consists of an anterior (= superior) and a posterior (= inferior) bridging leaflet, a left mural leaflet, a right inferior leaflet and a right anterior leaflet. The ventricular septum may shift to the right or left ventricle, thus creating unbalanced AVSD with one dominant and another hypoplastic ventricle.

According to the variability of only the anterior (superior) bridging leaflet to the crest of the ventricular septum or the right ventricle papillary muscles, complete AVSD can be divided into three categories:[1,2]

- Rastelli A: The superior bridging leaflet is tethered to the crest of the ventricular septum.
- Rastelli B: The superior bridging leaflet is attached to an anomalous papillary muscle in the right ventricle.
- Rastelli C: The superior bridging leaflet is not attached to the septum, but to the free wall of the right ventricle (free-floating leaflet).

Prevalence

AVSD accounts for about 4% of all congenital heart disease (CHD). In some cases, even this defect – and incomplete AVSD in particular – may not be recognized until adulthood. About 35% of AVSD patients have Down's syndrome. Among children with Down's syndrome, about 40–56%

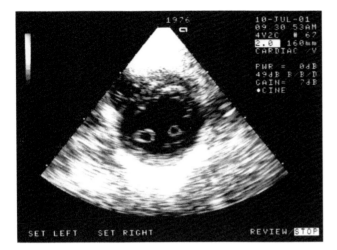

Figure 5.6
Double mitral orifice in incomplete atrioventricular septal defect, both orifices were incompetent. Transthoracic echo, short axis at the level of mitral valve.

have CHD, out of which proportion 40–44% have AVSD, usually the complete form.[3] AVSD appears to have a multifactorial inheritance pattern.

Complete AVSD may also be associated with the asplenia or polysplenia syndrome (see Chapter 23), or with conotruncal anomalies such as tetralogy of Fallot. AVSD may additionally involve a double mitral orifice (in 9%) (Figure 5.6), and mitral valve attachment into a single papillary muscle (in 3%).

Pathophysiology

In AVSD the shunt between the atria or ventricles is primarily a left-to-right one. In incomplete AVSD there is an increased pulmonary blood flow due to the left-to-right shunt. The right atrium, the right ventricle and the pulmonary vessels are volume loaded. In the case of left-sided AV valve regurgitation, the regurgitant volume is immediately shunted to the right atrium and the left atrium is decompressed.

In complete AVSD hemodynamic changes are the sum of an ASD and a VSD. Due to the left-to-right shunt, all cardiac chambers and the pulmonary vessels are volume loaded. The size of the left-to-right shunt is dependent on the level of the pulmonary arterial resistance. In contrast, in left ventricle to right atrium communication the shunt is obligatory and depends on the size of the defect.

The excessive pulmonary blood flow and elevated pulmonary artery pressure result rapidly in irreversible pulmonary vascular disease. Pulmonary hypertension does not develop in the case of concomitant pulmonary stenosis, severe enough to protect pulmonary vascular bed.

Clinical findings and diagnosis

In adult patients, one may see unoperated *incomplete or intermediate AVSD*, which may remain clinically silent for some time. Heart failure occurs in about 20% of unoperated incomplete AVSD.

Most untreated patients with *complete AVSD* develop congestive heart failure in early childhood, and only few survive the first 3 years of life without operation. After 6 months most patients (particularly those with Down's syndrome) develop rapidly severe pulmonary hypertension and irreversible pulmonary vascular obstructive disease (Eisenmenger syndrome). Pulmonary hypertension will not develop when associated with significant pulmonary artery stenosis, affording protection to the pulmonary vascular bed.

Most AVSD patients have had defect surgery during childhood and may have either no complaints, or their complaints are adequate to the residual findings.

Symptoms

- Symptoms of heart failure.
- Symptoms of pulmonary vascular disease.
- Dyspnea, exertional dyspnea.
- Fatigability.
- Palpitations.
- Respiratory tract infection.
- Arrhythmias.
- Complete heart block.

General examination

- Prominent and hyperactive precordium.
- Palpable S2 if pulmonary hypertension.
- Systolic thrill at the left lower sternal border.

Auscultatory findings

- Incomplete AVSD: There is a fixed splitting of the second sound over the pulmonary artery (increased blood flow) and a systolic ejection murmur over the pulmonary artery. In the rare presence of pulmonary hypertension, the second sound is enhanced over the pulmonary artery. Systolic regurgitant murmur of mitral insufficiency at the apex. Mid-diastolic rumble of relative AV valve stenosis.
- Intermediate AVSD: In addition to the findings for incomplete AVSD there is also a systolic VSD murmur.
- Complete AVSD: Auscultation will reveal the systolic murmur of AV valve regurgitation and, if significant, the mid-diastolic rumble of relative AV valve stenosis. The increased blood flow across the pulmonary outflow tract may cause a systolic crescendo–decrescendo murmur.

If there is associated pulmonary hypertension and balanced ventricular pressure, the second heart sound is single and accentuated, while the shunt may disappear, or may be silent and undetectable by auscultation and the Graham Steell diastolic murmur of pulmonary insufficiency may appear. In the case of concomitant pulmonary stenosis, a systolic ejection murmur will be heard over the pulmonary artery.

Electrocardiogram (ECG)

- The cardiac axis is tilted leftward in AVSD; superior frontal plane QRS wave with left-axis deviation (axis −30 to −180 degrees).
- AV conduction may be prolonged.
- Occasionally higher degree AV block.
- Right ventricular hypertrophy, additional left ventricular hypertrophy, incomplete or complete right bundle branch block (particularly after surgery).

Holter monitoring

This is indicated to identify potential transient AV block and supraventricular arrhythmias.

Chest X-ray

- Cardiomegaly in the presence of left and right ventricular dilatation or, possibly, left atrial dilatation.
- Enhanced pulmonary vasculature, prominent pulmonary artery.

Echocardiography

Definitive diagnosis will require echocardiography; in most adults, exact assessment will also require transesophageal echocardiography. The following parameters are assessed:

- Presence and magnitude of ostium primum defect.
- Presence and magnitude of the ventricular component of the defect or, alternatively, its spontaneous closure.
- Magnitude and direction of shunt at atrial and ventricular levels, and, possibly, shunt between ventricles and atria (most often between the left ventricle and right atrium).
- The pulmonary and systemic blood flow rates are determined (Qp/Qs).
- Morphology of AV valves, cusp attachment (septal cusps are attached at the same level), course and attachment of the chordae tendinae, cusp cleft, number of cusps. Rarely, a double mitral valve orifice can be found.
- Presence and degree of regurgitation at both AV valves (Figures 5.7–5.10).

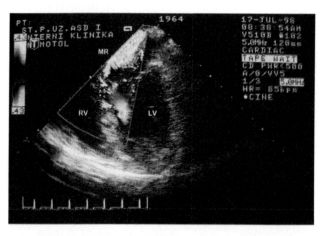

Figure 5.7
Severe residual mitral regurgitation (MR) after atrioventricular septal defect closure and suture of the cleft of mitral valve in childhood, notice the very eccentric jet of MR. Transesophageal echo, transversal plane, color Doppler. LV, Left ventricle; RV, right ventricle.

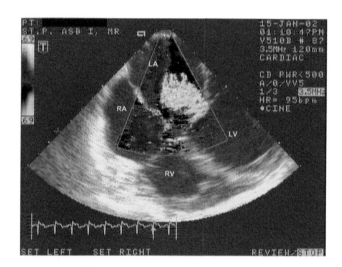

Figure 5.8
Severe residual mitral regurgitation after atrioventricular septal defect (AVSD) closure in childhood. Transesophageal echo, transversal plane. RA, Right atrium; RV, right ventricle; LA, left atrium; LV, left ventricle.

- AV valve 'straddling' (= attachment into an inappropriate ventricle) and atrioventricular annulus 'overriding'.
- Presence or absence of subaortic stenosis, which may develop even postoperatively and may be progressive.
- Pulmonary artery pressure is calculated noninvasively, preferably based on the gradient of tricuspid regurgitation; however, one should bear in mind the high flow rates associated with shunts between the left ventricle and right atrium, which may falsely overestimate the calculation.
- Size of ventricles (balance) = the ratio of cavities of either ventricle.

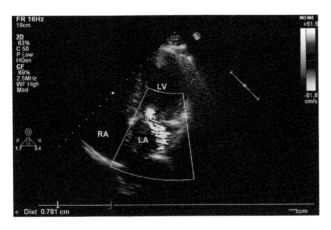

Figure 5.9
Incomplete atrioventricular septal defect, transthoracic echo, four-chamber apical view; severe mitral regurgitation with eccentric jet due to the cleft of the anterior mitral leaflet. Vena contracta is 7mm between the two marks. LV, Left ventricle; LA, left atrium; RA, right atrium.

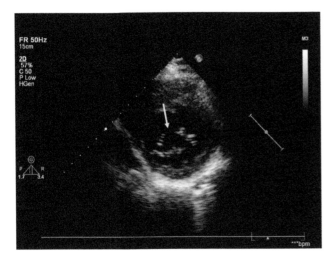

Figure 5.10
Incomplete atrioventricular septal defect, unoperated in adult patient. Transthoracic echo, short parasternal view at the level of mitral annulus, cleft of the anterior leaflet (arrow), severe mitral regurgitation, the same patient as in Figure 5.9.

- Associated CHD (e.g. tetralogy of Fallot, patent arterial duct, coarctation of the aorta, etc.).

Catheterization (not routinely used)

- Undertaken to exactly quantify intracardiac shunting.
- To rule out coexisting muscular VSD.
- To assess pulmonary artery pressure and pulmonary vascular resistance, and to test the reversibility of pulmonary vascular disease (O_2, NO, prostanoids).

- In cases requiring specification of regurgitation, or stenosis of the AV valves, or significance of the subaortic stenosis (possibly combined with provocation tests).
- To perform selective coronary arteriography prior to a cardiac surgical procedure in patients over 40 years of age, or younger if at risk for coronary artery disease or with the possibility of coronary artery anomalies or injury due to previous surgery.

Management

Correction of complete AVSD is performed, mostly as single-stage repair, as 'two-patch' or 'single-patch' repair.[4] For a two-patch repair a pericardial patch is used to close the interatrial defect, and a Dacron or Goretex patch to close the ventricular component of the defect. If possible, the AV valve is reconstructed, or it is replaced. Additional anomalies are fixed. In the case of atrial fibrillation or atrial flutter, the Maze procedure or cryo-ablation of cavo-tricuspid isthmus is performed during surgery.

The broad spectrum of malformations in AVSD requires experience and an individualized approach.[5] Surgery, or 're-do' surgery, of AVSD in adults should be performed by a cardiac surgeon experienced in CHD surgery, reoperations and corrections of the AVSD and mitral valve surgery.

Indications for surgical AVSD management:

- A significant left-to-right shunt at the level of atria and/or ventricles (Qp/Qs >1.5:1) or a major morphological defect (>15mm) associated with:
  o symptoms, or;
  o signs of right or left ventricular volume overload, or;
  o heart failure, or;
  o reversible pulmonary hypertension, or;
  o significant left AV valve regurgitation, or;
  o supraventricular arrhythmia, or;
  o incipient ventricular dysfunction (ejection fraction (EF) ≤ 60%).
- Paradoxical embolism in the presence of documented right-to-left shunt, regardless of the defect's magnitude (unless irreversible pulmonary hypertension is a contraindication to closure).

Contraindications to surgery are identical with those for ASD (see Chapter 3).

Residual postoperative findings

- *Residual left-sided AV valve regurgitation:* This is frequent after surgery in childhood and may be due to a variety of causes. It is determined by the degree of AV valve dysplasia, dilatation of the valve annulus, or may even be caused by loosening of sutures at the left AV valve cleft or, possibly, the operative technique. In >14% of cases, residual regurgitation requires reoperation in the long run (Figures 5.7 and 5.8).

The indication for reoperation is similar to that in acquired mitral regurgitation in view of a potential concomitant residual shunt, which may be enlarged by mitral regurgitation. Attention must be given to left ventricular size and systolic function. In the presence of severe residual left-sided AV valve (mitral) regurgitation, reoperation is indicated in the presence of symptoms or in asymptomatic patients, if the ejection fraction of the left ventricle decreases to 60% or if the left ventricle dilates (end-systolic diameter ≥40mm (24mm/m^2)). In the presence of favorable AV valve morphology, valve reconstruction can be undertaken; however, severe regurgitation often requires valve replacement.

- *Residual shunt* at the levels of atria, ventricles, a left-ventricle-to-right-atrium shunt or, alternatively, a right-ventricle-to-left-atrium shunt. Reoperation is indicated depending on the hemodynamic significance of the shunt.
- *Subaortic obstruction* is considered hemodynamically significant with a catheterization or mean echo-gradient >50 mmHg (at rest or following provocation by isoproterenol). In about 5% of cases, subaortic obstruction may develop and progress even after AVSD surgery.
- *Pulmonary vascular obstructive disease* occurs more often with complete AVSD.
- *Arrhythmias* are frequently seen after AVSD correction. A complete AV block may develop from intraoperative injury to the AV node region or the His bundle when suturing an atrial or ventricular patch; it is an indication for permanent cardiac pacing. A complete AV block may also develop at a longer postoperative interval, the same as atrial fibrillation and flutter.

Risks associated with an unoperated atrioventricular septal defect

- *Left-sided AV regurgitation* in the presence of a 'cleft' may progress and augment the left-to-right shunt at atrial level. AV valve regurgitation may be well tolerated for a long period of time. The risk of late indication of surgery with postoperative left ventricular dysfunction equals that of acquired mitral regurgitation.
- *Heart failure.*
- *Subaortic stenosis.*
- *Arrhythmia*: AV conduction disturbances, first-degree (or up to third-degree) AV block occur frequently, as do atrial fibrillation and flutter in elderly patients. Anticoagulation therapy is indicated in cases with chronic atrial fibrillation.

- Development and progression of *pulmonary hypertension.*
- *Transvenous stimulation* in an unclosed AVSD carries a risk because of potential paradoxical embolism into the systemic vascular bed.
- *Venous thrombosis* in an unclosed AVSD carries a risk because of potential paradoxical embolism.
- Generally, AVSD is a more serious defect compared to atrial septal ostium secundum defect.

Pregnancy and delivery

In unoperated cases, pregnancy and delivery may be risky because of paradoxical embolism or the development of heart failure. In operated AVSD, and in the absence of significant residual lesions, pregnancy and delivery are well tolerated, particularly if the patient is in NYHA Class I–II prior to delivery. However, pregnancy may result in hemodynamic deterioration.

Pregnancy poses a high risk in significant pulmonary hypertension and is contraindicated in Eisenmenger syndrome because of high maternal and fetal mortality rates. The occurrence rate of CHD in the offspring is about 14%.[6]

Infectious endocarditis

Compared with ASD, AVSD is associated with a significantly higher risk for the development of infectious endocarditis (IE) because of the concomitant involvement of the left-sided AV valve and, possibly, the ventricular septum defect. Considering the potential for residual shunts, morphologically abnormal AV valve, and patch calcification, prophylaxis of IE should be maintained even after successful surgery.

Follow-up of atrioventricular septal defect

Cardiologist with experience in ACHD.[7]

Prognosis

- AVSD is associated with an adverse prognosis because of the concomitant left AV valve regurgitation, conduction disturbances, and the more frequent and early development of pulmonary hypertension, particularly in complete AVSD. Without surgery, the mortality of children with complete AVSD patients is 80% in historical studies.

- Operative mortality rates in childhood are 3.7–4.2% with incomplete and intermediate AVSD, and up to 14.4–19.6% with complete AVSD.[8] Surgical success is dependent on the morphology of the left AV valve; its thickening and stenosis pose a risk factor for death and reoperation.
- Children with Down's syndrome usually have chronic nasopharyngeal obstruction with subsequent hypoventilation making the hemodynamic finding worse. Down's syndrome alone is not considered a risk factor; however, complications are due to the development of pulmonary vascular obstructive disease caused by late surgery. If a complete AVSD is repaired during the first year of life, Down's syndrome seems not to affect the long-term results negatively.[9]
- The prognosis of adults with AVSD operated on in childhood depends on the significance of residual findings, especially that of left AV valve (mitral) regurgitation and pulmonary hypertension. The 20-year survival following incomplete AVSD surgery in childhood was 96%.[10] During long-term follow-up, reoperation is required at least in 14–15.5% of patients: mostly for residual left AV valve regurgitation, with a small proportion of patients for a residual shunt or subaortic stenosis. As the time from surgery increases, the number of cases with significant left AV valve regurgitation requiring surgery will also rise. The cause of left AV valve regurgitation following primary valvuloplasty is usually dehiscence of 'cleft' suture in combination with fibrotic lesions and valve dysplasia, and also dilatation of the left AV valve annulus.
- Incomplete AVSD can usually be operated on in adulthood, unless there is severe, irreversible pulmonary hypertension or fairly significant left ventricular dysfunction and dilatation.[11] Some studies have shown that >50% of patients with incomplete AVSD undergoing surgery in their fifties have sustained or newly developed atrial arrhythmia.

References

1. Rastelli G, Kirklin JW, Titus JL. Anatomic observations on complete form of persistent common atrioventricular canal with special reference to atrioventricular valves. Mayo Clin Proc 1966; 41(5): 296–308.
2. Piccoli GP, Wilkinson JL, Macartney FJ, Gerlis LM, Anderson RH. Morphology and classification of complete atrioventricular defects. Br Heart J 1979; 42(6): 633–9.
3. Freeman SB, Taft LF, Dooley KJ et al. Population-based study of congenital heart defects in Down syndrome. Am J Med Genet 1998; 80(3): 213–17.
4. Lange R, Schreiber C, Gunther T et al. Results of biventricular repair of congenital cardiac malformations: Definitive corrective surgery? Eur J Cardiothorac Surg 2001; 20(6): 1207–13.
5. Crawford FA Jr, Stroud MR. Surgical repair of complete atrioventricular septal defect. Ann Thorac Surg 2001; 72(5): 1621–8; discussion 1628–9.
6. Digilio MC, Marino B, Cicini MP et al. Risk of congenital heart defects in relatives of patients with atrioventricular canal. Am J Dis Child 1993; 147(12): 1295–7.
7. Deanfield J, Thaulow E, Warnes C et al. Task Force on the Management of Grown Up Congenital Heart Disease, European Society of Cardiology; ESC Committee for Practice Guidelines. Management of grown up congenital heart disease. Eur Heart J 2003; 24(11): 1035–84.
8. Bando K, Turrentine MW, Sun K et al. Surgical management of complete atrioventricular septal defects. A twenty-year experience. J Thorac Cardiovasc Surg 1995; 110(5): 1543–52; discussion 1552–4.
9. Masuda M, Kado H, Tanoue Y et al. Does Down syndrome affect the long-term results of complete atrioventricular septal defect when the defect is repaired during the first year of life? Eur J Cardiothorac Surg 2005; 27(3): 405–9. (Epub 2004 Dec 30)
10. Formigari R, Gargiulo G, Picchio FM. Operation for partial atrioventricular septal defect: A forty-year review. J Thorac Cardiovasc Surg 2000; 119(5): 880–9; discussion 889–90.
11. El-Najdawi EK, Driscoll DJ, Puga FJ et al. Operation for partial atrioventricular septal defect: A forty-year review. J Thorac Cardiovasc Surg 2000; 119(5): 880–9.

6

Ventricular septal defect

Anatomical notes

In the normal heart, the interventricular septum has a fibrous component – the so-called membranous septum – and three muscular components: the inlet septum, the trabecular septum, and the outlet or infundibular septum. A ventricular septal defect (VSD) is a congenital communication between the two ventricles. VSD may be isolated or part of more complex congenital heart disease (CHD). This chapter addresses isolated VSD only.

There are several *classification systems*. Based on the location in the ventricular septum, VSD are divided into the following types (Figure 6.1):

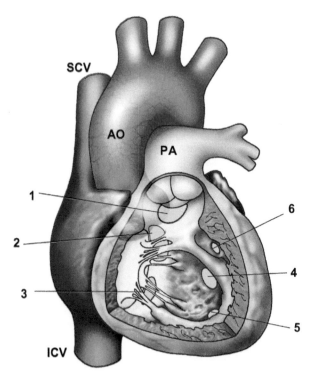

Figure 6.1
Anatomic location of ventricular septal defects (VSD), viewed from the right ventricle. 1, Outlet VSD; 2, perimembranous VSD; 3, inlet VSD; 4, muscular central VSD; 5, muscular apical VSD; 6, muscular marginal VSD. SCV, Superior caval vein; ICV, inferior caval vein; AO, aorta; PA, pulmonary artery.

- Perimembranous or membranous VSD – part of the defect occupies the area of membranous septum:
  - with extension to the inlet septum (atrioventricular septal defect (AVSD) or canal type);
  - with extension to the trabecular septum;
  - with extension to the outlet – (infundibular) septum (Fallot type).
- Muscular VSD – the defect is completely surrounded by a muscular rim:
  - in the inlet septum;
  - in the trabecular septum (central, marginal, apical);
  - in the outlet septum (infundibular).
- Doubly committed (subarterial) VSD.
- *Perimembranous* (membranous, infracristal) VSD accounts for about 60–80% of all VSD. The membranous septum is localized under the crista supraventricularis, immediately under the aortic valve and dorsally to the conal papillary muscle of the tricuspid valve (Figure 6.2). Perimembranous VSD extends to the adjacent parts of the inlet, muscular trabecular, or outlet septum.
- *Inlet VSD* (AVSD type): The inlet septum separates the inlet segment of both ventricles and is localized posteroinferior to the membranous septum. Inlet VSD are localized in the inlet part of the ventricular septum posterior to the tricuspid valve septal leaflet. They account for about 8% of all VSD.
- *Outlet VSD* (supracristal, subarterial, infundibular type) are localized in the outlet septal region beneath the pulmonary valve, and communicate with the right ventricular outflow tract above the crista supraventricularis. The outlet septum is localized between the crista supraventricularis and the pulmonary valve. This VSD type accounts for 5–7% of all VSD and is more frequent in Asia (up to 30% of all VSD).
- *The muscular type* is surrounded by the muscular ventricular septum from all sides. The defect is divided into an apical, central and a marginal defect (Figure 6.3); it may also be multiple ('Swiss cheese'). Muscular VSD account for some 5–20% of all VSD.
- *Gerbode defect* refers to a shunt between the left ventricle and right atrium; it is usually small and rare.[1]

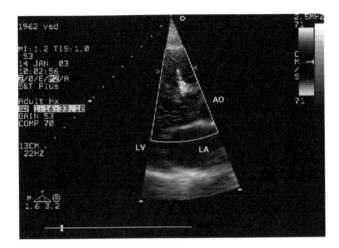

Figure 6.2
Small restrictive subaortic perimembranous ventricular septal defect with left-to-right shunt. Transthoracic echo, long-axis parasternal view with color Doppler.

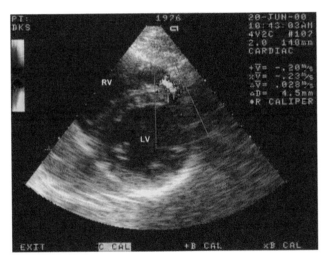

Figure 6.3
Small muscular marginal ventricular septal defect in the anterior part of the muscular ventricular septum. Transthoracic short-axis view at the level of papillary muscles, color Doppler. LV, Left ventricle; RV, right ventricle.

Physiological classification

The physiological classification defines:

- *Restrictive defect*: Right ventricular systolic pressure is lower than the left ventricular systolic pressure.
- *Non-restrictive defect*: Pressures in either ventricle are balanced in the absence of right ventricular outflow tract obstruction.

Hemodynamic significance

Shunt direction and size in isolated VSD are determined by the size of the defect and by the ratio of pulmonary to systemic vascular resistance. Based on their hemodynamic significance, VSD are divided according to the ratio of the pulmonary to systemic blood flow (Qp/Qs):

- *Small*: Pulmonary artery to systemic systolic pressure ratio <0.3 and Qp/Qs <1.4.
- *Moderate*: Ratio of systolic pressures <0.3 and Qp/Qs = 1.4–2.2.
- *Large*: Ratio of systolic pressures >0.3 and Qp/Qs >2.2.
- *VSD with Eisenmenger syndrome*: Ratio of systolic pressures >0.9 and Qp/Qs <1.5.

(Source: Canadian Consensus Conference, 2001[2])

Prevalence

VSD is the most common CHD in childhood, accounting for about 25% of all CHD as an isolated defect, and 50% of all CHD for all VSD (both isolated and part of other CHD).[3] In the adult population, VSD occur less often because of their frequent spontaneous closure. Often, associated anomalies are atrial septal defect, patent arterial duct, right aortic arch, and pulmonary stenosis.

Pathophysiology

- In a VSD the direction and the amount of shunt are determined by the size of the defect, and by the relationship of the systemic and pulmonary vascular resistance.
- The magnitude and direction of the shunt are determined by the pressure gradient between both ventricles in individual phases of the cardiac cycle.
- With small and moderate defects, a left-to-right shunt occurs during left ventricular ejection and isovolumic contraction. With large defects involving balanced pressure levels, the shunt is a left-to-right one during isovolumic contraction and a right-to-left one during isovolumic relaxation.
- In a *small VSD* (Qp/Qs <1.4:1; PAP_{sys}/Ao_{sys} <0.3), the shunt is left-to-right and its magnitude depends primarily on the defect size. The right ventricular pressure is normal. The main pulmonary artery, left atrium and left ventricle are only mildly enlarged and the vascular markings are not increased. The right ventricle is not volume or pressure loaded.
- A *moderate VSD* (Qp/Qs = 1.4–2.2:1; PAP_{sys}/Ao_{sys} >0.3) causes a significant enlargement of the main pulmonary artery, left atrium and left ventricle. The pulmonary vascular markings are increased. The right ventricle is not significantly pressure or volume overloaded. The

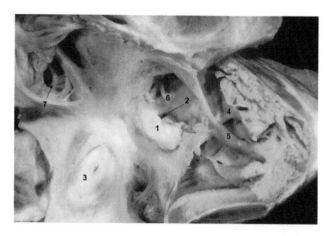

Figure 6.4

Spontaneous closure of ventricular septal defect by adherence of the septal cusp of the tricuspid valve (pseudoaneurysm); view from the right atrium and right ventricle. 1, Septal cusp of the tricuspid valve, closing the defect (pseudoaneurysm of the ventricular septum); 2, residual ventricular septal defect; 3, fossa ovalis; 4, trabecula septomarginalis; 5, anterior papillary muscle; 6, medial papillary muscle; 7, entry into the right auricle. (Courtesy of Dr Yen S Ho, Royal Brompton Hospital, London.)

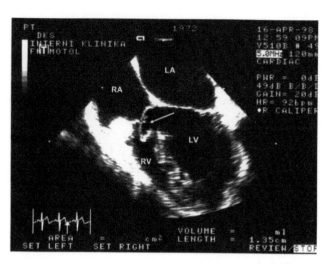

Figure 6.5

Pseudoaneurysm of the ventricular septum spontaneously closing a large ventricular septal defect (arrow). RA, Right atrium; RV, right ventricle; LA, left atrium; LV, left ventricle. Transesophageal echo, four-champer transversal projection.

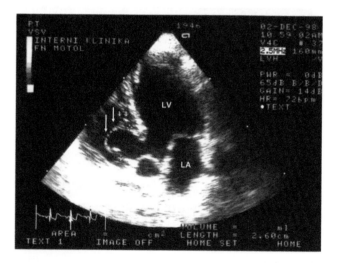

Figure 6.6

Large pseudoaneurysm of the ventricular septum closing perimembranous ventricular septal defect, marked with arrows. Transthoracic echo, apical four-chamber view. LV, Left ventricle; LA, left atrium.

pulmonary artery pressure may increase (reversible) to one third–one half of systemic pressure ($PAP_{sys}/Ao_{sys} = 0.5$).

- In a *large VSD* (Qp/Qs >2.2:1; PAP_{sys}/Ao_{sys} >0.3), the defect itself is unrestrictive, i.e. the left ventricular pressure is transmitted directly to the right ventricle and to the pulmonary arteries. The right ventricle develops hypertrophy. The right ventricular and pulmonary arterial pressures rise, mainly due to the high shunt volume and the increasing pulmonary artery resistance. The significant increase in pulmonary artery flow and pulmonary vascular resistance result – if untreated – in severe and sometimes irreversible pulmonary vascular obstructive disease. Pulmonary artery resistance will equal systemic vascular resistance and a right-to-left shunt will develop. In Eisenmenger reaction, Qp/Qs is <1.5:1, and PAP_{sys}/Ao_{sys} is >0.9.

Clinical findings and diagnosis

- Most adults with VSD have only a small left-to-right shunt.
- Major uncorrected VSD in adulthood are rare, as most of them have either had surgical defect closure during childhood or they have developed pulmonary vascular obstructive disease (Eisenmenger syndrome).
- In some, the shunt has diminished spontaneously, with the development of pseudoaneurysm (Figures 6.4–6.6), significant infundibular pulmonary stenosis, or prolapse of an aortic valve cusp into the defect (Figure 6.7).

Symptoms

- A minor VSD is usually asymptomatic.
- A moderate VSD may be associated with palpitations and exertional dyspnea.
- Syncope is a rare manifestation of right ventricular outflow tract obstruction due to a prolapse of the coronary cusp into the VSD.
- Eisenmenger syndrome is associated with cyanosis, dyspnea, palpitations, hemoptysis, and syncope (see Chapter 16).

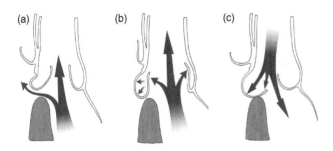

Figure 6.7
Prolapse of the aortic valve cusp into the ventricular septal defect with the development of aortic regurgitation. (a), (b) The aortic cusp and the wall of aortic sinus, which do not have the support of the ventricular septum, are pushed into the defect in systole; (c) in diastole, the prolapsing cusp bulges into the right ventricular outflow tract and is separated from the other aortic cusps, aortic regurgitation develops.

General examination

- Prominent and hyperactive precordium.
- Systolic thrill at the left lower sternal border.
- Palpable S2 if pulmonary hypertension.

Ausculatatory findings

- The systolic murmur from VSD, is loud, and is often located in the third to fourth left parasternal intercostal space. With minor muscular defects, the murmur is limited to the early systole, as the defect will close on myocardial contraction.
- The typical systolic murmur disappears if pulmonary hypertension develops.
- In a small VSD, the second heart sound is normal.
- With a moderate shunt, P2 will increase, and with obstructive pulmonary vascular disease the second sound will become single and loud.
- There may be a diastolic regurgitant murmur due to pulmonary regurgitation in pulmonary hypertension.
- Prolapse of the aortic valve cusp into the defect leads to the diastolic murmur of aortic regurgitation.
- A significant shunt is associated with S III and a diastolic rumble of relative mitral valve stenosis at the apex.
- Concomitant pulmonary artery stenosis is associated with systolic ejection murmur with a maximum over the pulmonary artery, while, in the presence of infundibular stenosis, the auscultatory maximum is lower, in the third left parasternal intercostal space.

Electrocardiogram (ECG)

- The ECG recording obtained in patients with a small VSD may be normal.

- With a moderate VSD, left atrial and left ventricular hypertrophy reflects left ventricular volume overload.
- A more than moderate VSD shows left and right ventricular hypertrophy.
- Eisenmenger ECG is dominated by right ventricular hypertrophy.
- Surgical closure of VSD is frequently followed by right bundle branch block.

Chest X-ray

- In a small VSD, heart size and pulmonary vasculature is normal.
- A moderate or large VSD is associated with enlargement of the left atrium, left ventricle and pulmonary artery. The central and peripheral pulmonary vascular markings are increased.
- In a large VSD with increased pulmonary vascular resistance, the heart size is normal. Due to the right ventricular hypertrophy the cardiac apex is rotated upward, to the left. The main pulmonary artery is prominent and the peripheral pulmonary vascular markings are increased in the outer third.

Echocardiography

Echocardiography is a sensitive technique with an excellent detection rate (up to 95%), depending on the size and location of the defect. It is particularly sensitive in perimembranous, inlet, or outlet VSD, if they are >5mm. The echo-sensitivity in apical muscular VSD is lower.

A complete echocardiographic examination should determine:

- The size, type and location of the defect. Transesophageal echocardiography is particularly useful in patients difficult to visualize, to specify the relation of the defect to other structures, e.g. to determine the distance between the defect and the aortic valve.
- Size and direction of the shunt and pulmonary to systemic flow ratio (Qp/Qs).
- Assessment of pulmonary artery pressure by means of tricuspid and pulmonary regurgitation.
- Assessment of the gradient across the defect to estimate the right ventricular pressure (blood pressure measured using a cuff on the arm – peak echo gradient = right ventricular systolic pressure); however, caution is necessary as the maximum gradient may be readily underestimated due to a narrow VSD jet.
- Size of cardiac chambers to estimate the hemodynamic significance of the defect.
- To assess spontaneous defect closure.
- To assess prolapse of the aortic cusp into the defect, presence and degree of aortic regurgitation.

- Presence of a right-to-left shunt using an echo-contrast media.
- Presence of associated CHD.

Catheterization

Catheterization is indicated:

- In the event of inconclusive results of noninvasive assessment to specify the presence and hemodynamic significance of a shunt.
- To obtain a more specific finding, e.g. in the presence of multiple muscular defects or concomitant peripheral pulmonary artery stenoses.
- To assess the severity of right ventricular outflow tract obstruction.
- To exactly determine pulmonary artery pressure and resistance.
- To test the response to vasodilating agents (e.g. O_2, NO, prostacyclin) in pulmonary hypertension.
- Selective coronary angiography is undertaken prior to cardiac surgery in patients over 40 years of age or in younger individuals with risk factors of coronary artery disease or reporting angina, or in the case of suspicion of congenital coronary artery anomalies or previous operative injury.

Pulmonary biopsy

This procedure is only rarely indicated. In adults, it is a matter of debate considering the associated risks. The procedure carries high risks and should, if ever, only be performed in selected centers. Classes I and II of the Heath-Edwards classification are considered reversible.

Natural history

- The natural history depends on the type and size of the VSD, and on associated anomalies.
- If untreated, VSD predispose to endocarditis, arrhythmias, cardiac failure, aortic regurgitation, and to obstructive pulmonary vascular disease.
- Defects close spontaneously in 40–60% of children, but only rarely in adulthood. Spontaneous closure results from growth of musculature around the VSD, ingrowth of fibrous tissue, or aneurysmatic transformation of the tricuspid valve leaflet adhering to the VSD (Figure 6.4).
- Inlet and subarterial defects seldom close spontaneously. Subarterial VSD can close due to a prolapse of the aortic valve into the defect (Figure 6.7).

- *Ventricular septal pseudoaneurysm*: A pseudoaneurysm is formed by abundant tissue of the tricuspid valve septal leaflet and its chordae, adhering to the surrounding area

of the defect. There may or may not be a residual shunt in the pseudoaneurysm (Figure 6.4).

- *Aortic valve cusp prolapse into the defect*: It occurs in supracristal or perimembranous defects extending into the outlet septum. There is usually a deficiency of muscular or fibrous support below the aortic valve. Subsequently the right or the noncoronary aortic cusp may prolapse. While the defect itself remains unchanged in size, the shunt may get smaller or disappear at the expense of aortic valve regurgitation (Figure 6.7 a–c).
- *Pulmonary stenosis*: It usually occurs subvalvular, in the infundibular region; less frequently at pulmonary valve level, and it may progress over lifetime. It may result in an increase in right ventricular pressure and a reduction of the left-to-right shunt.
- *Pulmonary hypertension*, secondary to pulmonary vascular obstructive disease, will also diminish, (or even eliminate), the left-to-right shunt.

- In the era before VSD closure became routine during childhood, Eisenmenger syndrome was relatively often diagnosed, even in adults (9.4% of all VSD).[3]
- The prognosis of patients with a small VSD, and a normal pulmonary artery pressure and resistance, is good. The main potential risk is infectious endocarditis (IE), with a reported incidence of up to 11%.[4,5]
- Historically, unoperated patients with a major VSD showed high mortality (80% in their late forties).[4]
- If VSD closure is performed before 2 years of age, even patients with major defects have a good prognosis.

Risks associated with an unclosed ventricular septal defect

- Underestimation of the defect size and development of irreversible pulmonary vascular obstructive disease (Eisenmenger syndrome).
- Risk of paradoxical embolism in transvenous stimulation and deep vein thrombosis in patients with right-to-left shunt.
- Arrhythmia: Atrial fibrillation occurs in the presence of significant left atrial dilatation; Eisenmenger syndrome may be associated with malignant arrhythmia.
- Heart failure with predominant right-heart failure in Eisenmenger syndrome (left-heart failure usually present in children with a major left-to-right shunt, and is virtually absent in adults).

Management

- The treatment of isolated VSD depends on the type, size and location of the defect, the amount of shunt, pulmonary vascular resistance, functional ability, and on associated or acquired anomalies.

- Operative treatment is intended to increase long-term prognosis, to lower pulmonary artery pressure and resistance, to improve the functional status, and to minimize the risk of endocarditis.
- Surgical treatment is performed by closing the defect directly or with a patch.
- Usually, perimembranous and inlet defects are repaired transatrial; outlet septum defects through the pulmonary valve; and muscular defects through an apical left ventriculotomy.
- Major defects are closed surgically in the first year of life when pulmonary hypertension is usually still reversible.

Surgical treatment is principally indicated in:

- Symptomatic VSD.
- Significant VSD with Qp/Qs ≥2:1.
- VSD in the presence of reversible pulmonary hypertension with a systolic pulmonary artery pressure >50mmHg.
- Deteriorating left ventricular function due to chronic volume overload.
- Deteriorating right ventricular function due to pressure overload.
- VSD in the presence of concomitant significant right ventricular outflow tract obstruction (mean gradient >50mmHg).
- VSD in the presence of a perimembranous defect with moderate or severe aortic regurgitation.
- Recurrent endocarditis.
- In the presence of severe pulmonary hypertension (PAP >2/3 systemic arterial blood pressure (SABP); Rp >2/3 Rs), there must be a net left-to-right shunt of ≥1.5:1; or preserved pulmonary artery resistance reactivity at a pulmonary vasodilator; or lung biopsy gives evidence that pulmonary arterial changes are potentially reversible.

(Source: Canadian Consensus Conference, 2001[2])

Pulmonary hypertension with increased pulmonary vascular resistance (PVR ≥4 Wood units) is associated with a considerably increased operative risk and a poor postoperative prognosis. The upper limit of pulmonary vascular resistance where surgery is still possible, is not generally defined. Factors such as the patient biological age, concomitant diseases, conversion of pulmonary vascular resistance to body surface area, as well as the conditions and reliability of pulmonary vascular resistance determination and its response to pharmacological testing, have to be taken into account. In many centers, surgical closure is considered *contraindicated* if PVR ≥7 WU (nonindexed value), respectively 10WU × m² (indexed value), if the systolic pulmonary artery pressure is >2/3 of systemic arterial pressure, unless there is a significant response of the pulmonary vascular bed to pulmonary vasodilating agents.

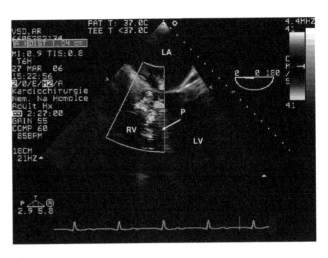

Figure 6.8
Two residual defects after ventricular septal defect (VSD) closure; two jets form LV to RV seen in color Doppler, due to the dehiscence of the patch. Transesophageal echo, four-chamber view in transversal plane. LV, Left ventricle; RV, right ventricle; LA, left atrium; P, Dacron patch on VSD.

Catheter-based VSD closure: Today, catheter-based closure is an option in trabecular *muscular VSD* and in some residual VSD after surgery.[6,7] Given the proximity of the aortic valve, catheter-based closure of a perimembranous VSD is currently still considered experimental. Catheter-based closure of these defects usually requires a 5mm septal margin below the aortic valve. The procedure should only be performed in specialized centres. The device currently mostly used for closure is the Amplatzer occluder.[8–9]

In addition to congenital VSD, catheter-based closure can also be performed in acquired postinfarction VSD. Postinfarction defect closure differs from closure of congenital muscular defects in terms of size, and also in the presence of necrotic tissue around the defect.[10,11] Mortality after acute myocardial infarction is higher compared to those with a congenital form of VSD.

Residual findings after ventricular septal defect surgery

The most important residua after VSD surgery include residual VSD (Figure 6.8), residual pulmonary hypertension, decreased exercise capacity, arrhythmia and conduction disturbances (right bundle-branch block, complete heart block, sinus node dysfunction, ventricular and supraventricular arrhythmias), infective endocarditis, and ventricular dysfunction.

- Most patients on long-term follow-up after VSD closure are in functional NYHA Class I.[12]
- *Residual shunts*, or recanalized defects, occur in up to 30% of cases:[12] they are usually small, and reoperation is only required with hemodynamically significant shunts.

- *Residual pulmonary hypertension* may persist even after successful surgery for VSD. Patients with a major VSD, operated on later than at 2 years of age, may have pulmonary vascular obstructive disease – even without a residual shunt.
- *Residual aortic regurgitation* may progress even after defect closure and aortic valvuloplasty.
- *Arrhythmia and conduction disturbances*: Ventricular arrhythmia with a risk of sudden cardiac death may appear in defects operated on late in life. A complete AV-block may develop immediately after surgery, in rare cases even later; right bundle branch block (RBBB) or left anterior hemiblock (LAH) occur more often.
- *Conduction disturbances* (right bundle-branch block, left anterior hemiblock, complete AV block), supraventricular *arrhythmia* as well as *sudden death* were reported during long-term follow-up after VSD surgery.[5,12,13]
- Patients with *Eisenmenger* syndrome have a grim prognosis but, by adhering to lifestyle limitations and with reasonable professional care, they may live to their forties, and even beyond (see Chapter 16).
- *Aortic regurgitation* in the presence of aortic cusp prolapsing into a perimembranous or subarterial defect is reported to be 5–20%.[4,14–16] Aortic regurgitation may progress, and its incidence rises with age. The rate of progression is often slow and variable. Therefore, the proper timing and type of operation are still controversial.[16]

Pregnancy and delivery

Delivery is well tolerated in small and moderate VSD:

- with good ventricular function;
- in functional NYHA Class I–II;
- after VSD closure;
- in the absence of significant pulmonary hypertension, significant right ventricular outflow tract obstruction.

Prevention of IE prior to delivery is mandatory in patients with a history of IE; it is also provided to patients with unoperated defects and residual shunts.

- Pregnancy is contraindicated in Eisenmenger syndrome considering the high maternal and fetal mortality.

Infective endocarditis

- The risk for IE after surgical closure is nearly half that in medically treated patients. The reported incidence varies from 0.8 to 1.7 per 1000 patient years. On long-term follow-up, the incidence of IE even after VSD surgery has been reported to be 0–2.7%.[18,19]
- IE has been reported, on long-term follow-up, in 3–4% of patients with known VSD or undergoing surgery, and in up to 15% of adults unaware of their defect.[15]
- IE prevention is critical with all VSD, including trivial residual shunts after surgery.
- The risk of IE is particularly high in patients with small (residual) VSD, and if there is also aortic regurgitation.
- After surgery without a residual shunt, prevention of IE is continued for 6 months.

Follow-up

- All patients with residual findings after VSD closure or with a suspected VSD should be followed by a cardiologist. Also on follow-up by a cardiologist should be patients in whom a major VSD was closed after 2 years of age, and all undergoing catheter-based defect closure.
- Patients with a hemodynamically insignificant defect may be followed by a general practitioner or internist in cooperation with a cardiologist.

References

1. Gerbode F, Hultgren H, Melrose D, Osborn J. Syndrome of left ventricular–right atrial shunt. Successful surgical repair of defect in five cases, with observation of bradycardia on closure. Ann Surg 1958; 148: 433.
2. Therrien J, Dore A, Gersony W et al. Canadian Cardiovascular Society Consensus Conference 2001 update: Recommendations for the management of adults with congenital heart disease. Part I. Can J Cardiol 2001; 17(9): 940–59.
3. Keith JD, Rose V, Collins G, Kidd BSL. Ventricular septal defect. Incidence, morbidity, and mortality in various age groups. Br Heart J 1971; 33(Suppl): 81–7.
4. Campbell M. Natural history of ventricular septal defect. Br Heart J 1971; 33: 246–57.
5. Neumayer U, Stone S, Somerville J. Small ventricular septal defects in adults. Eur Heart J 1998; 19(10): 1573–82.
6. Van der Velde ME, Sanders SP, Keane JF, Perry SB, Lock JE. Transesophageal echocardiographic guidance of transcatheter ventricular septal defect closure. J Am Coll Cardiol 1994; 23(7): 1660–5.
7. Moodie DS. VSD closure device in the setting of adult congenital heart disease. Catheter Cardiovasc Interv 2005; 64(2): 213.
8. Hijazi ZM, Hakim F, Al-Fadley F, Abdelhamid J, Cao QL. Transcatheter closure of single muscular ventricular septal defects using the Amplatzer muscular VSD occluder: Initial results and technical considerations. Catheter Cardiovasc Interv 2000; 49(2): 167–72.
9. Thanapoulos BD, Tsaoulis GS, Konstadopoulou GN, Zarayelyan AG. Transcatheter closure of muscular ventricular septal defects with the Amplatzer ventricular septal defect occluder: Initial clinical applications in children. J Am Coll Cardiol 1999; 33(5): 1395–9.
10. Chessa M, Carminati M, Cao QL et al. Transcatheter closure of congenital and acquired muscular ventricular septal defects using the Amplatzer device. J Invasive Cardiol 2002; 14(6): 322–7.

11. Pesonen E, Thilen U, Sandstorm S et al. Transcatheter closure of post-infarction ventricular septal defect with the Amplatzer Septal Occluder device. Scand Cardiovasc J 2000; 34(4): 446–8.

12. Moller JH, Patton C, Varco RL, Lillehei CW. Late results (30 to 35 years) after operative closure of isolated ventricular septal defect from 1954 to 1960. Am J Cardiol 1991; 68: 1491–7.

13. Kidd L, Driscoll DJ, Gersony WM et al. Second natural history study of congenital heart defects. Results of treatment of patients with ventricular septal defects. Circulation 1999; 87(Suppl I): I-38–I-51.

14. Brauner R, Birk E, Sahar L, Vidbe BA. Surgical management of ventricular septal defect with aortic valve prolapse: Clinical considerations and results. Eur J Cardiothorac Surg 1995; 9: 315–19.

15. Otterstad JE, Nitter-Hague S, Myrhe E. Isolated ventricular septal defect in adults. Clinical and haemodynamic findings. Br Heart J 1983; 50: 343–8.

16. Perloff JK. The Clinical Recognition of Congenital Heart Disease, 4th edn. Philadelphia, PA: WB Saunders Company, 1994.

17. Ammash N, Warnes CA. Ventricular septal defect in adults. Ann Intern Med 2001; 135: 812–24.

18. Morris CD, Reller MD, Menashe VD. Thirty year incidence of infective endocarditis after surgery for congenital heart defect. JAMA 1998; 279: 599–603.

19. Li W, Somerville J. Infective endocarditis in the grown-up congenital heart (GUCH) population. Eur Heart J 1998; 19(1): 166–73.

7

Tetralogy of Fallot

Anatomical notes

The tetralogy of Fallot (TOF) defect originates from a deviation of the infundibular septum to the right and anterocephalad, resulting in a hypoplasia of the right ventricular outflow tract (RVOT) and the pulmonary artery system, a subaortic malalignment ventricular septal defect (VSD), and an aortic overriding. Right ventricular hypertrophy is consecutive (Figures 7.1–7.5).

In the past, the classical criteria of TOF were:

1. Right ventricular outflow tract obstruction (RVOTO) (infundibular stenosis, often in combination with valvular and supravalvular pulmonary artery stenosis).
2. A large (nonrestrictive) perimembraneous VSD with extension to the outlet septum (malalignment VSD).

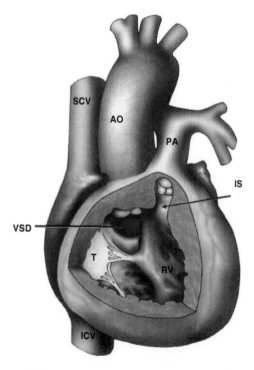

Figure 7.1
Tetralogy of Fallot. AO, Aorta; SCV, superior caval vein; ICV, inferior caval vein; VSD, ventricular septal defect; IS, infundibular septum; T, tricuspid valve; RV, right ventricle; PA, pulmonary artery.

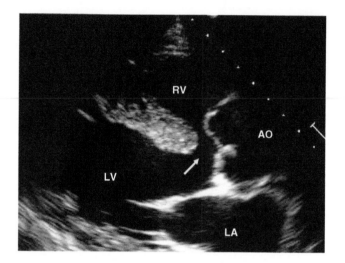

Figure 7.2
Unoperated tetralogy of Fallot in adult patient, transthoracic echo, parasternal view, longitudinal axis. AO, Dilated aorta, overriding the ventricular septal defect (arrow); RV, right ventricle; LV, left ventricle; LA, left atrium.

3. Aortic overriding (<50%; at a higher degree of overriding, the defect is classified as a double-outlet right ventricle).
4. Consecutive right ventricular hypertrophy.

As with all cyanotic defects, bronchopulmonary and aortopulmonary collaterals may develop in TOF, although not to the extent seen in pulmonary atresia. About 25% of patients with TOF have a right-side aortic arch, frequently seen in patients with TOF and microdelection on chromosome 22q11. In about 5% of TOF patients, the left anterior descending coronary artery originates from the right coronary artery, and crosses the RVOT anteriorly (Figure 7.6).[1]

Pathophysiology

Critical considerations in unoperated TOF are the size of the VSD, shunt direction and amount, the severity of the RVOTO, and the degree of pulmonary artery hypoplasia. The clinical spectrum of TOF ranges from mild forms with left-to-right shunt ('pink Fallot'), over the 'classical' form (right-to-left shunt through the VSD, resulting in cyanosis and chronic hypoxia), up to extreme forms with pulmonary atresia.

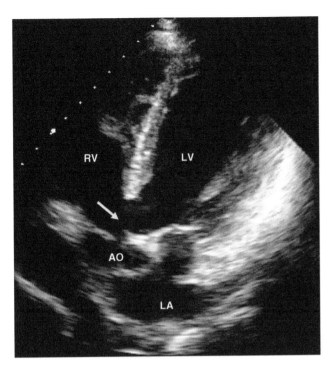

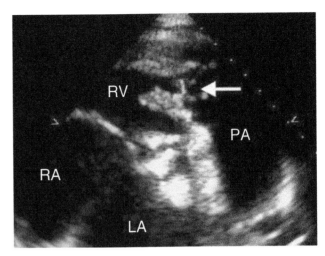

Figure 7.5
Transthoracic echocardiography of unoperated patient with tetralogy of Fallot. Modified short axis view focusing on the right ventricular outflow tract. Severe infundibular and valvular pulmonary stenosis is marked by arrow, stenotic pulmonary valve. PA, Pulmonary artery; RA, right atrium; RV, right ventricle; LA, left atrium.

Figure 7.3
Transthoracic echocardiography, modified apical view with aorta in unoperated patient with tetralogy of Fallot. Aorta (AO) is overriding the ventricular septal defect (arrow). LA, Left atrium; LV, left ventricle; RV, right ventricle.

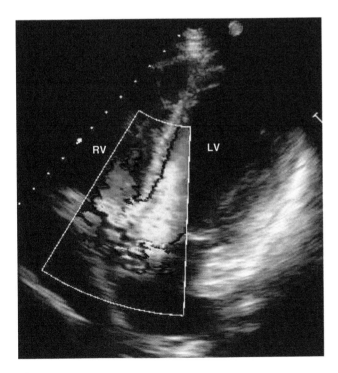

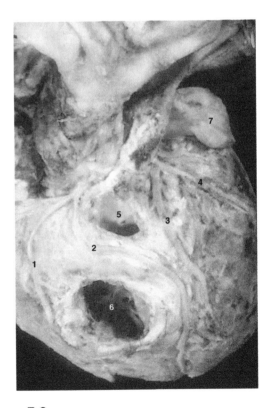

Figure 7.4
Unoperated patient with tetralogy of Fallot. Transthoracic echocardiography apical 4-chamber view, color flow shows that both right and left ventricles eject blood in systole into the dilated overriding aorta. That causes cyanosis and low pulmonary flow.

Figure 7.6
Anomalous left coronary artery crossing the right ventricular outflow tract (RVOT). 1, Right coronary artery (RCA); 2, anomalous aberrant left anterior descending (LAD) from RCA, crossing RVOT; 3, normal LAD from left coronary artery (LCA); 4, diagonal branch of the LCA; 5, pulmonary valve and surgical orifice for dostal anastomosis of the conduit; 6, surgically created orifice for proximal anastomosis of the conduit, which bypasses the RVOT; 7, left atrial auricle. (Courtesy of Dr SY Ho, Royal Brompton Hospital, London, UK.)

After corrective surgery, circulation in TOF becomes physiological, with the cyanosis resolving.

Prevalence

TOF is the most common cyanotic cardiac anomaly in adulthood, present in 4–10% of all congenital heart diseases (CHD). Some 15% of patients with TOF have chromosome 22q11 deletion (CATCH-22 syndrome).

TETRALOGY OF FALLOT AFTER CORRECTIVE SURGERY

Description of the operative technique

For repair, a patch is placed over the VSD and the right ventricular outflow tract obstruction is relieved. A narrow infundibulum is resected, a stenotic pulmonary valve is incised, a patch may be placed across the RVOT (not disrupting the pulmonary valve annulus), and narrow pulmonary arteries are widened.

In cases of a restrictive pulmonary valve annulus, a transannular patch is used, disrupting the integrity of the pulmonary valve annulus. Under certain circumstances (e.g. in coronary artery anomalies), the RVOT is reconstructed using an extracardiac conduit from the right ventricle to the pulmonary artery (Figure 7.6).

Clinical findings and diagnosis after repair

Repair of TOF is followed by a dramatic change in the patient's clinical status, with remission of cyanosis, exertional dyspnea, and hypoxic spells.

Symptoms

These are dependent on the severity of residual findings:

- Palpitation.
- Fatigability, exertional dyspnea, deteriorated exercise tolerance.
- Right-heart decompensation with hepatomegaly and lower limb edema (= late findings).

Auscultatory findings

- Split second pulmonary heart sound (due to right bundle branch block (RBBB)).
- Systolic ejection murmur in the second left intercostal space in the presence of RVOTO.
- Diastolic decrescendo murmur in the second left intercostal space in the presence of pulmonary valve regurgitation.
- Diastolic decrescendo murmur in the third intercostal space on the right in the presence of aortic valve regurgitation.
- Systolic murmur on the left parasternal border in the presence of a residual VSD.
- In the stenosis of the peripheral pulmonary artery, the murmur radiates into the posterior lung fields and the axilla.

Electrocardiogram (ECG), ECG Holter monitoring

- Right bundle branch block is almost a rule following TOF repair. QRS duration may increase over time. In particular, a progressive QRS duration >180ms may be ominous (Figure 7.7).
- Left anterior hemiblock may develop postoperatively.
- Supraventricular and ventricular arrhythmias are frequent.
- Intraoperative injury to a coronary artery may result in pathological QS pattern (Figure 7.7).

Chest X-ray

- The cardiac shadow may increase in size in the presence of right ventricular dilatation due to pulmonary regurgitation.
- Calcified outflow tract patch.
- RVOT aneurysm (with calcification).
- Calcified right vertricular–pulmonary artery conduit.
- A right-side aortic arch.

Echocardiography

Regular echocardiographic examination after repair of TOF should focus on:

- Detection, quantification, and evaluation of progression of *residual pulmonary regurgitation*. The velocity of the regurgitation flow is low; severe pulmonary regurgitation will manifest itself by laminar 'free-flow' in the RVOT (Figures 7.8–7.10).
- In the presence of *restrictive right ventricular physiology*, there is forward flow in the pulmonary artery in late diastole, at the time of atrial systole, which can be detected by pulsed Doppler in the pulmonary artery trunk during the entire respiratory cycle, or at least five consecutive cardiac contractions.[2,3] This forward diastolic flow in the pulmonary artery will shorten the duration of pulmonary regurgitation (Figure 7.8).
- Detection, quantification, and evaluation of any progression of *residual pulmonary stenosis*.
- Detection of a *residual ventricular septal defect*.

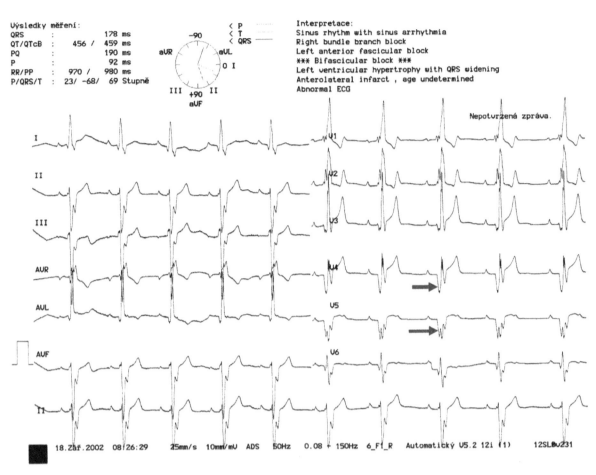

Figure 7.7
Electrocardiogram in a patient after corrective surgery of tetralogy of Fallot. Sinus rhythm, right bundle branch block with QRS 178ms, left anterior hemiblock, right ventricle hypertrophy. Except that there are typical pathological Q waves in the leads V4–V5 (arrows), indicating necrosis (scar) after operative injury of the left coronary artery.

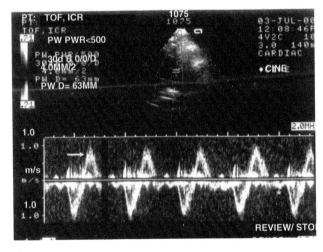

Figure 7.8
Tetralogy of Fallot, pulsed Doppler echocardiography in the pulmonary artery. Laminar diastolic backflow due to the free-flow severe pulmonary regurgitation (arrow). Forward flow in the pulmonary artery during atrial contraction (*) shortens the duration of pulmonary regurgitation (restrictive physiology of the right ventricle).

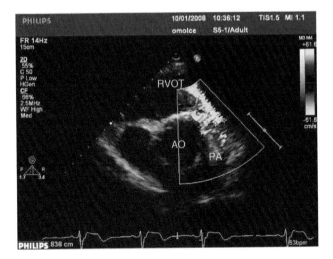

Figure 7.9
Tetralogy of Fallot, transthoracic echo, short-axis at the level of great arteries, color jet indicates severe pulmonary regurgitation remaining after intracardiac repair in childhood. PA, Pulmonary artery; AO, aorta; RVOT, right ventricular outflow tract.

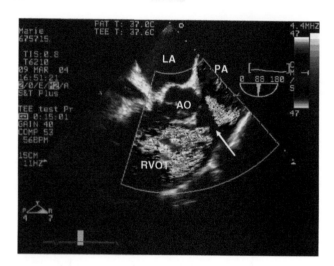

Figure 7.10

Tetralogy of Fallot, transesophageal echo, 88 degrees.
Color jet in the RVOT in diastole indicates residual severe
pulmonary regurgitation after intracardiac repair in childhood
(pulmonary valvulotomy and transannular patch). The
severity of pulmonary regurgitation may be in some patients
better evaluated by transesophageal echocardiography.
LA, Left atrium; AO, aorta; RVOT, aneurysmatically
dilated right ventricular outflow tract; PA, pulmonary artery;
arrow, site of the pulmonary valve.

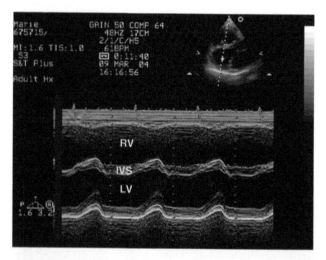

Figure 7.11

Tetralogy of Fallot with severe residual pulmonary regurgitation
and volume overload of the right ventricle (RV), with paradoxical
septal movement. LV, Left ventricle; IVS, interventricular septum.

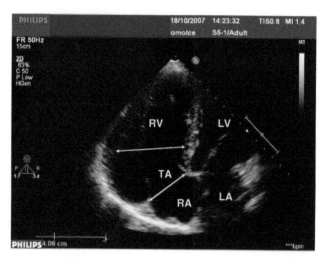

Figure 7.12

Tetralogy of Fallot transthoracic echo, apical four-chamber view,
severely dilated right ventricle (RV; 62mm) and tricuspid annulus
(TA; 41mm) due to severe pulmonary regurgitation.
RA, Right atrium; LV, left ventricle; LA, left atrium.

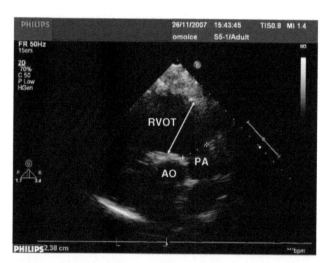

Figure 7.13

Tetralogy of Fallot, transthoracic echo, short-axis parasternal
view, aneurysm of the right ventricular outflow tract
(RVOT, yellow arrow; 45mm). AO, Aorta; PA, pulmonary artery,
pulmonary annulus: 24mm.

- Evaluation of *right ventricular function and size* (Figures 7.11 and 7.12).
- Presence and size of a *RVOT aneurysm* (Figure 7.13).
- Evaluation of *left ventricular size and function.* An aneurysm on the left ventricular apex is found if the left coronary artery, atypically crossing the RVOT, was damaged during repair. Further, systolic and diastolic left ventricular function may be affected by mutual change in the geometry of both ventricles, with asynchronous contraction and relaxation of a dilated and pressure-overloaded right ventricle in the presence of significant pulmonary regurgitation.
- Evaluation of the *aortic root diameter* and any *aortic valve regurgitation.*
- Detection of any *associated CHD*, even if previously unrecognized (e.g. atrial septal defect (ASD)).
- Residual stenoses of central pulmonary artery segments.

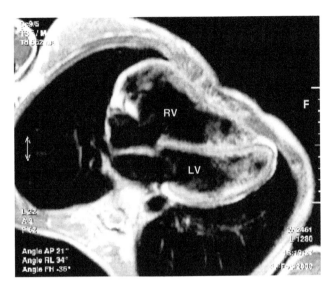

Figure 7.14
Tetralogy of Fallot, magnetic resonance imaging, dilated inflow part of the right ventricle (RV), which is situated just behind the sternum. LV, small left ventricle.

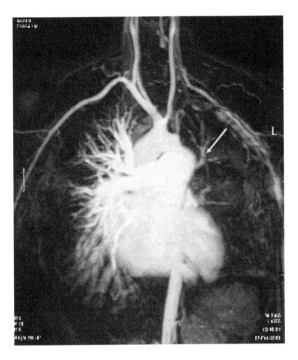

Figure 7.15
Tetralogy of Fallot, magnetic resonance imaging. Dilated right pulmonary artery, agenesis of the left pulmonary artery, from which there is only the tiny hypoplastic branch for the apical segment of the left upper lobe (arrow). The left subclavian artery is also lacking after Blalock–Taussig anastomosis in childhood, which closed spontaneously. Patient is asymptomatic.

Exercise testing, spiroergometry

Exercise testing should ideally be performed using the same method in the same center. This allows the longitudinal comparison of functional exercise capacity and peak oxygen consumption, and the assessment of the presence of any exercise-induced arrhythmia.

Electrophysiological examination

This may be indicated in the presence of supraventricular or ventricular arrhythmias.

Magnetic resonance imaging (MRI)

This may be indicated to identify anomalies of the pulmonary artery and its branches, to determine right ventricular size and function (Figures 7.14 and 7.15), to quantify pulmonary regurgitation on longitudinal follow-up, and to assess aortic diameter.

Radionuclide angiography

This may be indicated to assess right ventricular function.

Perfusion lung scintigraphy

This may be indicated in case of suspected peripheral pulmonary artery stenosis or atresia.

Computerized tomography (CT) scan

A CT scan shows morphology of the pulmonary trunk and excludes peripheral pulmonary stenosis. It is very important before reoperation to show the relation of the structures in the retrosternal space.

Catheterization

Catheterization is indicated to determine hemodynamic status, if not clarified by a noninvasive procedure, and to perform selective coronary angiography before elective surgery. In addition to atherosclerotic lesions, coronary arteries may also be damaged during surgery in childhood.

Residual findings after repair of tetralogy of Fallot and their management

Course and prognosis

At a time when surgery was unavailable, only 11% of TOF patients survived beyond 20 years of age, with only 3% of patients living to 40 years of age.[4]

Palliative surgery alleviated cyanosis and symptoms and allowed longer survival.

The prognosis of TOF patients substantially improved with the advent of repair.

Today, most patients with TOF have had corrective surgery in childhoods, uncorrected or only palliated adults with TOF are rare (see 'Tetralogy of Fallot after palliative surgery').

The operative mortality of TOF repair in childhood is currently <3% in experienced centers. Repair in adults has a higher operative mortality (3–9% in small series).

The long-term prognosis after TOF repair is good. Long-term survival is 94% after 25 years, 89% after 30 years, and 76% after 40 years.

Most patients are doing well and are in functional class II or I.

However, there are residual findings, which may require reoperation even decades after the primary repair.

- *Residual pulmonary regurgitation* is present, to a certain extent, in all patients after TOF repair and is well clinically tolerated in the long run. Significant pulmonary regurgitation is particularly present with the use of a transannular patch.[5,6] Protracted significant pulmonary regurgitation leads to an aneurysmal RVOT, right ventricle volume overload and dilatation, right ventricle dysfunction, and, eventually, a low cardiac output syndrome. It may lead, through slowing of electrical activation, to a significant QRS prolongation.

- Dilatation of the right ventricle and tricuspid annulus results in *secondary tricuspid regurgitation* (Figure 7.16).

- *Aneurysm of the RVOT* is dyskinetic and worsens the right ventricular function (Figure 7.13).

- A dilated and volume-overloaded right ventricle (with residual severe pulmonary regurgitation) causes a change in the mutual geometry of both ventricles with interventricular septal dislocation. The interventricular septal movement becomes paradoxical (Figure 7.1 and 7.14), resulting in secondary *systolic and diastolic left ventricular dysfunction*. While residual pulmonary regurgitation may be tolerated well by patients for prolonged periods of time, it is necessary to longitudinally monitor exercise tolerance and to look for any deterioration in performance, which may signal the need for reoperation.

- After TOF repair, the condition with appreciably reduced diastolic compliance of the right ventricle is referred to as *restrictive right ventricular physiology*.[2] On atrial contraction, the right ventricle acts as a rigid conduit between the right atrium and the pulmonary artery. In restrictive right ventricular physiology, late diastolic forward flow on atrial contraction is transmitted up to the pulmonary artery, thus limiting the duration of pulmonary regurgitation (Figure 7.8).

- Residual valvular *pulmonary stenosis* is less frequent than regurgitation; however, residual peripheral stenoses of the right or left pulmonary arteries are quite frequent. They may be either congenital or due to the previous palliative Blalock–Taussig shunt.

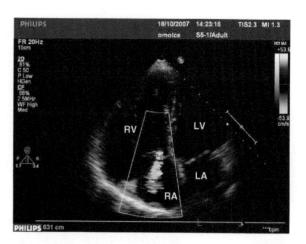

Figure 7.16
Tetralogy of Fallot, transthoracic echo, four-chamber apical view, color flow shows moderate tricuspid regurgitation due to the right ventricle and tricuspid annulus dilatation in a patient with severe pulmonary regurgitation. RV, right ventricule; RA, right atrium; LV, left ventricle; LA, left atrium.

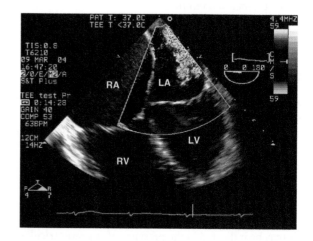

Figure 7.17
Tetralogy of Fallot after repair in childhood, transesophageal echo, 0 degrees, color flow shows moderate mitral regurgitation, loss of coaptation of the mitral leaflets with prolapse of the anterior leaflet and dilatation of the mitral annulus. LA, Left atrium; LV, left ventricle; RA, right atrium; RV, right ventricle. This patient has also severe tricuspid regurgitation and severely dilated right atrium.

- Left ventricular dysfunction after TOF repair may particularly occur in the case of injury to the left coronary artery with an atypical course.

- *Mitral regurgitation* may be occasionally seen in older patients with mitral valve degeneration, mitral valve prolapse and left ventricular dysfunction (Figure 7.17).

- With increasing age, there may be progressive *dilatation of the aortic root* due to previous long-standing volume overload, and possibly to intrinsic properties with development of *aortic regurgitation* (Figure 7.18).[7–9]

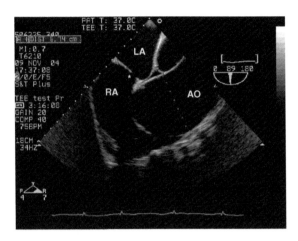

Figure 7.18
Severely dilated aorta (AO; 67mm) in adult patient with unoperated pentalogy of Fallot, transesophageal echo, 89 degrees. AO, Aorta; LA, left atrium; RA, right atrium. Small atrial septal defect between the atria (*).

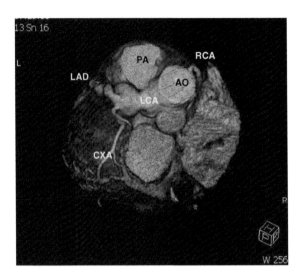

Figure 7.19
Adult patient with tetralogy of Fallot, computerized tomography angio with 3D reconstruction. Huge aneurysm of the left main coronary artery (LCA), dilated left anterior descending coronary artery (LAD). Normal circumflex coronary artery (CXA) and right artery (RCA). AO, Aorta; PA, pulmonary artery.

- Regurgitation of all valves may be present in older patients after TOF repair – pulmonary, tricuspid, aortic and mitral regurgitation.

- *Coronary artery anomalies* should be expected, especially in patients with severe pulmonary stenosis or pulmonary atresia in childhood with the anamnesis of surgical suture of the coronary fistula (Figure 7.19).

- *Ventricular arrhythmias* are frequent, even after repair.[10]

- *Supraventricular arrhythmias* are also frequent after repair, and a main reason of morbidity.

- RBBB occurs in 59–100% of cases and is usually also present prior to surgery: RBBB + LAH in 7–25%; complete atrioventricular block in 1–2%; supraventricular tachyarrhythmia in 10–30%; ventricular arrhythmia in 46–67%; ventricular tachycardia in 10–15%; sustained monomorphous tachycardia in 4–10%.[11]

- *QRS prolongation* ≥180ms is regarded a potential marker of right ventricular dilatation, ventricular tachycardia occurrence, and sudden death.[5] A longer QRS duration can be associated with an increased risk in developing malignant ventricular arrhythmias in asymptomatic patients after Fallot repair.[12]

- *Sudden death* on long-term follow-up after TOF repair was noted in 1.8–6% of cases.[5,13–15] The reported cumulative risk is 1.2% after 10 years, 2.2% after 20 years, 4.0% after 25 years, and 6.0% after 35 years. Sudden death is mostly connected to sustained ventricular tachycardia, and less often with complete heart block or a sick-sinus syndrome. Significant arrhythmias may be associated with abnormal hemodynamics, most often with significant pulmonary regurgitation. Potential predictors of sudden death include a QRS complex width ≥180ms on ECG, inhomogeneous QRS- and QT-dispersion.

- *Atrioventricular conduction disturbances* may deteriorate ventricular filling while shortening total ventricular filling time.

- *Interventricular conduction disturbance* in the right ventricle (in the presence of RBBB) may deteriorate right ventricular ejection secondary to desynchronization of the right ventricular contraction. A negative correlation between QRS duration and right and left ventricular ejection rate on one hand, and peak left ventricular filling rate in patients after TOF repair on the other, was demonstrated.[7] A dilated right ventricle with asynchronous septal contraction may thus even have an adverse effect on left ventricular systolic and diastolic function.[7,16,17]

- In addition, *left ventricular function* is also affected by the operative technique, including the potential for damage to a coronary artery, duration of cyanosis in childhood, and other factors.

Management strategies after TOF repair

Reoperation

Reoperation is necessary in some 25% of patients after TOF repair during a 20-year follow-up, or even more. Reoperation after TOF repair may be indicated in the following conditions:

- Residual *ventricular septal defect* with a left-to-right shunt if Qp/Qs >1.5:1.
- Residual *pulmonary artery stenosis* with a right ventricular systolic pressure ≥2/3 of systemic systolic pressure.
- Significant *pulmonary regurgitation* associated with significant or progressive right ventricular dilatation,

tricuspid regurgitation, supraventricular or ventricular arrhythmia, or declining physical performance.

- Significant *aortic regurgitation* associated with symptoms and/or progression of left ventricular dilatation and worsening left ventricular ejection fraction (LVEF) (as in acquired heart diseases).
- *Aortic root dilatation* >55–60mm associated with symptoms or with aortic regurgitation.
- A large *aneurysm of the RVOT.*
- Any *combination* of the above residual findings of a mild degree, resulting in progressive right ventricular dilatation and dysfunction, or in clinical symptoms.

When indicating a patient for reoperation, consideration should be taken of symptomatic worsening of exertional dyspnea and fatigability, progressive right ventricular dilatation, progression of QRS duration, significance of pulmonary and tricuspid regurgitation, arrhythmias, and other residual findings.[18,19]

In most TOF patients, reoperation with pulmonary valve replacement results in symptom relief, reduction in right ventricular end-diastolic and end-systolic volume, and an increase in functional exercise capacity.[6,20,21] Reversibility of right ventricular dilatation and dysfunction is dependent on the degree of histological changes in the right ventricle.

The best time for reoperation in patients after TOF repair with significant pulmonary regurgitation is a matter of controversy given the limited life of the newly implanted prostheses and the risk of another reoperation.

An MRI study in adults with repaired TOF revealed postoperatively a significant decrease in right ventricular volumes after pulmonary valve replacement, while right ventriclar systolic function remained unchanged. In patients with a right ventricle end-diastolic volume >170ml/m^2 or a right ventricle end-systolic volume >85ml/m^2 before pulmonary valve replacement, right ventricle volumes did not normalize.[19]

Long-term survival rates after TOF reoperation with pulmonary valve replacement were 95 and 76% after 5 and 10 years, respectively, with implanted pulmonary valve reoperation required by 30% of patients at 10 years.[22]

Catheterization-based interventions

- *Balloon angioplasty* of peripheral stenoses, possibly with stent implantation, is indicated in significant peripheral pulmonary artery stenoses.
- *Catheter-based closure of a residual ASD or patent foramen ovale (PFO)* is performed in cyanotic patients or after paradoxical embolism.
- *Percutaneous implantation of a bovine jugular valve into the pulmonary position* is possible in certain cases.[23]

Management of arrhythmias

- *In ventricular tachycardia,* a hemodynamic cause of right ventricular dilatation should be eliminated (e.g. by pulmonary homograft implantation in pulmonary

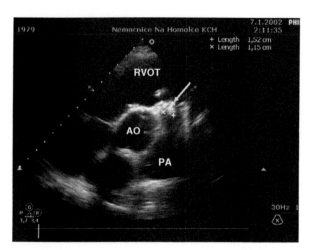

Figure 7.20
Tetralogy of Fallot, transthoracic echo, short-axis, parasternal view. Large vegetation on calcified pulmonary homograft (arrow), which subsequently embolized to pulmonary artery (PA). AO, Aorta; RVOT, right ventricular outflow tract.

regurgitation; resection of a RVOT aneurysm). Catheter-based ablation of the arrhythmogenic focus or intraoperative cryoablation are increasingly used. Only if this fails, is drug therapy instituted and/or an implantable cardioverter/defibrillator (ICD) is implanted.

- *In atrial flutter and fibrillation,* it is critical to eliminate hemodynamic causes of atrial dilatation, to perform cryoablation or radiofrequency ablation of arrhythmogenic pathways, or to initiate antiarrhythmic drug therapy.

Pregnancy and delivery

If, after TOF repair, the patient is free of significant residua, and if she is in functional Class I or II, pregnancy and delivery are usually well tolerated. Women with significant residual findings, particularly with RVOTO, severe pulmonary regurgitation and right ventricular dysfunction, arrhythmias, or in functional Class III, are at risk. Correction of the residual findings should be performed before pregnancy.

Infectious endocarditis

The risk of infectious endocarditis (IE) persists after repair. Prevention of IE is indicated in all TOF patients throughout their lifetime (Figure 7.20).

Follow-up

All TOF patients require lifelong follow-up by a cardiologist.

TETRALOGY OF FALLOT AFTER PALLIATIVE SURGERY

Rarely, one can encounter an adult with TOF who has had only palliative surgery.[24] The most frequent procedure

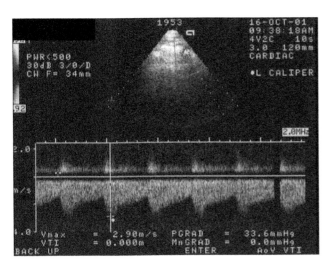

Figure 7.21
Continuous Doppler, suprasternal view, systolic and diastolic flow in Blalock–Taussig shunt.

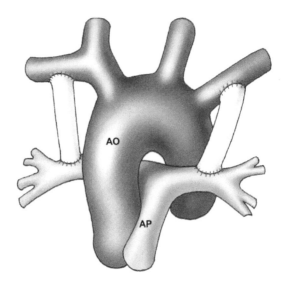

Figure 7.23
Palliative modified Blalock–Taussig shunt (subclavio-pulmonary anastomosis) with vascular prosthesis. AO, Aorta; AP, pulmonary artery.

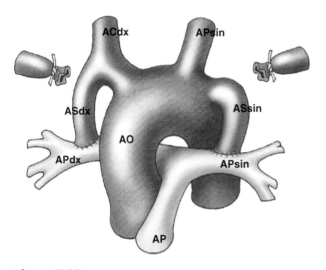

Figure 7.22
Palliative classical Blalock–Taussig shunt. ASdx, Right subclavian artery; ASsin, left subclavian artery; AO, aorta; PA, pulmonary trunk; ACdx, right common carotid artery; ACsin, left common carotid artery; APsin, left branch of the pulmonary artery; APdx, right branch of the pulmonary artery.

performed was a classical or modified suclavio-pulmonary shunt as proposed by Blalock–Taussig (Figures 7.21–7.23), or, alternatively, an aortopulmonary anastomosis (Waterston or Potts anastomosis) or a central aortopulmonary shunt.

Clinical findings

Physical examination may reveal mild central cyanosis with clubbing; however, this may not be present in all cases. Advanced stages may show signs of left-heart decompensation or pulmonary hypertension.

Auscultatory findings

- If the patient had a subclavio-pulmonary shunt procedure according to Blalock–Taussig (Figures 7.21–7.23), one can hear a continuous systolic–diastolic murmur in the left or right subclavian space.
- In the presence of other forms of an aortopulmonary shunt, a continuous murmur can be heard in the second to third parasternal intercostal space.
- If after a shunt operation the typical murmur cannot be heard, the reason may be a tight stenosis or complete closure, or development of pulmonary hypertension with balanced diastolic pressure levels in the aorta and pulmonary artery. Both conditions may result in clinical deterioration in a previously compensated patient.

Further diagnosis

A thorough examination, including transesophageal echocardiography and, possibly, MRI, multislice CT (MS-CT) and exercise testing, and a catheter-based examination should be performed, preferably in a specialized adult CHD center.

Prognosis

Shunt surgery was used as the only palliative therapeutic method when extracorporal circulation was unavailable. Later, shunt surgery represented phase one of a two-step surgical management, allowing infants to survive the critical period. The shunt was removed later during repair.

After palliative surgery alone, the prognosis is appreciably worse compared with repair. In historical studies, 60% of patients operated on between their third and fifth year of life became adults; 50% survived to 25 years of age.

Over the course of time, patients often grew out of their shunt and the effect of the shunt degraded. Moreover, there was a significant volume load on the left ventricle. In particular, patients after Waterston or Potts shunt were prone to pulmonary hypertension due to pulmonary overperfusion, or to shunt-kinking due to tension on the pulmonary artery.

Management

Pregnancy and delivery
Pregnancy is not advisable in patients after palliative surgery because of the significantly increased risk for maternal and newborn.

Infective endocarditis
The risk for IE is high, and there is a need for lifelong IE prophylaxis.

Follow-up
Patients should be followed-up at specialized centers.

TETRALOGY OF FALLOT WITHOUT SURGERY

It is rare to see a TOF patient without previous surgery (Figures 7.2–7.5, 7.18). TOF can be managed surgically even in adulthood;[25] however, the operative risk depends significantly on the experience of the cardiac surgical center. The risk associated with the procedure is high, particularly in individuals over 50 years of age. It is therefore appropriate to assess the degree of complaints and risk on an individual basis. The decision of whether to operate or not is a difficult one, particularly in patients with minor complaints.

Pregnancy and delivery

Pregnancy is not advisable in unoperated patients because of the significantly increased risk for maternal and newborn.

Infective endocarditis

The risk for IE is high, and there is a need for lifelong IE prophylaxis.

Follow-up

Patients should be followed-up at a specialized center.

References

1. Dabizzi RP, Teodori G, Barletta GA et al. Associated coronary and cardiac anomalies in the tetralogy of Fallot. An angiographic study. Eur Heart J 1990; 11: 692–704.
2. Gatzoulis MA, Clark AL, Cullen S, Newman CGH, Redington AN. Right ventricular diastolic function 15 to 35 years after repair of tetralogy of Fallot. Restrictive physiology predicts superior exercise performance. Circulation 1995; 91: 1775–81.
3. Munkhammar P, Cullen S, Jögi P et al. Early age at repair prevents restrictive right ventricular physiology after surgery for tetralogy of Fallot. J Am Coll Cardiol 1998; 32: 1083–7.
4. Perloff JK. The Clinical Recognition of Congenital Heart Disease, 4th edn. Philadelphia, PA: WB Saunders Company, 1994.
5. Gatzoulis MA, Balaji S, Webber SA et al. Risk factors for arrhythmia and sudden cardiac death late after repair of tetralogy of Fallot: A multicentre study. Lancet 2000; 356: 975–81.
6. Hazekamp MG, Kurvers MMJ, Schoof PH et al. Pulmonary valve insertion late after repair of Fallot's tetralogy. Eur J Cardiothorac Surg 2001; 19(5): 667–70.
7. Niwa K, Siu SC, Webb GD, Gatzoulis MA. Progressive aortic root dilatation in adults late after repair of tetralogy of Fallot. Circulation 2002; 106(11): 1374–8.
8. Niwa K. Aortic root dilatation in tetralogy of Fallot long-term after repair – histology of the aorta in tetralogy of Fallot: Evidence of intrinsic aortopathy. Int J Cardiol 2005; 103(2): 117–19.
9. Ishizaka T, Ichikawa H, Sawa Y et al. Prevalence and optimal management strategy for aortic regurgitation in tetralogy of Fallot. Eur J Cardiothorac Surg 2004; 26(6): 1080–6.
10. Daliento L. Total correction of tetralogy of Fallot: Late clinical follow-up. Ital Heart J 2002; 3(1): 24–7.
11. Vetter VL. Arrhythmias in congenital heart disease. In: Crawford MH, Dimarco JP. Cardiology, 1st edn. London: Mosby International Ltd, 2001: 7.21.1–7.21.14.
12. Russo G, Folino AF, Mazzotti E, Rebellato L, Daliento L. Comparison between QRS duration at standard ECG and signal-averaging ECG for arrhythmic risk stratification after surgical repair of tetralogy of fallot. J Cardiovasc Electrophysiol 2005; 16(3): 288–92.
13. Garson A Jr. Ventricular arrhythmias after repair of congenital heart disease: Who needs treatment? Cardiol Young 1991; 1: 177–81.
14. Murphy JG, Gersh BJ, Mair DD et al. Long-term outcome in patients undergoing surgical repair of tetralogy of Fallot. N Engl J Med 1993; 329: 593–9.
15. Harrison DA, Harris L, Siu SC et al. Sustained ventricular tachycardia in adult patients late after repair of tetralogy of Fallot. J Am Coll Cardiol 1997; 30(5): 1368–73.
16. Sunakawa A, Shirotani H, Yokoyama T, Oku H. Factors affecting biventricular function following surgical repair of tetralogy of Fallot. Jpn Circ J 1988; 52: 401–10.
17. Schamberger MS, Hurowitz RA. Course of right and left ventricular function in patients with pulmonary insufficiency after repair of tetralogy of Fallot. Pediatr Cardiol 2000; 21: 244–8.
18. Graham TP Jr. Management of pulmonary regurgitation after tetralogy of Fallot repair. Curr Cardiol Rep 2002; 4(1): 63–7.
19. Therrien J, Provost Y, Merchant N et al. Optimal timing for pulmonary valve replacement in adults after tetralogy of Fallot repair. Am J Cardiol 2005; 95(6): 779–82.
20. Therrien J, Siu S, McLauglin PR et al. Pulmonary valve replacement in adults late after repair of tetralogy of Fallot: Are we operating too late? J Am Coll Cardiol 2000; 36: 1670–5.
21. Thierren J, Siu SC, Harris L et al. Impact of pulmonary valve replacement on arrhythmia propensity late after repair of tetralogy of Fallot. Circulation 2001; 103: 2489–94.
22. Discigil B, Derani JA, Puga FJ et al. Late pulmonary valve replacement after repair of tetralogy of Fallot. J Thorac Cardiovasc Surg 2001; 121(2): 344–51.
23. Bonhoeffer P, Boudjemline Y, Qureshi SA et al. Percutaneous insertion of the pulmonary valve. J Am Coll Cardiol 2002; 39: 1664–9.
24. Popelová J, Slavík Z, Škovránek J. Are cyanosed adults with congenital cardiac malformation depressed? Cardiol Young 2001; 11: 379–84.
25. Hu DCK, Seward JB, Puga FJ, Fuster V, Tajik AJ. Total correction of tetralogy of Fallot at age 40 years and older: Long-term follow-up. J Am Coll Cardiol 1985; 5: 40–4.

8

Coarctation of the aorta

Anatomical notes

Coarctation of the aorta (CoA) is usually a localized narrowing of the aortic isthmus with a shelf-like infolding of the posterior wall of the aorta, in most cases opposite to the origin of the ductus arteriosus or the ligamentum arteriosum (Figure 8.1). CoA is most often localized immediately below the origin of the left subclavian artery, but may even be localized before the origin of the left subclavian artery (whose orifice may be stenotic) (Figure 8.2), or, rarely, in the abdominal aorta. The right subclavian artery may originate separately, atypically, below the site of coarctation (Figure 8.3).

Although usually CoA is a localized narrowing, it may be accompanied by aortic arch hypoplasia and/or a prolonged tubular narrowing of the isthmus. The poststenotic descending aorta is usually dilated below the coarctation site.

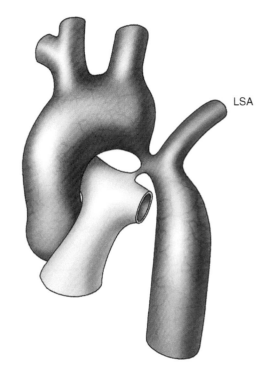

Figure 8.2
Coarctation of the aorta in front of the left subclavian artery (LSA).

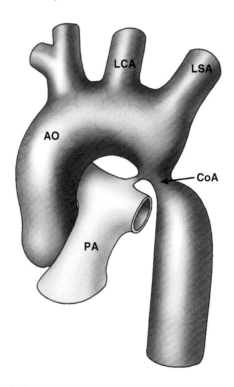

Figure 8.1
Coarctation of the aorta (CoA). AO, Aorta; PA, pulmonary artery; LCA, left carotid artery; LSA, left subclavian artery.

The real cause of CoA is not known. Postnatal constriction of aberrant ductal tissue and intrauterine alterations of blood flow through the aortic arch are under discussion. Simple CoA refers to coarctation in the absence of other relevant lesions. Complex CoA is used to describe coarctation in the presence of other important intracardiac and/or extracardiac lesions.

CoA is often (in 46–85% of cases) associated with a bicuspid aortic valve (see Chapter 9).[1,2] Concomitant mitral valve anomalies have been reported in 26–58% of patients with CoA.[2] Aortic aneurysm has been reported both in the ascending and descending aorta. An association between the bicuspid aortic valve and aortic wall fragility with a tendency to spontaneous rupture was described by Maude Abbott as early as 1928.[3] Cerebral berry aneurysms tend to form in the region of circle of Willis and may constitute the morphological basis of intracranial bleeding.[2,4]

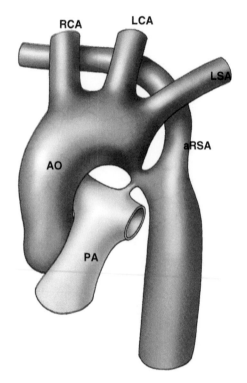

Figure 8.3
Anomalous right subclavian artery (aRSA) below coarctation. RCA, Right carotid artery; LCA, left carotid artery; LSA, left subclavian artery; AO, aorta; PA, pulmonary artery.

Most adult patients with CoA have had surgery in childhood. Unoperated significant CoA is rare, and is usually associated with significant collateral circulation. The collateral vessels develop from the subclavian, axillary, internal thoracic, scapular and intercostal arteries. In rare cases, the small lumen of the aorta may even develop aortic atresia.

Prevalence

CoA accounts for 5–8% of all congenital heart diseases (CHD), and occurs two to three times more often in men than in women.[2] A higher incidence of CoA has been reported in women with Turner's syndrome (in up to 35% of cases).

Pathophysiology

A hemodynamically significant CoA has an invasive peak gradient ≥20mmHg. However, a morphologically significant coarctation may be associated with a smaller gradient between the upper and lower extremities in the presence of significant collaterals.

In adulthood, untreated coarctation results in hypertension in the precoarctation region, hypotension in the postcoarctation region, in notable left ventricular myocardial hypertrophy, and in advanced cases even in left ventricular dilatation and systolic left ventricular dysfunction. In the presence of a dysfunctional bicuspid aortic valve, the above may be accompanied by left ventricular volume overload or pressure overload.

While surgery of coarctation in childhood will remove a mechanical obstacle, a variety of abnormalities will persist in these patients into adulthood. These are primarily altered vascular reactivity in the precoarctation arterial bed, which is less capable of vasodilation compared with the postcoarctation vascular bed.[5] In the precoarctation vascular bed, there is impaired endothelium-dependent and -independent vasodilatation and hyperreactivity to vasoconstrictor stimuli.[6–8] Scarring occurs at the site of surgery. Still, a reduced aortic wall compliance can be seen not only at the site of surgery, but also proximally to it.[9] In young adults after coarctation surgery in childhood, these changes lead to a frequent exercise-induced hypertensive response in the upper limbs, and the incidence of resting hypertension also rises with advancing age.[10,11]

Clinical findings and diagnosis

Rarely, unoperated CoA may be found as a cause of secondary hypertension in adulthood. The diagnosis described here refers mainly to states after CoA surgery.

Symptoms

- Hypertension-related headache.
- Weakness in the lower limb, fatigability, and pain.
- Abdominal angina.
- Exertional dyspnea due to heart failure in the presence of significant coarctation or recoarctation, valve disease or decompensated hypertension, or a combination thereof.
- Chest pain suggestive of angina pectoris.
- Epistaxis.
- Dysphagia in the presence of an anomalous course of the right subclavian artery beyond the esophagus.
- Cerebral hemorrhage.
- Infective endocarditis (IE).
- Aortic dissection or rupture.

Clinical examination

In addition to a standard examination by a cardiologist, it is mandatory to assess:

- Blood pressure on all four limbs.
- Determination of the upper-to-lower limb gradient. Blood pressure at lower limbs can be taken with the patient lying prone, a tonometer with a larger cuff on the thigh, and auscultation in the popliteal fossa or using Doppler echo.

- Pulsation on both femoral and radial arteries. However, adults rarely show absent or clearly reduced pulsation on their femoral arteries because of the collateral circulation in patients with significant unoperated coarctation or recoarctation. One would rather find a slower rise in pulse in the femoral arteries, or its delayed peak on simultaneous pulse palpation on the radial and femoral arteries.
- After subclavian flap repair (i.e. Waldhausen plastic), blood pressure in the left upper limb is inadequate, and pulse in the left upper limb is also weak or absent.
- A thrill in the suprasternal notch or the neck vessels, and a heaving but not displaced apex beat (concentric left ventricular hypertrophy) may be present.

Auscultatory findings

- Auscultation reveals a loud aortic closure sound and, in patients with a bicuspid aortic valve, an aortic ejection click. Systolic ejection murmur over the aorta with propagation into the carotids in the presence of a stenotic bicuspid aortic valve or arterial hypertension.
- Diastolic murmur over the aorta in the presence of aortic regurgitation.
- Systolic vascular murmur between the scapulae in coarctation and recoarctation. With critically tight coarctation, a continuous murmur may be present between the scapulae, which disappears after development of isthmus atresia.
- Collaterals manifest by late systolic, crescendo–descrescendo murmur (occasionally referred to as continuous), audible on the chest, above the scapulae, and in the intercostal spaces.
- Systolic regurgitant murmur on the apex with propagation into the axilla in the presence of mitral regurgitation.

Electrocardiogram (ECG)

- Left atrial enlargement and left ventricular hypertrophy.
- Left ventricular hypertrophy with strain (ST-segment depression and T-wave inversion) is usually associated with significant aortic stenosis.

Chest X-ray

- A sign of '3' on the aorta (notch at the site of coarctation).
- Rib notching – at the posteroinferior borders of the third and fourth (to eighth) ribs.

Echocardiography

- Suprasternal approach focusing on aortic arch morphology, the descending aorta gradient, and the diastolic run-off (Figures 8.4 and 8.5).

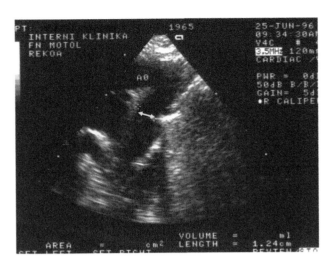

Figure 8.4
Suprasternal view in adult patient wtih gothic aortic arch and mild residual coarctation after resection with end-to-end anastomosis in childhood.

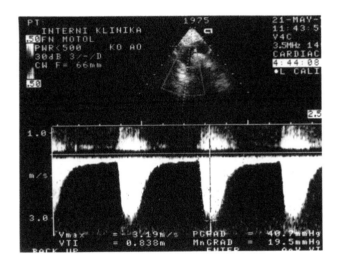

Figure 8.5
Mild coarctation, suprasternal view, maximal gradient by continuous Doppler (CW) 41mmHg.

- Doppler echo in the descending aorta is more accurate when using a pencil probe with continuous Doppler examination (Figure 8.6). Patients after CoA surgery often show higher systolic velocities in the descending aorta compared with those in healthy controls (flow rate acceleration). The simplified Bernoulli formula cannot be used for gradient calculation as the potential for velocity acceleration in the aorta before the point of narrowing has also to be taken into account: $\Delta P = 4(V_2^2 - V_1^2)$. The increase in velocity may likewise reflect reduced compliance of the aortic wall. The gradient is dependent on the aortic flow rate.[12]

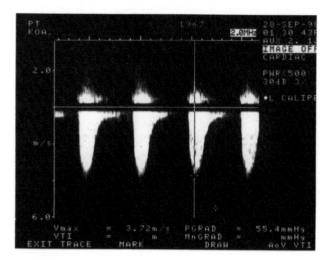

Figure 8.6
Unoperated adult with coarctation of the aorta with Doppler gradient of 55mmHg.

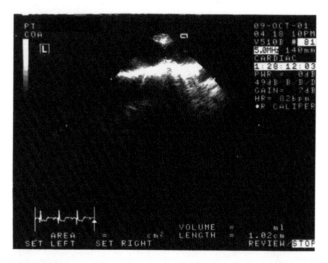

Figure 8.7
Mild recoarctation of the aorta with narrowing of the lumen to 10mm at the site of resection and anastomosis end-to-end. Transesophageal echo, longitudinal view.

- Velocities of up to 3m/s at rest need not imply significant recoarctation as suggested by the corresponding gradient.[6,12] A resting peak systolic velocity ≥3.2m/s and a diastolic velocity ≥1.0m/s may be suggestive of significant coarctation.
- In the presence of (re)coarctation, a diastolic forward flow ('run-off') is found in the descending aorta.
- In addition, CoA requires examination of the aortic valve morphology and function, of the whole course of the aorta (aneurysms or dilatation), assessment of left ventricular size and function, elimination of mitral valve abnormalities and other associated CHD.
- The role of transesophageal echocardiography is a minor one, unless the patient has a bad quality of the suprasternal view (Figures 8.7 and 8.8).

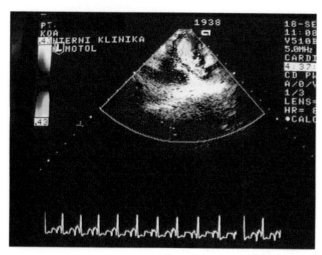

Figure 8.8
Older lady with unoperated coarctation of the aorta; turbulent color flow and narrowing of aorta could be seen on the transesophageal echo only, modified longitudinal view.

Magnetic resonance imaging (MRI) and computerized tomography (CT)

- MRI as well as CT show site, extent and degree of the aortic narrowing, the aortic arch, which may be hypoplastic, the prestenotic and poststenotic aorta, and the collateral vessels, if present. State-of-the-art MRI methods provide information on coarctation blood flow, the pressure gradient across the stenosis, and collateral flow.[14]
- MRI and CT detect complications related to the natural history, or to therapeutic procedures (e.g. aneurysm of the ascending aorta or at the operative site, aortic dissections, a residual stenosis or hypoplastic aortic arch).[14]
- Narrowing of the aorta at the site of coarctation or recoarctation >30–40% of the width of the descending aorta over the diaphragm is considered pathological (Figures 8.9 and 8.10). The aortic dimensions on angiography correlate better with MRI dimensions then with echocardiographic dimensions of aorta.[15]

Catheterization

- Cardiac catheterization delineates the anatomy of the aorta and supraaortic vessels, reveals the pressure gradient across the coarctation, recognizes associated cardiac defects, and evaluates left ventricular function and coronary status.
- A significant coarctation is defined as a gradient >20mmHg across the coarctation site in the absence of well-developed collaterals around the coarctation site.
- Selective coronary arteriography is mandatory because of the increased risk for coronary artery lesions, even in younger individuals, particularly in the presence of clinical symptoms, signs of heart failure, prior to scheduled intervention, or at ages over 40 years.

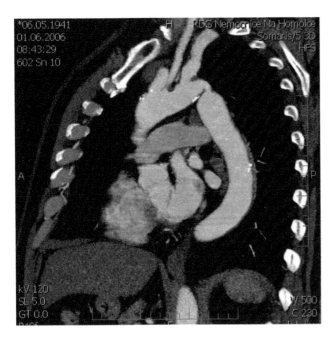

Figure 8.9
Computerized tomography angiography of 65-year-old man with unoperated severe coarctation of the aorta, coronary artery disease and severe and resistant hypertension.

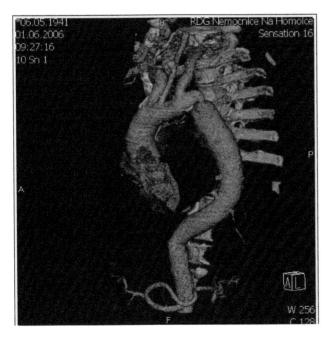

Figure 8.10
Computerized tomography scan with 3D reconstruction; the same patient as in Figure 8.9.

Management

The following situations may warrant consideration for intervention or reintervention:[16]

- All symptomatic patients with a gradient >30mmHg across the coarctation.

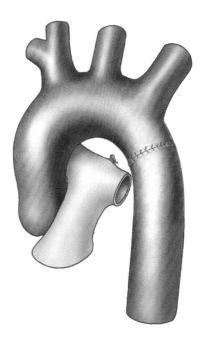

Figure 8.11
Resection of the coarctation and anastomosis end-to-end.

- Asymptomatic patients with a gradient >30mmHg across the coarctation and upper limb hypertension, pathologic blood pressure response during exercise, or significant left ventricular hypertrophy.
- Independent from the pressure gradient, some patients with ≥50% stenosis of the aorta (on MRI, CT or angiography).
- Significant aortic valve stenosis or regurgitation.
- Aneurysm of the ascending aorta.
- Aneurysm at the site of previous treatment.
- Symptomatic aneurysms of the circle of Willis.

Surgery

Several different *surgical techniques* have been designed for coarctation and recoarctation repair. Most often, CoA can be managed by resection of the involved segment and an end-to-end anastomosis (Figure 8.11). If the resected segment is too long, a vascular Goretex or Dacron prosthesis is implanted (Figure 8.12). Aortoplasty according to Vossschulte enlarges the involved segment either directly (rarely used) or indirectly with a patch (Figures 8.13 and 8.14). However, the latter type of surgery has been reported to be associated, on long-term follow-up, with a high incidence of aneurysms and with a risk of fatal rupture.[17] Under certain circumstances in adulthood, an extra-anatomical bypass between the pre- and poststenotic aortic segment can be implanted (Figures 8.15 and 8.16).

The choice of procedure depends on the nature, site and extent of the coarctation, and on the patient's age. Surgical management in adults with coarctation or recoarctation carries a significantly higher risk compared with children, and should be undertaken in a center with adequate experience and good outcomes in this area.

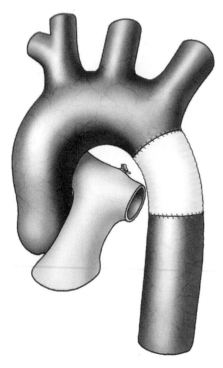

Figure 8.12
Resection of the coarctation and replacement of the long resected part of narrowed aorta by the vascular prosthesis.

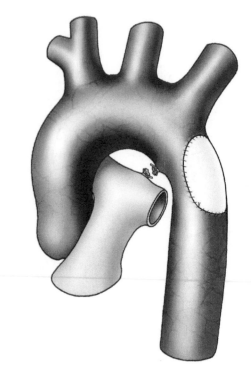

Figure 8.14
Aortoplasty of the coarctation of aorta according to Vossschulte, using a patch.

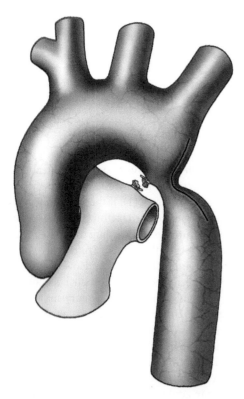

Figure 8.13
Aortoplasty of the coarctation hof aorta according to Vossschulte.

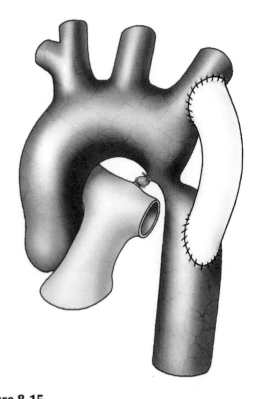

Figure 8.15
Coarctation of the aorta; repair by bypass from the left subclavian artery to descending aorta.

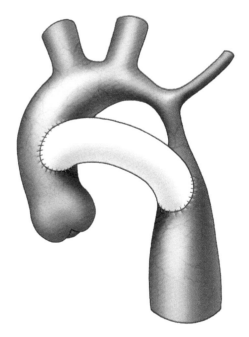

Figure 8.16
Coarctation of the aorta with hypoplastic arch. Correction by extraanatomical bypass from ascending to descending aorta.

A concomitant significant valve defect can be an indication for surgery together with or after CoA treatment. More significant defects are operated on first.

Interventional therapy

Angioplasty, with or without *stent implantation* (Figure 8.17) is the preferred approach to recoarctation or residual coarctation after previous surgery.[18] Considering the potential for serious complications (e.g. aortic dissection, aneurysm formation, rupture), the method should only be used in centers with an adequate body of experience and facilities for cardiac surgery.

It is increasingly used, but not generally accepted, for the management of unoperated coarctation in adulthood.

Conservative therapy

Conservative therapy is used primarily in the treatment of hypertension, which can be very difficult. While ACE inhibitors and beta blockers are the most often used drugs, other commonly used antihypertensive agents can also be applied. In the presence of coarctation or recoarctation, properly controlled hypertension may result in inadequate blood pressure below the coarctation site, sometimes manifesting itself as lower limb pain. This phenomenon may occasionally also be experienced by hypertensive patients without recoarctation, most likely because of altered vascular reactivity of the pre- and postcoarctation vascular beds. Prevention of atherosclerosis, developing prematurely in the coarctation vascular bed, is another important consideration.

Residual findings and risks

- *Recoarctation* may occur on long-term follow-up with all known surgical and interventional techniques. The prevalence after surgery is between 3 and 41% of cases. It is an important cause of morbidity due to induced or aggravated systemic arterial hypertension, increased left ventricular wall mass, coronary artery disease or congestive heart failure.

- *Arterial hypertension*, either at rest or during exercise, is common, even after successful primary treatment. Its incidence rises up to 52%, particularly decades after the operation.[10,19–22] Structural vascular abnormalities and alterations in vascular reactivity are causative for the development of raised blood pressure at rest and during exercise after CoA repair.[23] Affected patients are at risk of premature coronary artery disease, ventricular

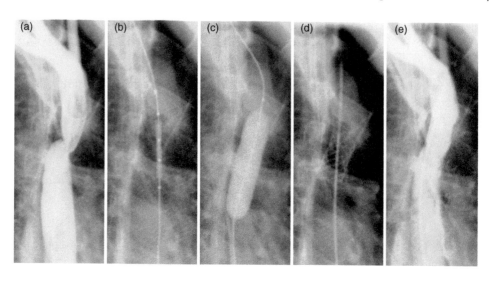

Figure 8.17
Recoarctation treated by stent implantation. (a) Angiography confirming recoarctation; (b) introdution of nonexpanded Palmaz stent into the site of recoarctation; (c) dilatation of balloon; (d) expanded stent; (e) angiographic result without residual recoarctation. (Courtesy of Oleg Reich, MD, and Petr Tax, MD, Children Kardiocentrum, Prague, Czech Republic.)

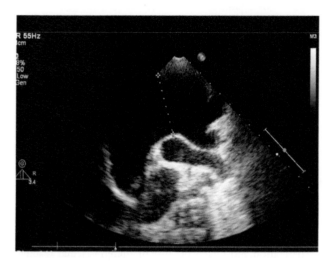

Figure 8.18
Dilatation of distal aortic aorta and brachiocephalic trunk in a 27-year-old woman with Turner syndrome and mild recoarctation. Echocardiography, suprasternal view.

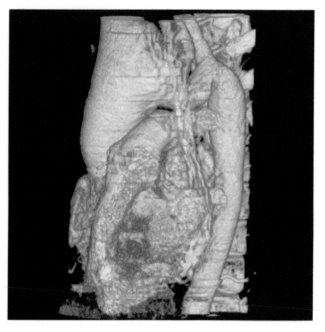

Figure 8.19
Computerized tomography scan with 3D reconstruction of recoarctation and dilatation of distal ascending aorta; the same patient as in Figure 8.18.

dysfunction, and rupture of aortic or cerebral aneurysms, particularly in the third and fourth decades of life. Patients operated on in early childhood have a higher rate of normal blood pressure postoperatively. Several studies also suggest an increase in the prevalence of systemic hypertension with increasing length of follow-up after CoA repair.

- *Systemic hypertension* in the upper limbs, either exacerbated by exercise or only during exercise, is seen in up to 30% of operated CoA patients.[7,11,24]

- *Aneurysms* of the ascending aorta, or in the region of the aortic isthmus, are dangerous complications (Figures 8.18–8.20). Practically all surgical and interventional techniques carry this risk. Their occurrence depends on the era of the operation, the patient's age at the time of surgery, the postoperative interval, and the technique of treatment. Recent studies show postoperative aortic aneurysms in only 5–9% of patients, whereas older studies reported aneurysm in 33–51% of patients (mostly after Dacron patch aortoplasty[25]). Aneurysms have been found after a postoperative interval of >30 years. In many patients aneurysms are detected incidentally, as their development seldom produces symptoms.

- *Aneurysms after angioplasty* occur immediately or after a lag of several months. In native adult coarctation the frequency is 4–12%, and after previous surgical repair 5%.

- A *bicuspid aortic valve* occurs in up to 85% of cases of CoA; the occurrence and significance of aortic valve disease rises with age. Besides valvular lesions, 11–15% will acquire *dilatation of the ascending aorta*, which may progress to aortic aneurysm, and even dissect and rupture (Figure 8.21).

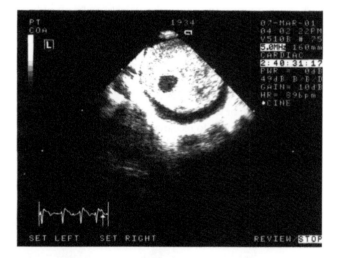

Figure 8.20
Severe dilatation of ascending aorta (80mm) in a patient with coarctation of the aorta. The aneurysm is filled with recanalized huge thrombus. Transthoracic echo.

- *Premature atherosclerosis* and functional abnormalities in the precoarctation vascular bed.

- *IE* at the site of coarctation, or an abnormal aortic valve.

- *Cerebrovascular event* (stroke) in hypertensive patients, or associated with *rupture of cerebral artery aneurysm*.

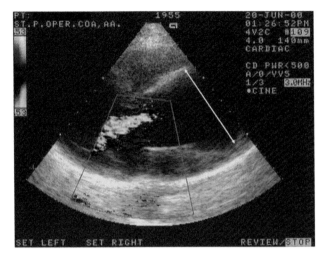

Figure 8.21
Woman after successful operation of coarctation of the aorta with bicuspid aortic valve, mild aortic regurgitation and large dilatation of ascending aorta (68mm, arrow); transthoracic echo, parasternal long-axis view.

Pregnancy and delivery

After successful treatment of CoA, pregnancy should be tolerated without major problems although hemodynamic. Nevertheless, hormonal changes during pregnancy may pose an increased risk to both mother and fetus, particularly in patients with unoperated significant coarctation or with severe recoarctation, where pregnancy can even be contraindicated. Maternal death due to aortic dissection and rupture of a cerebral aneurysm has been reported.

Treatment of hypertension in the precoarctation region may result in hypotension in the postcoarctation region, abortion, or fetal death. When important coarctation, recoarctation or aortic aneurysm is diagnosed in pregnant woman, cesarean section may be appropriate for delivery. Before pregnancy, the aforementioned findings should be corrected (usually surgically).

The recurrence risk of CoA increases in the offspring of parents with CoA and with the number of affected relatives. Women with a history of coarctation repair, who contemplate pregnancy, should have hemodynamic assessment and genetic counseling before conception.[26]

Infectious endocarditis

The risk of IE persists even after CoA surgery because of the frequent occurrence of aortic valve disease. The risk of IE also exists at the site of coarctation, especially if vascular prostheses were used. Therefore, lifelong endocarditis prophylaxis is recommended after surgical or interventional treatment of CoA.

Follow-up

Lifelong follow-up by a cardiologist, even of asymptomatic patients in good clinical state, is important.[27] Follow-up care should include a search for late complications, including arterial hypertension, recurrent obstruction, aneurysm formation or other associated anomalies.

In addition to the clinical examination, the use of imaging techniques (particularly MRI and CT) is essential.[28,29] Treatment, if necessary, should take place in centers with extensive experience in coarctation.

Prognosis

In the past, patients with CoA had a very grim prognosis, dying without surgery at a mean age of 35, with only 10% of patients surviving to the age of 50.[30,31] Surgery in childhood significantly improved the prognosis: the rates of 24- and 44-year survival after surgery were 81 and 73%, respectively.[20,32] At 33 years postoperatively, 88% of patients were in functional NYHA Class I–II.[10]

Still, some 9–12% of those undergoing surgery die prematurely at a young age from cardiovascular causes: most often from heart failure, aortic aneurysm rupture or dissection, complications of significant aortic valve disease or hypertension, cerebral hemorrhage, IE, coronary lesions, and also during reoperation for recoarctation.[10,20,33,34]

CoA cannot be considered a simple CHD which can be eliminated by surgery. Even after successful surgery, development of premature atherosclerosis involving the precoarctation arterial bed, frequent hypertension, higher incidence of aortic valve disease, recoarctation, and structural and functional abnormalities of the aortic wall (aneurysm) and of other arteries in the precoarctation region can be expected in adulthood.

References

1. Valdes-Cruz LM, Cayre LO. Echocardiographic Diagnosis of Congenital Heart Disease. An Embryologic and Anatomic Approach, 1st edn. Philadelphia, PA: Lippicott-Raven Publishers, 1999.
2. Perloff JK. The Clinical Recognition of Congenital Heart Disease, 4th edn. Philadelphia, PA: WB Saunders Company, 1994.
3. Abbott ME. Coarctation of the aorta of adult type; statistical study and historical retrospect of 200 recorded cases with autopsy: of stenosis or obliteration of descending aortic arch in subjects above age of two years. Am Heart J 1928; 3: 574.
4. Connolly HM, Huston J 3rd, Brown RD Jr et al. Intracranial aneurysms in patients with coarctation of the aorta: a prospective magnetic resonance angiographic study of 100 patients. Mayo Clin Proc 2003; 78(12): 1491–9.
5. Šámánek M, Goetzová J, Fišerová J, Škovránek J. Differences in muscle blood flow in upper and lower extremities of patients after correction of coarctation of the aorta. Circulation 1976; 54(3): 377–81.
6. Gardiner HM, Celemajer DS, Sorensen KE et al. Arterial reactivity is significantly impaired in normotensive young adults after successful repair of aortic coarctation in childhood. Circulation 1994; 89: 1745–50.

7. Guenthard J, Wyler F. Exercise-induced hypertension in the arms due to impaired arterial reactivity after successful coarctation resection. Am J Cardiol 1995; 75: 814–17.

8. Gidding SS, Rocchini AP, Moorehead C, Schork MA, Rosenthal A. Increased forearm vascular reactivity in patients with hypertension after repair of coarctation. Circulation 1985; 71: 495–9.

9. Rees S, Somerville J, Ward C. Coarctation of the aorta: Magnetic resonance imaging in the late post-operative assessment. Radiology 1989; 173: 499–502.

10. Popelová J, Dostálová P, Telekes P, Škovránek J, Belšan T. What is the status of patients operated on for coarctation of the aorta 33 years ago? Cor Vasa 2002; 44(4): 169–74.

11. Kaemmerer H, Oelert F, Bahlmann J et al. Arterial hypertension in adults after surgical treatment of aortic coarctation. Thorac Cardiovasc Surg 1998; 46: 121–5.

12. Tan JL, Babu-Narayan SV, Henein MY, Mullen M, Li W. Doppler echocardiographic profile and indexes in the evaluation of aortic coarctation in patients before and after stenting. J Am Coll Cardiol 2005; 46(6): 1045–53.

13. Chan KC, Dickinson DF, Wharton GA, Gibbs JL. Continuous wave Doppler echocardiography after surgical repair of coarctation of the aorta. Br Heart J 1992; 68: 192–4.

14. Kaemmerer H, Stern H, Fratz S et al. Imaging in adults with congenital cardiac disease (ACCD). Thoracic Cardiovasc Surg 2000; 48: 328–35.

15. Muhler EG, Neuerburg JM, Ruben A et al. Evaluation of aortic coarctation after surgical repair: Role of magnetic resonance imaging and Doppler ultrasound. Br Heart J 1993; 70(3): 290–5.

16. Kaemmerer H. Aortic coarctation and interrupted aortic arch. In: Gatzoulis M, Webb G, Daubeney P, eds. Management of Adult Congenital Heart Disease. New York: Churchill Livingstone, 2003.

17. Parks WJ, Ngo TD, Plauth WJ et al. Incidence of aneurysm formation after dacron patch aortoplasty repair for coarctation of the aorta: Long-term results and assessment utilizing magnetic resonance angiography with three-dimensional surface rendering. J Am Coll Cardiol 1995; 26: 266–71.

18. Pilla CB, Fontes VF, Pedra CA. Endovascular stenting for aortic coarctation. Expert Rev Cardiovasc Ther 2005; 3(5): 879–90.

19. Hager A, Kanz S, Kaemmerer H, Schreiber C, Hess J. COArctation Long-term Assessment (COALA-Study): Incidence of restenosis and hypertension after surgical repair. JACC 2004; 43(5, Suppl A): 31A [A].

20. Clarkson PM, Nicholson MR, Barrat-Boyes BG, Neutze JN, Whitlock RM. Results after repair of coarctation of the aorta beyond infancy: A 10 to 28 year follow-up with particular reference to late systemic hypertension. Am J Cardiol 1983; 51: 1481–8.

21. Kappetein AP, Zwinderman AH, Borges AJJC, Rohmer J, Huysmans HA. More than thirty-five years of coarctation repair. J Thorac Cardiovasc Surg 1994; 107: 87–95.

22. Fišerová J, Šámánek M, Tůme S, Padovcoá H, Hučín B. Clinical findings and hemodynamic parameters in adults surgically treated for coarctation of aorta in childhood. Cardiology 1980; 65: 205–13.

23. Vriend JW, de Groot E, Bouma BJ et al. Carotid intima–media thickness in post-coarctectomy patients with exercise induced hypertension. Heart 2005; 91(7): 962–3.

24. Cyran SE, Grzesciak M, Kaufman K et al. Aortic 'recoarctation' at rest versus at exercise in children as evaluated by stress Doppler echocardiography after a 'good' operative result. Am J Cardiol 1993; 71: 963–70.

25. von Kodolitsch Y, Aydin MA, Koschyk DH et al. Predictors of aneurysmal formation after surgical correction of aortic coarctation. J Am Coll Cardiol 2002; 39(4): 617–24.

26. Vriend JW, Drenthen W, Pieper PG et al. Outcome of pregnancy in patients after repair of aortic coarctation. Eur Heart J 2005; 26(20): 2173–8. (Epub 2005 Jun 9).

27. De Bono J, Freeman LJ. Aortic coarctation repair – lost and found: The role of local long term specialised care. Int J Cardiol 2005; 104(2): 176–83.

28. Hager A, Kaemmerer H, Hess J. Comparison of helical CT scanning and MRI in the follow-up of adults with coarctation of the aorta. Chest 2005; 127(6): 2296.

29. Didier D, Saint-Martin C, Lapierre C et al. Coarctation of the aorta: Pre and postoperative evaluation with MRI and MR angiography; correlation with echocardiography and surgery. Int J Cardiovasc Imaging 2005; Nov 3: 1–19.

30. Campbell J. Natural history of coarctation of the aorta. Br Heart J 1970; 32: 633–40.

31. Maron BJ. Aortic isthmic coarctation. In: Roberts WC, ed. Adult Congenital Heart Disease, 1st edn. Philadelphia, PA: FA Davis Co, 1987: 443–53.

32. Brouwer RMHJ, Erasmus ME, Ebels T, Eijgelaar A. Influence of age on survival, late hypertension, and recoarctation in elective aortic coarctation repair. J Thor Cardiovasc Surg 1994; 108(3): 525–31.

33. Bobby JJ, Emami JM, Farmer RDT, Newman CGH. Operative survival and 40 years follow up of surgical repair of aortic coarctation. Br Heart J 1991; 65: 271–6.

34. Presbitero P, Demarie D, Villani M et al. Long term results (15–30 years) of surgical repair of aortic coarctation. Br Heart J 1987; 57: 462–67.

9

Bicuspid aortic valve and diseases of the aorta

Anatomical notes

A bicuspid aortic valve (BAV) has two cusps, which may be symmetrical or asymmetrical. The most frequently proposed mechanism for the development of this anomaly is commissural fusion during an inflammatory process in embryonic development.[1,2] A thickened connective tissue at the site of the original commissure is called the 'raphe'. In childhood, a BAV may be stenotic or insufficient; however, its function is normal in most cases, resulting in underestimation of the incidence of BAV in childhood. A bicuspid orifice is often eccentric and flow is usually turbulent. The abnormal dynamics of bicuspid valve flow leads to its premature degeneration with cusp thickening and calcification (Figure 9.1). Over years, BAV function tends to deteriorate, be that in terms of stenosis, insufficiency or a combination of both. The factors contributing to insufficiency are elongation and prolapse of the cusps, or shortening of thickened cusps, or dilatation of the aortic annulus and aortic root. Bicuspid aortic valves, which are only insufficient, seldom calcify before the age of 50 (Figure 9.2). A BAV may be associated with other defects, most often with mitral valve prolapse and with coarctation of the aorta (CoA).[1] Of importance is the association between a congenital BAV with

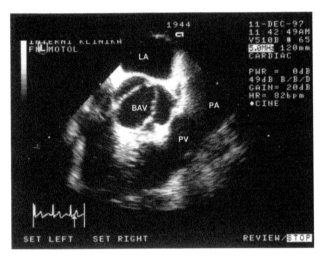

Figure 9.2
Transesophageal echo, longitudinal view. Bicuspid aortic valve (BAV) with mild thickening of the margins of the cusps, no calcification; moderate aortic insufficiency; male, 53 years of age. LA, Left atrium; PA, pulmonary artery; PV, pulmonary valve.

an abnormal histological structure of the aortic root, where the picture of cystic media necrosis has been reported.[3,4] This condition may predispose to aortic aneurysm formation or to aortic dissection.[5,6] Dilatation of the ascending aorta in BAV is out of proportion to the valvular lesion, and appears also in normally functioning BAV (Figure 9.3).[7–10]

CONGENITAL AORTIC STENOSIS

Left ventricular outflow tract obstruction (LVOTO) may occur at several levels, including combinations thereof:

Valvular aortic stenosis

Aortic valvular stenosis represents the most frequent cause of LVOTO (80–91%). Aortic valve stenosis below 60 years of age occurs most often secondary to congenital BAV, which degenerates earlier than aortic valve with three cusps (Figure 9.1). Aortic stenosis (AS) in BAV may be present at birth, or may develop in childhood, adolescence or adulthood, and is usually of progressive nature. AS present at birth is usually

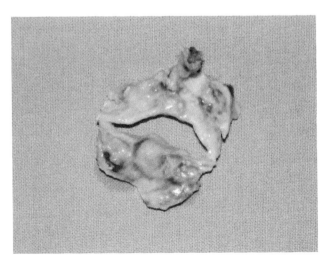

Figure 9.1
Bicuspid aortic valve with severe degenerative changes after surgical excision. (Courtesy of Associate Professor Dr T Honek, Cardiac Surgery, Faculty Hospital Motol, Prague, Czech Republic.)

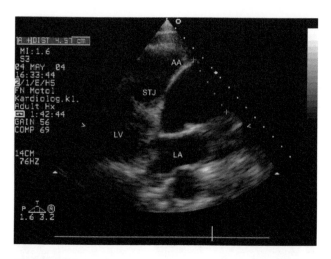

Figure 9.3
Transthoracic echo, modified parasternal long-axis view from the higher intercostal space for better visualization of the ascending aorta. Bicuspid aortic valve with normal function; normal size aortic annulus, bulbus and sinotubular junction (STJ); however, the ascending aorta (AA) is dilated to 46mm. LA, Left atrium; LV, left ventricle.

associated with aortic annular hypoplasia. *This chapter deals not only with AS in childhood but also with AS developed secondary to congenital BAV at any point of one's life.*

Supravalvular aortic stenosis

Supravalvular aortic stenosis *(SVAS)* is the rarest obstructive lesion of the LVOT (0.5%). It usually takes the shape of an hourglass with a localized membrane, or narrowing, over the sinuses of Valsalva at the sino-tubular junction (Figure 9.4), or it is a diffuse narrowing due to the aortic wall thickening involving the whole ascending aorta and, possibly, even the aortic arch (Figure 9.5). Approximately 60% of patients with SVAS have Williams' syndrome (= SVAS, mental retardation, facial dysmorphism).[11] This syndrome is caused by a deletion for the elastin gene in chromosome 7, which may be detected by fluorescent in situ hybridization (FISH). Patients with SVAS may also have stenoses of the other major vessels, e.g. peripheral stenoses of the pulmonary artery branches, carotid, subclavian, coronary arteries, or, occasionally, stenoses of the renal arteries with subsequent hypertension. In supravalvular AS, the coronary arteries are usually dilated; however, as they are in a region of high pressure, accelerated atherosclerosis occurs.

Subvalvular aortic stenosis

Subvalvular *AS* account for 8–10% of all LVOTO. The lesion is usually discrete, made up by either a fibrotic or fibromuscular membrane encircling the LVOT (Figures 9.6–9.8) or a long tunnel-like fibromuscular narrowing involving the

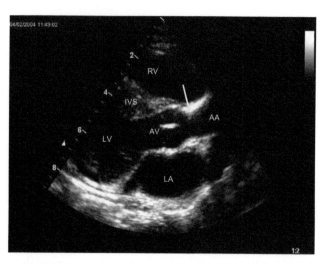

Figure 9.4
Transthoracic echo, parasternal long-axis view, supravalvular aortic stenosis with narrowing in the sino-tubular junction, hour-glass type (arrow). LV, Left ventricle; IVS, interventricular septum, which is hypertrophic; AV, aortic valve; LA, left atrium; RV, right ventricle; AA, ascending aorta. (Courtesy of Drs V Tomek and J Skovranek, Kardiocentrum and Cardiovascular Research Centre, University Hospital Motol, Prague, Czech Republic.)

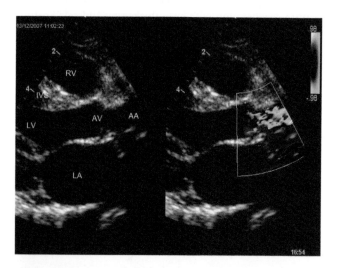

Figure 9.5
Supravalvular aortic stenosis, tubular type with narrowing of the whole ascending aorta; transthoracic echocardiogram, parasternal long-axis view. AA, Ascending aorta; AV, aortic valve; LV, left ventricle; LA, left atrium; IVS, interventricular septum; RV, right ventricle. Color Doppler on the right-hand image shows turbulent flow behind the stenosis. (Courtesy of Drs V Tomek and J Skovranek, Kardiocentrum and Cardiovascular Research Centre, University Hospital Motol, Prague, Czech Republic.)

entire LVOT. This condition is usually associated with aortic annular hypoplasia. Rarely, the cause of LVOT obstruction may be an abnormal or accessory mitral apparatus.

Predisposition for subvalvular AS is sharp aortoseptal angle, posterior deviation of the outlet septum, increased

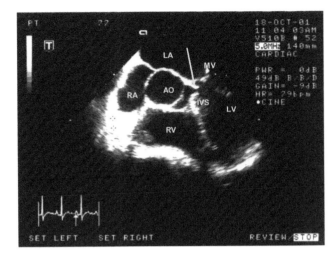

Figure 9.6
Subvalvular aortic stenosis; transesophageal echo, transversal projection. Below bicuspid aortic valve, there is a hypertrophic interventricular septum (IVS) bulging into left ventricular outflow tract (LVOT). The fibrous membrane encircles and narrows the LVOT. It originates from the aortomitral fibrous continuity (arrow). This patient had surgical excision of the membrane, partial myectomy of the interventricular septum, valvotomy of the stenotic bicuspid valve and plication of the dilated ascending aorta. AO, Aorta; LA, left atrium; MV, mitral valve; IVS, interventricular septum; LV, left ventricle; RV, right ventricle; RA, right atrium.

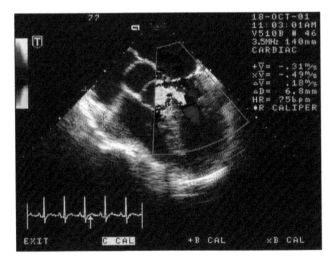

Figure 9.7
Subvalvular aortic stenosis; the same patient as in Figure 9.6. Transesophageal echo, color Doppler mapping shows turbulent stenotic flow in the left ventricular outflow tract.

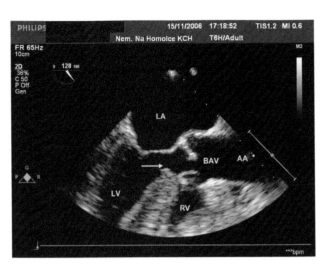

Figure 9.8
Subvalvular and valvular aortic stenosis; transesophageal echo, 128 degrees. Fibromuscular membrane narrowing the left ventricular outflow tract (arrow), stenotic bicuspid aortic valve (BAV), normal size of ascending aorta (AA). LV, left ventricle; LA, left atrium; RV, right ventricle. Lady, 71 years old, after surgery (resection of the membrane and partial septal myectomy and aortic bioprosthesis) is feeling well, without residual obstruction.

- *Shon's syndrome* refers to the left ventricular inflow and outflow tract obstruction (supramitral membrane, parachute-like mitral valve, subvalvular aortic stenosis, bicuspid aortic valve with stenosis, coarctation of the aorta).

Prevalence

LVOTO accounts for some 8% of all congenital heart disease (CHD) in children. The incidence in adulthood is not known, as many aortic valvular stenoses developing in adulthood secondary to BAV are not classified as congenital. BAV is the most frequent congenital anomaly occurring in 1–2% of the population at large with predominance in men (4:1).[12] SVAS is usually part of Williams' syndrome, with multisystem involvement in chromosomal deletion.

Pathophysiology

The left ventricular work against increased resistance results in left ventricular pressure overload. A compensatory response is left ventricular concentric hypertrophy. Early after birth, the ability of myocyte multiplication (hyperplasia) is still maintained; later, the myocardium responds to pressure overload merely by myocyte hypertrophy (enlargement). The combination of hyperplasia (early after birth) and hypertrophy (later in life) results in extremely thick myocardium in some congenital obstructions of the LVOT (Figure 9.9).

shear stress in the LVOT, and genetic predispositions for cell proliferation in this area. Turbulent flow in subvalvular AS damages the aortic valve and results in aortic insufficiency. Subvalvular AS is progressive disease and often recurs, even after surgical treatment.

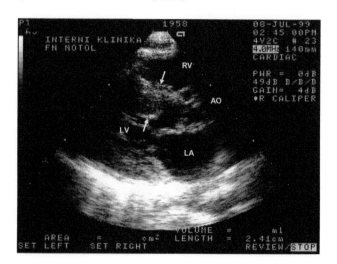

Figure 9.9
Extremely thick interventricular septum (24mm in diastole, arrows) in 41-year-old lady with unrecognized supravalvular and valvular aortic stenosis. The echocardiographic picture could be mistaken for hypertrophic cardiomyopathy. Transthoracic echo, parasternal long-axis view. LV, Left ventricle; LA, left atrium; AO, aorta; RV, right ventricle.

The left ventricular concentric hypertrophy allows preservation of normal systolic wall stress. Hence, in the presence of a nondilated left ventricle with a significantly hypertrophic myocardium, there is no increase in left ventricular work even with an increased afterload in AS.

Compensated aortic stenosis is associated with:

- A nondilated left ventricle with a hypertrophied myocardium.
- Normal myocardial contractility, and a normal ejection fraction.
- A reduced compliance of the hypertrophied myocardium.
- A slightly increased end-diastolic left ventricular pressure.
- Coronary blood flow may be reduced, even in the presence of normal coronary anatomy. An increased diastolic left ventricular pressure may result in a decrease in coronary perfusion pressure and coronary blood flow. A hypertrophied myocardium shows reduced coronary reserve. Hypertrophy is not associated with capillary proliferation, and the pathway of oxygen diffusion into the center of the myocyte is longer.
- Exercise cannot result in a physiological increase in stroke volume, and cardiac output can only be increased by an increase in heart rate. The result is shortening of diastole and further deterioration in left ventricular filling.
- Exercise may be associated with subendocardial ischemia even without coronary artery disease. Different degrees of subendocardial fibrosis occur.

Decompensated AS (the compensatory mechanism of hypertrophy becomes exhausted):

- Is not associated with further myocardial hypertrophy.
- Is associated with left ventricular cavity dilatation resulting in an increased 'wall stress'.
- Is associated with a decrease in ejection fraction, which, however, need not always be associated with a disorder of actual myocardial contractility.
- In the presence of significantly reduced left ventricular systolic function, there is a decrease of the systolic gradient at the site of stenosis.
- There is a further increase in left ventricular diastolic pressure and deterioration of coronary perfusion.
- Signs of subendocardial ischemia ('left ventricular overload') are evident even at rest.
- Atrial fibrillation results in the absence of atrial contraction, in a significant deterioration of left ventricular filling, and a decrease in cardiac output.

Clinical findings and diagnosis

Symptoms

Even a significant aortic stenosis may be associated with a long, completely asymptomatic period with patients experiencing no problems at all, even during exercise. However, if a patient with a significant AS complains of problems, then surgical management is imperative as the patient is at risk of sudden death.

Critical symptoms of a significant AS include:

- Syncope or, possibly, exercise-induced vertigo.
- Exertional dyspnea.
- Exercise-induced chest pain.

Clinical examination

Peripheral pulse in significant AS usually features poor filling (pulsus parvus, tardus), with blood pressure being low with significant AS, although this is not a rule. A patient with significant AS may also have hypertension, which tends to raise the left ventricular pressure overload even more.

Auscultatory findings

- An ejection systolic murmur with a maximum in the second right intercostal space parasternally, and propagating into both carotids; a second auscultatory maximum may be on the apex; the murmur has a crescendo–decrescendo nature and does not immediately pick up on the first sound.
- An early systolic click may be heard after the first sound with a stenotic, yet compliant aortic valve, fused in commissures.
- A palpable vortex may be present over the aorta and over the carotids.

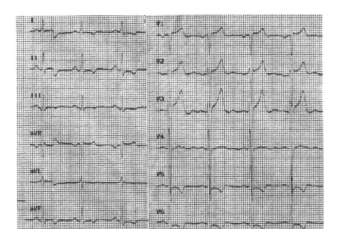

Figure 9.10
ECG in a patient with severe aortic stenosis. Signs of left ventricular hypertrophy and overload with ST segment depression and negative T waves in leads I, II, aVF, V5–V6.

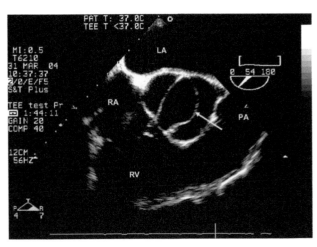

Figure 9.11
Transesophageal echo, 54 degrees, typical bicuspid aortic valve with thin leaflets without degenerative changes (arrow). LA, Left atrium; RA, right atrium; RV, right ventricle; PA, pulmonary artery.

Electrocardiogram (ECG)

- Left ventricular hypertrophy with isoelectrical ST segments (in compensated AS).
- Left ventricular hypertrophy with 'overload' signaling subendocardial ischemia. This manifests itself by ST segment depressions in leads over the left ventricle: V4–V6, I, aVL. Signs of subendocardial ischemia may be evident either only during exercise or, in more advanced stages, also in resting ECG (Figure 9.10).

Chest X-ray

- Left ventricular hypertrophy with a rounding and bulging of the left cardiac border.
- Dilatation of the ascending aorta may be present.
- Aortic valve calcifications may be evident.
- In advanced stages, cardiomegaly with congestion in the lungs.

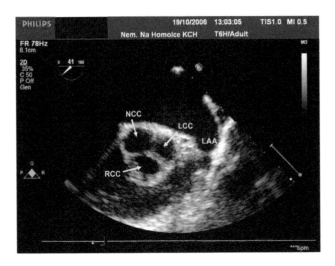

Figure 9.12
Transesophageal echo, 41 degrees. Aortic valve in diastole with apparently three cusps; however, the systolic phase has always to be evaluated (Figure 9.13). LAA, Left atrial auricle; NCC, noncoronary cusp; RCC, right coronary cusp; LCC, left coronary cusp.

Echocardiography

The parameters to be assessed:

- Aortic valve morphology, number of cusps, calcifications, width of the annulus, aortic root, sino-tubular junction and ascending aorta (Figures 9.11–9.14).
- Aortic valve gradient. In the presence of a tight AS, the high-speed flow is very narrow and sometimes eccentric, thus creating the potential for gradient underestimation with subsequent underestimation of the severity of AS (Figures 9.15 and 9.16). Conversely, mistaking the aortic

flow for the high-speed flow from mitral regurgitation could result in false overestimation of the aortic valve gradient (Figure 9.17).
- Aortic valve orifice area (AVA) using the continuity formula (Figures 9.16 and 9.18), or using planimetry. Transesophageal echocardiography is employed in patients with poor visualization.
- Presence of left ventricular hypertrophy, whose severity, however, need not be fully proportionate to the severity of AS.

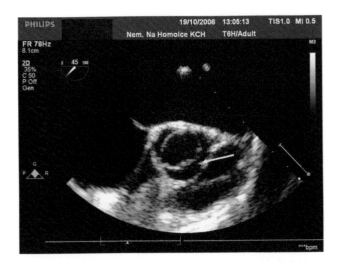

Figure 9.13
Transesophageal echo, 45 degrees; the same patient as in Figure 9.12. This aortic valve is functionally bicuspid with fused commissure between the left and right coronary cusp forming the raphe (arrow). This can be evaluated in the systolic phase.

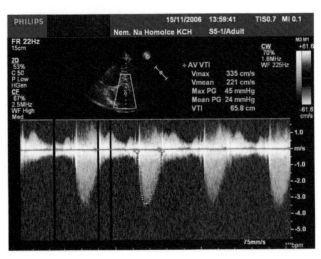

Figure 9.15
Continuous Doppler examination from the apical five-chamber view, showing clear signal from the aortic stenosis indicating apparently only moderate aortic stenosis with the maximal/mean gradient 45/24mmHg. (See also Figure 9.16.)

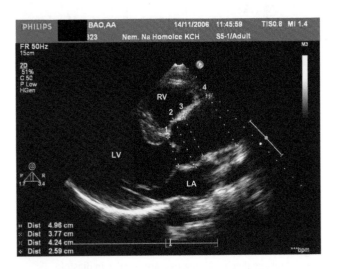

Figure 9.14
Transthoracic echo, parasternal long-axis view. 1, Annulus; 2, aortic bulbus (sinuses); 3, sino-tubular junction; 4, ascending aorta; LV, left ventricle; LA, left atrium; RV, right ventricle.

- Left ventricular systolic and diastolic function.
- Morphological and Doppler examination of the LVOT, ascending aorta, aortic arch (Figures 9.19 and 9.20), and descending aorta to rule out simultaneous subvalvular (Figures 9.6–9.8), or supravalvular obstruction, or dilatation (Figures 9.4 and 9.5).
- To assess the morphological cause of subvalvular obstruction.
- To rule out simultaneous CoA (Figures 9.20 and 9.21) and other associated defects (mitral valve prolapse, ventricular septal defect, etc.).

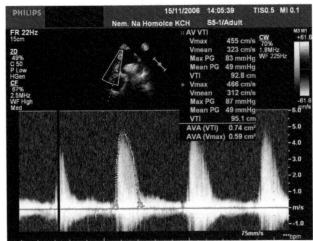

Figure 9.16
Continuous Doppler from the same patient as in Figure 9.15, suprasternal view. The velocity is much higher, indicating the maximal/mean gradient 87/49mmHg, the aortic stenosis is in fact severe. The difference between the velocities measured from the apical and suprasternal approach is caused by the very eccentric jet in aortic stenosis in bicuspid aortic valve.

- To assess, prior to elective Ross procedure (aortic valve replacement by a pulmonary autograft), pulmonary valve function and pulmonary annular size.
- The extreme left ventricular myocardial hypertrophy, which is most often seen in unoperated SVAS, may be misdiagnosed for hypertrophic cardiomyopathy (Figure 9.9).

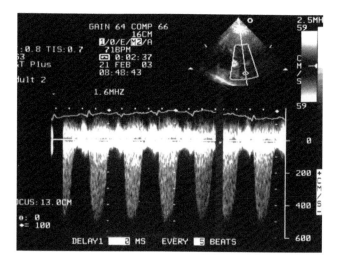

Figure 9.17

Continuous Doppler from the apical five-chamber view in a patient with severe aortic stenosis. Turbulent systolic flow has the maximal velocity of approximately 5m/s, indicating severe aortic stenosis, with the maximal systolic gradient 125mmHg. Appropriate control on the 2D echocardiogram should be done because of the flow with similar velocities and direction from mitral regurgitation.

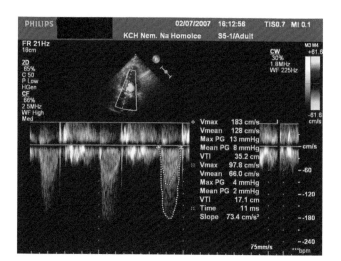

Figure 9.18

Continuous Doppler examination from the apical five-chamber approach. For assessing the aortic valve area by continuity equation in atrial fibrillation, the velocity from the left ventricular outflow tract and aortic valve must be evaluated from the same beat.

Dobutamine stress echocardiography

Dobutamine stress echocardiography is used to distinguish a significant AS with a low gradient due to secondary systolic left ventricular dysfunction (Figures 9.22 and 9.23)

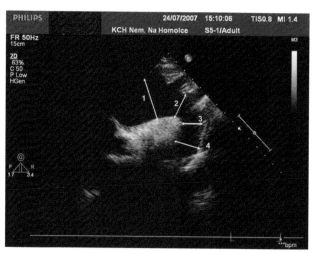

Figure 9.19

Transthoracic echo, suprasternal view, aortic arch. 1, Distal ascending aorta; 2, aortic arch; 3, isthmus; 4, descending aorta.

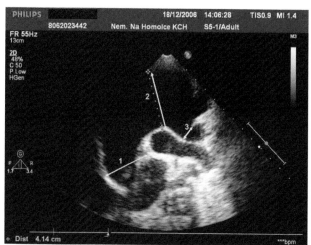

Figure 9.20

Suprasternal echocardiographic view. Patient with Turner's syndrome, bicuspid aortic valve with aortic stenosis, normal size of the aortic bulbus 32mm (1), dilatation of the distal ascending aorta 41mm (2), and recoarctation 10mm (3).

from a mild aortic stenosis with left ventricular dysfunction due to another cause (coronary artery disease, myocarditis, dilating cardiomyopathy). The technique also tests the left ventricular contractile reserve. Low-dose dobutamine (5–20μg/kg/min) is used in continuous infusion with progressive dose increments and simultaneous monitoring of echocardiographic parameters, blood pressure, ECG, and the patient's clinical status. An increase in the aortic valve gradient after low-dose dobutamine signals a significant AS if the aortic flow rate is at least four times the rate in the LVOT (Figure 9.24). In cases where there was no rise in the gradient but an increase in aortic orifice size, a

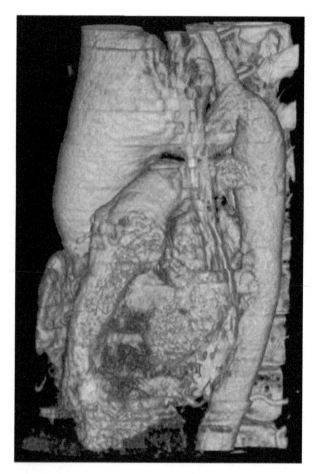

Figure 9.21
Three-dimensional reconstruction of the computerized tomography angiography; the same patient as in Figure 9.20 with Turner's syndrome, dilatation of the distal ascending aorta, and brachiocephalic trunk and recoarctation.

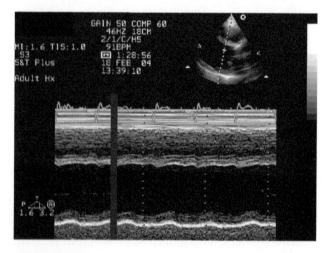

Figure 9.22
Transesophageal echo, parasternal long-axis view, M-mode; 56-year-old man with unoperated aortic stenosis on bicuspid aortic valve and severely depressed left ventricular systolic function, ejection fraction of the left ventricle was 12%.

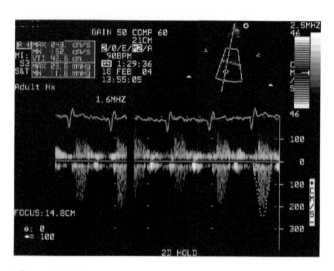

Figure 9.23
Pulsed Doppler examination in the same patient as in Figure 9.22. The rest gradient on the aortic valve is 23/11mmHg (maximal/mean).

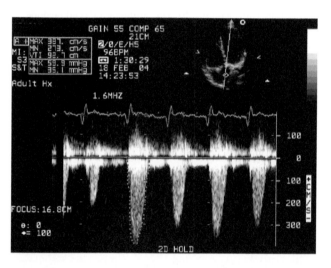

Figure 9.24
Continuous Doppler examination in aortic valve stenosis during dobutamine echocardiography in the same patient as in Figures 9.22 and 9.23. The systolic gradient on the aortic valve incresed from 23/11mmHg up to 60/35mmHg (maximal/mean) during low-dose dobutamine infusion. This examination confirms severe aortic stenosis with low gradient due to the left ventricular dysfunction. The gradients are variable due to the atrial fibrillation.

low-rate 'pseudostenosis' was involved. If there is no increase in cardiac output in inotropic stimulation, the patient has no contractile reserve, implying the worst prognosis.[13] If there was a decrease in the gradient associated with deteriorated kinetics, myocardial ischemia without a contractile reserve was involved. This examination is important when indicating surgery.

Table 9.1   *Guidance values for assessment of the significance of aortic valve stenosis (AVS) (modified according Bonow, 2006[15])*

Aortic stenosis	Aortic orifice area (cm^2)	Indexes orifice area (cm^2/m^2)	Catheter-based 'peak-to-peak' gradient (mmHg)	Doppler maximum gradient (mmHg)	Mean gradient (mmHg)
Mild	1.5–2	>0.8	<30	<36	<25
Moderate	1–1.5	0.6–0.8	30–60	36–64	25–40
Significant	<1–0.75	<0.6	>60	>64	>40

Computerized tomography (CT) angiography

This is a useful examination, especially for the morphology of the ascending aorta, aortic arch with the big arteries, and descending aorta (Figure 9.21; see also Figure 8.10).

Exercise ECG

Exercise ECG using bicycle ergometry or a treadmill is contraindicated in patients with *symptomatic* AS. However, it can be performed in *completely asymptomatic patients* with significant AS for proper timing of surgery.[14–16] With significant AS, exercise testing may carry potential risks; it can only be undertaken in centers with adequate facilities and a sufficient body of experience.

In patients with AS, exercise testing is considered positive if it is associated with:

- Development of symptoms: dyspnea, angina pectoris, syncope, presyncope.
- A decrease in the systolic blood pressure during exercise, or an increase <20mmHg.
- ST-segment depression on the ECG occurring during exercise, horizontal or descending, >2mm, which can be explained by no other reason than significant AS.
- Complex ventricular arrhythmia (ventricular tachycardia, more than four premature consecutive ventricular beats).
- The patient failing to reach 80% of maximum age- and sex-predefined workload.

An abnormal result of exercise testing in a patient with significant AS is an indication for surgical management even if the patient is asymptomatic.[14] If negative, exercise testing is repeated in patients with significant asymptomatic AS at regular intervals, most often every 6 months.

Catheterization

Catheter-based examination in AS is performed:

- To assess the coronary bed using selective coronary arteriography prior to elective surgery in patients over 40 years of age, or in younger individuals at increased risk for premature atherosclerosis, in left ventricular dysfunction, or in the case of suspected congenital or postoperative coronary anomalies.
- To evaluate the significance of AS only in cases where echocardiographic results are nondiagnostic, or at variance with clinical data, or in cases of multilevel obstructions, unless the hemodynamic significance is clear.

Evaluating the significance of aortic stenosis

The orifice of a normal aortic valve in an adult has an area of 2–4cm^2. A range to serve as guidance for determining the significance of AS is shown in Table 9.1. The values apply to a hemodynamically balanced status with a normal heart rate and normal flow rates. The gradient itself is very much dependent on the magnitude of the flow rate. A low gradient will be found even in a tight AS in patients with low cardiac output, left ventricular systolic dysfunction and a low ejection fraction (Figures 9.22 and 9.23).

Management

In childhood, *aortic valve stenosis* is most often managed by balloon valvuloplasty and/or surgical valvulotomy. The Ross procedure is performed rarely. Prosthetic valves are used only exceptionally in older children. In contrast, prosthetic valves are used predominantly in adult patients given the progression of degenerative changes involving the aortic valve. The prostheses may be mechanical (most often bileaflet); biological, made from a porcine aortic valve or pericardium (heterograft, xenograft); or human aortic valves (homograft, allograft). In some cases, the Ross procedure, with implantation of the patient's own pulmonary autograft into the aortic position and a homograft into the pulmonary position, is also performed in adults. The advantage of this operation is that patients do not need anticoagulation.

Unlike childhood and adolescence, balloon valvuloplasty in adulthood is not indicated, even in congenital aortic valvular stenoses, because of the unsatisfactory outcomes due to degenerative changes in the aortic valve. Balloon valvuloplasty can be undertaken in adolescents or young adults with a morphologically appropriate finding of a compliant valve fused in commissures.

Transcatheter percutaneous aortic valve implantation is still a clinical experiment preserved for inoperable high-risk patients in the end-stage of AS.[17]

Supravalvular AS is managed by extended aortoplasty with a Dacron or Goretex patch sutured.

Subvalvular AS is managed by resection of the fibrotic membrane or, possibly, aberrant mitral valve tissue. It can be complemented by ventricular septal myectomy, which should prevent recurrence of fibromuscular obstruction. The recurrence of subvalvular stenosis is frequent even after surgical treatment, with reoperation required in 20% of cases.[18] Aortoventriculoplasty according to Konn is performed in tunnel-like fibromuscular subaortic stenosis with a hypoplastic aortic annulus.

Indication for surgical management of aortic stenosis[15,16,19]

Valvular AS

A significant *symptomatic* AS (accompanied by dyspnea, angina pectoris, presyncope or syncope during exercise) requires expedite surgery, as soon as possible after the onset of symptoms.

A significant *asymptomatic* AS (area <0.6cm^2/m^2, mean gradient >40mmHg) requires careful regular follow-up by a cardiologist for proper timing of surgery. It is mandatory to look for symptoms as the patient may be unaware of their severity. Surgery (intervention) in a patient with significant asymptomatic AS is indicated in the presence of prognostically adverse findings, which include:

- a positive exercise test;
- deterioration of left ventricular systolic function (EF <50%);
- severe left ventricular myocardial hypertrophy (≥15mm) due to AS;
- critical AS with an AVA <0.6cm^2;
- rapid progression of peak flow rate on the aortic valve by >0.3m/s per year at a total flow rate >4m/s, and simultaneously significantly calcified aortic valve;
- a simultaneous other cardiac surgical procedure;
- before planned pregnancy.

Mild and moderate AS are monitored on a regular basis because of the potential progression.

Supravalvular AS

The intervention is indicated in symptomatic patients or in asymptomatic patients with a catheter-based or mean echocardiographic gradient >50mmHg. As the procedure does not carry risks associated with valve implantation, there is no reason to postpone the procedure.

Subvalvular AS

The indication for intervention:

- Symptoms.
- In asymptomatic patients a resting catheter-based or mean echocardiographic gradient >50mmHg, maximal echocardiographic Doppler gradient >85mmHg.
- Presence of aortic regurgitation, which is either progressive or moderate to significant.
- In the presence of a ventricular septal defect, the subvalvular stenosis gradient may be underestimated, not manifesting itself until after ventricular septal defect closure.

Subvalvular AS and SVAS should be managed surgically in a center specializing in the treatment of CHD.

Residual findings

- Aortic valve stenosis after a valvuloplasty or valvulotomy in childhood carries a risk of progression of restenosis, or progression of residual aortic regurgitation requiring aortic valve replacement.
- The recurrence of subvalvular fibromuscular stenosis after surgery is up to 20% over a 10-year period, especially in patients with a small aortic annulus. If only the fibrotic annulus has been removed, the fibrosis may recur at the same site, or a more complex tunnel-shaped fibromuscular stenosis of the LVOT may develop.
- Aortic regurgitation on the aortic valve, damaged by turbulent flow, may persist or progress after removal of a subvalvular AS.
- In patients after the Ross procedure, a pulmonary homograft in the pulmonary position may degenerate, whereas a pulmonary autograft in the aortic position may regurgitate.
- The risks and residual findings with mechanical prostheses and bioprostheses are identical to those with acquired defects.
- Aortic dilatation after BAV replacement.

Pregnancy and delivery

In patients with a significant uncorrected AS, pregnancy and delivery are associated with an increased risk of maternal and fetal mortality, regardless of the presence of symptoms before pregnancy. A mechanical prosthesis in pregnancy poses the risk of anticoagulation therapy. Therefore, in young women planning to conceive, it is appropriate to consider the possibility of balloon valvuloplasty, valve reconstruction, bioprosthesis implantation, or the Ross procedure (a pulmonary autograft). However, these procedures also have their shortcomings, particularly a risk of further reoperation.

Infectious endocarditis

Given the nonlaminar pattern of flow, BAV carries a high risk of infectious endocarditis (IE) even without major dysfunction. While mechanical aortic prostheses are associated with a high risk of IE, IE may also affect biological prostheses, subvalvular AS, and patches or conduits in the ascending aorta.

Follow-up

Regular cardiological and echocardiographic follow-up should be performed, depending on the significance of the defect, every 6 months to 2 years. If IE is suspected, the examination must be performed immediately, including transesophageal echocardiography and blood cultures.

Prognosis

Aortic valvular stenosis has a progressive nature. Over a period of 20 years, surgical intervention is required by about half of patients with mild AS in childhood. As regards AS in adulthood, a decrement in AVA by average of 0.1–0.3cm² per year, an increment of maximum gradient by 10–15mmHg per year, and mean gradient by about 7mmHg per year, were described.[14,20] With BAV, the rate of progression of AS is slower compared with degenerative AS.[14] The risk factors for AS progression include age, body weight, hypertension, sex (males at greater risk), smoking and increased levels of low-density lipoprotein (LDL) cholesterol and lipoprotein(a), i.e. risk factors similar to those with vascular wall atherosclerosis.

The prognosis of AS is affected adversely by the development of symptoms. With asymptomatic patients with AS and aortic blood flow rates >4m/s (consistent with a maximum gradient of 64mmHg), symptoms are experienced by some 40% of patients per year, at rates of 3–4m/s in 17% of patients annually, and at rates <3m/s (36mmHg), development of symptoms has been reported in 8% of patients per year.[21]

Asymptomatic patients with AS have significantly lower overall mortality, cardiovascular mortality, and incidence of sudden death compared with symptomatic patients. The 5-year survival rate of symptomatic patients with AS is 15–50%.[21] The mean time from onset of symptoms to death in patients with AS and exertional syncope was 2 years; with AS and heart failure, 3 years; and with AS and angina pectoris, 5 years.[21]

The operative mortality of aortic valve replacement is in the range of 2–5% in adults below 70 years of age, rising to 5–24% in older patients and those who undergo combined procedures. Surgery is followed by regression of left ventricular hypertrophy, whose rate is rapid in the first months (decreasing myocyte diameter) and slower in the ensuing years (regression of interstitial changes). In cases where myocardial contractility has not been impaired, surgery is followed by an increase in left ventricular ejection fraction.

After balloon valvuloplasty or surgical valvulotomy of AS in childhood, residual findings (restenosis or regurgitation) should be anticipated in adulthood, which will require, sooner or later, reoperation in many patients. Valvuloplasty failure occurred in long-term follow-up in 42% of patients 15 years after aortic valvuloplasty in childhood. Independent predictors of unfavorable outcome were small aortic annulus, BAV, and poor left ventricular function.[22] Among patients undergoing surgical valvulotomy of AS in childhood, reoperation was required by 40% of patients by 25 years.[23]

The early operative mortality in *subvalvular aortic stenosis* is 3.1–3.4%, residual stenosis or restenosis is found in 27%, and reoperation-free survival is 88% in 5 years and 75% in 12 years.[24,25]

AORTIC REGURGITATION IN CONGENITAL HEART DISEASE

Chronic aortic regurgitation is caused by malcoaptation of the aortic cusps due to the aortic valve involvement, or normal aortic valve with dilatation of the aortic annulus and sino-tubular junction, or a combination of both. In terms of etiology, CHD accounts for 13% of cases of chronic aortic regurgitation, and for 25% of connective tissue disease with aortic root dilatation.[26] Congenital causes of aortic regurgitation include:

- Degeneration of a congenital BAV (the most frequent cause) with dilatation of the sino-tubular junction and ascending aorta (Figure 9.25).
- Residual regurgitation after valvulotomy or valvuloplasty of a congenital AS in childhood.
- Aortic valve prolapse into the LVOT (Figure 9.26).
- Aortic valve cusp prolapse into a ventricular septal defect (with prolapse of the right coronary or noncoronary cusp into a subarterial outflow defect, or into a perimembranous ventricular septal defect (Figure 9.27; see Chapter 6).
- A subaortic stenosis causes, by turbulent flow, aortic valve damage with subsequent aortic regurgitation (see 'Congenital aortic stenosis', p. 63).
- IE is frequent with a BAV, and may lead to acute or chronic aortic regurgitation by cusp perforation or aortic valve destruction (Figure 9.28).
- Connective tissue disease, e.g. in Marfan's syndrome, leads to aortic root and annulus dilatation (aortoannular ectasia) with subsequent aortic regurgitation (see 'Marfan's syndrome', p. 79).
- Degeneration of the aortic homograft may cause acute or chronic aortic regurgitation (Figure 9.29).

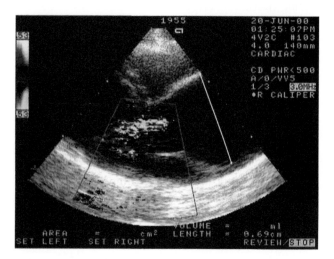

Figure 9.25
Transthoracic echo, longitudinal parasternal view. Bicuspid aortic valve with mild aortic regurgitation, normal dimension of the annulus and bulbus, mild dilatation of the sino-tubular junction and severe dilatation of the ascending aorta (76mm) distal to sino-tubular junction (arrow).

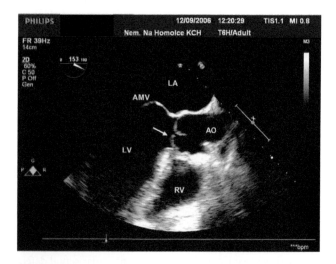

Figure 9.26
Transesophageal echo, 153 degrees, prolapse of the right coronary aortic cusp (arrow), causing severe eccentric aortic regurgitation. AO, Aorta; LV, left ventricle; LA, left atrium; AMV, anterior cusp of the mitral valve; RV, right ventricle.

- An aorto-left ventricular tunnel is a rare CHD. Aortic regurgitation occurs as a result of a communication bypassing the proper aortic valve and connecting the region of the right or left coronary sinus with the LVOT, under the aortic valve cusps. The aortic orifice is usually dilated, whereas the ventricular orifice is narrower and tubular. The coronary arteries are usually not affected by the malformation. Most cases are associated with ascending aorta and aortic annulus dilatation, aortic

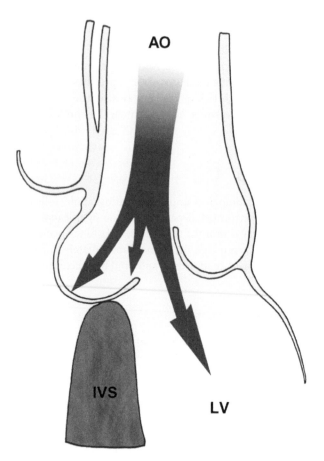

Figure 9.27
Aortic regurgitation due to the prolapse of the aortic cusp into the ventricular septal defect. AO, Aorta; LV, left ventricle; IVS, interventricular septum.

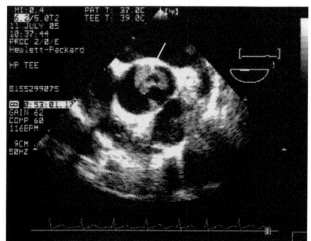

Figure 9.28
Transesophageal echo, 0 degrees. Large vegetation on a bicuspid aortic valve (arrow).

valve thickening, and subsequent simultaneous intra-valvular aortic regurgitation.[1]

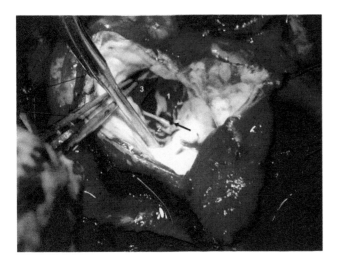

Figure 9.29
Rupture of the aortic homograft, leading to severe acute aortic regurgitation, surgical view. 1, Left coronary cusp; 2, right coronary cusp; 3, intact noncoronary cusp; arrow, rupture of right and left coronary cusp in the commissure due to degeneration of the aortic homograft in a young man. (Courtesy of Dr J Spatenka, Dept of Cardiac Surgery, University Hospital Motol, Prague, Czech Republic.)

Pathophysiology

The regurgitation volume represents volume overload for the left ventricle, resulting in a compensatory increase in left ventricular diastolic volume. The increased stroke volume in the presence of significant aortic regurgitation leads to a rise in systolic pressure in the aorta with a concomitant left ventricular pressure overload. Consequently, significant aortic regurgitation represents combined left ventricular volume and pressure overload, usually resulting in eccentric left ventricular hypertrophy. This results in chamber dilatation as well as left ventricular wall thickening.

Tachycardia leads to diastole shortening with a subsequent decrease in aortic regurgitation. A reduced peripheral vascular resistance will also diminish the regurgitation fraction. Both these mechanisms are involved in exercise, and explain the good exercise tolerance even in patients with significant aortic regurgitation. Aortic root and annular dilatation is a consequence of increased stroke volume, which leads to further progression of aortic regurgitation.

Progression and decompensation of aortic regurgitation are associated with a decrease in myocardial contractility, systolic dysfunction with a reduction in ejection fraction, and an increase in left ventricular end-systolic volume. This is accompanied by myofibril loss while the proportion of connective tissue increases. This stage is also associated with increased left ventricular end-diastolic pressure, increased pressure in left atrium, and in pulmonary veins. A low diastolic aortic pressure and an increased diastolic left ventricular pressure are associated with a reduction in coronary blood flow. Starting with a certain degree of left ventricular dilatation in systole, myocardial changes become irreversible and surgery will no longer be able to improve left ventricular function or survival.

Clinical findings and diagnosis
Symptoms

- Typical features include a long-term asymptomatic course with good exercise tolerance, even in patients with significant aortic regurgitation.
- Exertional dyspnea.
- Fatigability.
- Chest pain.

Clinical examination

- Palpable apex beat with a lateral shift.
- Increase in pulse pressure, i.e. increased systolic and decreased diastolic pressure. The bigger the pressure amplitude, the more significant the aortic regurgitation.
- Corrigan's pulse, i.e. bounding, surging and rapid (pulsus magnus, celer, frequens).
- Musset's symptom results in head shaking on each systole.
- Quincke's symptom refers to visible capillary pulsation at the nailbed at the interface occurring between the perfused and nonperfused areas on exerting pressure on the nail.

Auscultatory findings

- Diastolic murmur above the aorta with propagation along the sternum; with significant regurgitations, the murmur is holodiastolic, it may be quiet.
- Significant aortic regurgitation may also be associated with systolic murmur above the aorta, with propagation into the carotids due to the increased stroke volume or a combined defect.

ECG

- Left ventricular hypertrophy and overload may be present.

Chest X-ray

- Cardiomegaly.
- An elongated and tortuous aorta.
- Pulmonary circulation congestion on decompensation.

Echocardiography

Etiology of aortic regurgitation

- Morphology of the aortic valve, number of cusps (Figures 9.2 and 9.11), thickening, shortening, perforation or elongation, and prolapse of the cusps (Figure 9.26), width of the anulus, aortic root, sino-tubular junction and the ascending aorta (Figure 9.14). Dilatation of the aorta in BAV typically affects the ascending aorta distal from sino-tubular junction (Figure 9.25). In Marfan's syndrome there is often also dilatation of the aortic annulus and bulbus (see 'Marfan's syndrome', page 79, and Figures 9.43 and 9.44).

- Assessment of any prolapse of an aortic valve cusp into a ventricular septal defect, which may be almost closed by the cusp prolapse (Figure 9.27).
- Evaluation of vegetation (and/or periannular abscess) on the aortic or mitral valves in the case of suspected IE (Figure 9.28).
- Exclusion of another cause of aortic regurgitation, e.g. an aorto-left ventricular tunnel, subvalvular AS, etc.

Quantification of aortic regurgitation

- Aortic regurgitation in BAV may be difficult to quantify, because of the slit-like regurgitation orifice and, frequently, very eccentric regurgitation flow. This results in a high risk of underestimation of the severity of the regurgitation; transesophageal echocardiography is appropriate (Figures 9.30 and 9.31).
- Just as guidance, aortic regurgitation can be quantified as the percentage of the width of the regurgitation jet and the width of the LVOT:
    - ≤25% = mild aortic regurgitation;
    - 25–45% = moderate aortic regurgitation;
    - 45–65% = intermediate aortic regurgitation;
    - >65% = severe aortic regurgitation.
- Prolonged diastolic reversed flow in the descending aorta or abdominal aorta signals significant aortic regurgitation (Figures 9.32–9.34).
- Rapid deceleration of the regurgitation flow (>3.5m/s²) occurs in significant, and usually acute, aortic regurgitation.

Longitudinal follow-up

- Comparison of the left ventricular size with carefully assessed end-systolic size, which is one of the critical considerations in indicating surgery.
- Ejection fraction monitoring.

Catheterization

- Selective coronary angiography in patients prior to elective surgery over 40 years of age, or with risk factors for premature atherosclerosis.
- In the case of mismatch between the clinical and echocardiographic findings, and inadequately reliable noninvasive quantification of the aortic regurgitation, left ventricular size and function, aortography, pulmonary artery and wedge pressure.

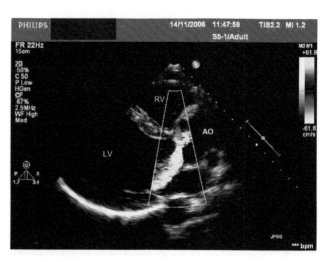

Figure 9.30
Transthoracic echo, long-axis parasternal view with color Doppler mapping. Bicuspid aortic valve, moderate eccentric aortic regurgitation, dilatation of the left ventricle (LV). AO, Aorta; RV, right ventricle.

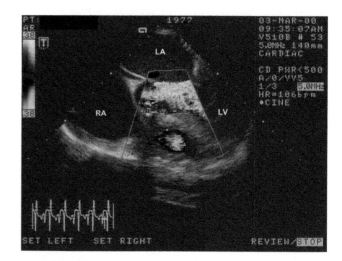

Figure 9.31
Transesophageal echo, transversal projection, bicuspid aortic valve with severe aortic regurgitation (color flow). The severity of the aortic regurgitation may sometimes be better appreciated in transesophageal than transthoracic echo. LV, Left ventricle; LA, left atrium; RA, right atrium.

Management
Medical therapy

Patients with severe chronic aortic regurgitation and symptoms, decreasing exercise capacity, decreasing ejection fraction or asymptomatic dilatation of the left ventricle should be operated on, not treated medically. Vasodilator agents (ACE inhibitors, nifedipine) may be used, particularly for

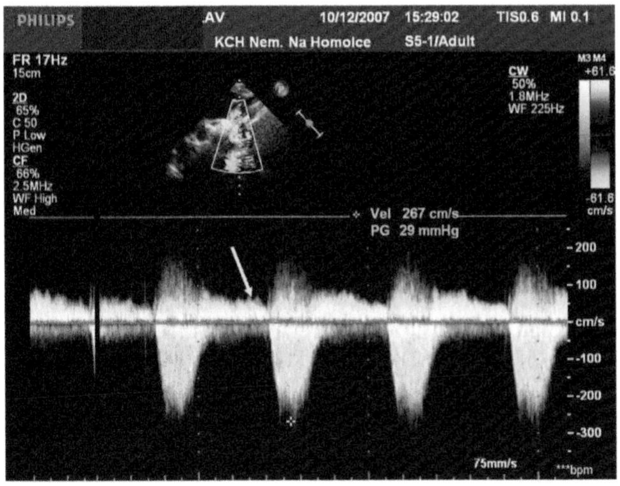

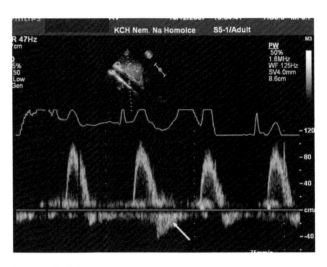

Figure 9.32
Continuous Doppler examination in the descending
aorta from the suprasternal approach. There is
accelerated systolic flow (velocity 267cm/s) in the descending
aorta and reversed holodiastolic flow
(velocity 50–100cm/s) indicating severe aortic
regurgitation (arrow).

Figure 9.34
Pulsed Doppler flow in the abdominal aorta, subcostal
approach. Systolic normal laminar flow towards the
transducer and reversed diastolic flow in the abdominal
aorta (arrow) due to significant aortic regurgitation.

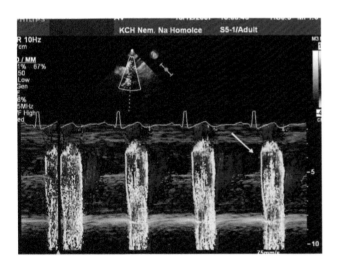

Figure 9.33
Color flow M-mode of the flow in descending aorta,
suprasternal view; the same patient as in Figure 9.31.
Systolic forward flow and diastolic reversed flow
during the whole diastole indicates severe aortic
regurgitation (arrow).

Surgical therapy

Aortic valve replacement is carried out using a mechanical
prosthesis, a biological valve (xenograft), a human valve
(allograft), or Ross procedure (pulmonary autograft). In
some cases, aortic valvuloplasty retaining the patient's own
valve is possible. Aortic root dilatation requires root reconstruction, or aortic root and valve replacement by a homograft (allograft), or a composite graft with mechanical
prosthesis (Bentall's procedure), or a valve-sparing operation (root remodeling technique or reimplantation of the
own aortic valve into the prosthesis).

Indications for surgical management of chronic aortic regurgitation
(modified according Bonow, 2006;[15] Vahanian, 2007[16])

- Significant aortic regurgitation, and;
- Symptoms, deteriorating exercise tolerance, exertional
  dyspnea, or;
- A decrease in left ventricular ejection fraction, which,
  however, should not fall below 55%, in which case even
  fully asymptomatic patients should be indicated.
- Left ventricular dilatation; the end-systolic dimension
  should not exceed 50–55mm (25–26mm/m² of the body
  surface area); exceeding these values results in higher
  postoperative mortality. These patients can be fully
  asymptomatic.

correction of systolic hypertension. The role of vasodilating
treatment in aortic regurgitation without hypertension in
order to delay surgery is not proved.[15,16]

Patients with Marfan's syndrome, or BAV and ascending
aorta dilatation, receive beta blockers to slow down progression of aortic dilatation; however, the bradycardizing effect
may worsen aortic regurgitation.[14]

- Exceeding the end-diastolic dimension of 70–75mm is associated with worse operative outcomes and higher postoperative mortality.
- If left ventricular myocardial hypertrophy (with reduced compliance) is present, the left ventricle usually does not dilate, even in the presence of significant aortic regurgitation; worsening of the left ventricular diastolic dysfunction with increased diastolic pressure is usually present.
- Aortic root replacement or reconstruction is indicated in patients with aortic root dilatation >55–60mm. In Marfan's syndrome, or patients with BAV, surgical management is indicated earlier, on aortic root dilatation >50mm, especially in those with a positive family history or with documented progressive dilatation >2mm/year, or in the presence of significant aortic regurgitation (see also 'Marfan's syndrome', page 79).
- Aortic regurgitation in the presence of cusp prolapse into a ventricular septal defect (see Chapter 6).

Residual findings and complications

- Residual aortic regurgitation following aortic valvuloplasty.
- Persistent left ventricular dilatation and systolic dysfunction after surgery in cases of late indication for surgery.
- Aortic homograft, autograft or bioprosthesis degeneration.
- Thrombosis or pannus involving a mechanical aortic valve prosthesis.

Risks

- BAV is usually associated with an abnormal structure of the aortic wall carrying a risk for aneurysmal dilatation and dissection; concomitant significant aortic regurgitation with an increased stroke volume raises the risk.
- Late indication for surgical management in patients with an asymptomatic course.
- IE.

Pregnancy and delivery

In patients with aortic regurgitation, pregnancy is usually well tolerated provided the woman was asymptomatic with good exercise tolerance before pregnancy. A decrease in systemic vascular resistance in pregnancy will alleviate aortic regurgitation. In patients with aortic root dilatation >40–45mm, the use of beta blockers and delivery by cesarean section, with minimizing of the blood pressure increase, is recommended because of the risk of aortic dissection or rupture.[27] In patients with aortic dilatation (especially Marfan's syndrome or BAV) it is reasonable to perform valve-sparing surgery before pregnancy (see 'Marfan's syndrome', page 79).

Infectious endocarditis

BAV may be affected by fatal IE even in patients with previously negligible functional impairment (Figure 9.28). IE may lead to acute aortic regurgitation, resulting in the development of pulmonary edema and cardiogenic shock as there is no time factor of left ventricular adaptation to volume overload. IE prevention is recommended in all BAV irrespective of the severity of functional impairment, in all mechanical and biological aortic valve prostheses, when using patches and conduits, in cusp prolapse into a ventricular septal defect and, also, in all other types of aortic valve functional and morphological impairment.

Follow-up

Given the potential for its progression, aortic regurgitation is to be followed by a cardiologist, with longitudinal echocardiographic follow-up performed at time intervals depending on the severity of the aortic regurgitation. Patients undergoing, in childhood, aortic valvuloplasty in the presence of cusp prolapse into the defect, aortic valvulotomy or balloon aortic stenosis valvuloplasty are at risk of development of progressive aortic regurgitation, and should also be on echocardiographic follow-up even if the primary outcome is good.

Prognosis

Patients with chronic significant aortic regurgitation who start to show symptoms, usually die within 2 years if the symptom is dyspnea (NYHA Class II or higher), and within 4 years if the symptom is angina.[26] In asymptomatic patients with chronic severe aortic regurgitation, the necessity of valve replacement is about 5% per year. Surgical management, if indicated in time, results in remission of symptoms. In asymptomatic patients, surgical management prevents irreversible systolic left ventricular dysfunction. A mechanical prosthesis raises the risk of thromboembolism and bleeding complications, whilst biological prostheses, including human ones, carry a higher risk of degeneration, especially in young adults. Valve-sparing operation with reimplantation has good long-term results with 94% freedom from moderate or severe aortic regurgitation at 10 years.[28]

A BAV is associated, regardless of the degree of functional impairment, with a risk of the development of aortic aneurysm and dissection.[3,5,6] The risk of dissection with a BAV is reported to be up to nine times that seen with a normal aortic valve.[29]

Aortic regurgitation in the presence of cusp prolapse into a ventricular septal defect in childhood is managed by defect closure and aortoplasty, requiring reoperation at 10 years in some 15% of cases (see Chapter 6).

SINUS OF VALSALVA ANEURYSM

Anatomical notes

Sinus of Valsalva aneurysm develops in patients with a congenitally absent media in the aortic wall at the site of junction with the aortic annulus. Consequently, part of the sinus of Valsalva is made up by collagenous tissue without smooth muscle and elastic fibers. The most often affected sinus is the right coronary sinus (73–83%), followed by the noncoronary sinus (17–25%); left coronary sinus involvement is rare (≤6%).[30,31] Right coronary sinus aneurysm usually protrudes into the right ventricle, less often into the right atrium (Figure 9.35). A noncoronary sinus aneurysm will protrude into the right atrium (Figure 9.36). Aneurysm rupture results in a communication between the aorta and these cardiac chambers. There have also been rare reports about aneurysm prolapse and rupture into the pulmonary artery, left ventricle, left atrium, or the pericardial cavity. A large aneurysm without rupture may hinder the right ventricular outflow tract (RVOT), right atrium, vena cava superior, and coronary arteries; it may also dissect the interventricular septum. A sinus of Valsalva aneurysm may be the cause of aortic regurgitation: blood from the aorta will regurgitate both through the perforated aneurysm into the right-heart chambers and, occasionally, intravalvularly into the left ventricle. Coronary artery compression may result in myocardial ischemia, whereas conduction system compression may lead to conduction disturbances.[30] In 30–50% of cases, it is associated with a ventricular septal defect, most often a supracristal one, and with aortic valve prolapse into the defect, with a BAV and other CHD.[1,30] A sinus of Valsalva aneurysm frequently features a typical stocking-like shape (Figures 9.35 and 9.36), yet it may also be spherical (Figures 9.37 and 9.38).

Prevalence

Congenital aneurysms of the sinus of Valsalva account for <0.1% of all CHD, it is present in 0.05% of autopsy findings in the population at large. These aneurysms occur more frequently in Asians (2–3.5% of all CHD). These aneurysms develop four times more often in males compared with females.

Clinical findings

A sinus of Valsalva aneurysm may be fully asymptomatic and may be found incidentally by echocardiography or autopsy. In the presence of oppression of the adjacent structures, the clinical signs and symptoms are consistent with the localization (e.g. typical systolic murmur associated with the RVOT obstruction (RVOTO)). The symptoms specified below apply to *the sinus of Valsalva aneurysm rupture.*

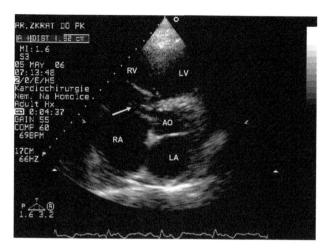

Figure 9.35
Transthoracic echo, modified apical view with aorta. Aneurysm of the right Valsalva sinus (arrow), prolapsing into the right atrium (RA). Due to the rupture of the aneurysm there is a shunt between aorta and right atrium, causing continuous murmur and right heart decompensation; see also Figures 9.39–9.41. AO, Aorta; RV, right ventricle; LA, left atrium; LV, left ventricle; RA, right atrium.

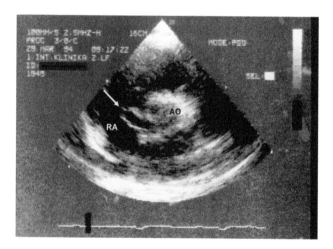

Figure 9.36
Transthoracic echo, short-axis parasternal view on the level of aorta, older picture with clear aneurysm of the noncoronary Valsalva sinus (arrow), prolapsing into the right atrium (RA). AO, Aorta.

Symptoms associated with sinus of Valsalva aneurysm rupture

- Sudden death.
- Retrosternal pain.
- Dyspnea.
- Palpitations.
- Signs of heart failure.
- Cardiogenic shock.

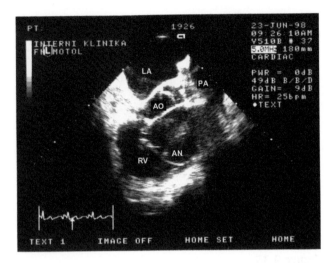

Figure 9.37
Transesophageal echo, longitudinal projection. Large aneurysm (50mm) of the right sinus of Valsalva (AN), protruding into right ventricle (RV), causing obstruction of the right ventricular outflow tract. PA, Pulmonary artery; AO, aorta; LA, left atrium.

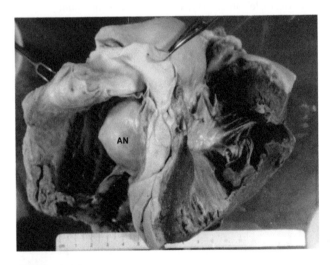

Figure 9.38
Large aneurysm of the right sinus of Valsalva (AN) protruding into the right ventricular outflow tract; the same patient as in Figure 9.37. (Courtesy of Professor J Stejskal, Institute of Pathology and Molecular Medicine, University Hospital Motol, Prague, Czech Republic.)

- In about 20% of cases, a small rupture may remain asymptomatic for some time, manifesting itself by murmur only, with signs of heart failure developing progressively.

Auscultatory findings

- Continuous systolic–diastolic murmur in the presence of aneurysm rupture into the right-heart chambers or into the left atrium.

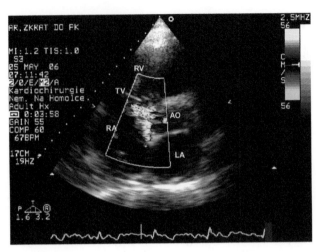

Figure 9.39
Transthoracic echo, modified apical view. Color Doppler identifies shunt from aorta (AO) to the right atrium (RA) due to the rupture of the aneurysm of the right sinus of Valsalva; the same patient as in Figures 9.35, 9.40 and 9.41. LA, Left atrium; RV, right ventricle; TV, tricuspid valve.

- Diastolic murmur in the rare case of rupture into the left ventricle.

Echocardiography

- Morphologically, a sinus of Valsalva aneurysm will visualize in standard transthoracic projections depending on the direction of prolapse; in case of doubt, transesophageal echocardiography will be helpful.
- The shape of a sinus of Valsalva aneurysm very often typically resembles a long finger (Figures 9.35 and 9.36), occasionally, it may be spherical and enormously large (Figures 9.37 and 9.38).
- In cases of rupture, the perforation is usually at the aneurysm top; Doppler echo will document a communication (Figures 9.39 and 9.40), and a continuous systolic–diastolic shunt flow (Figure 9.41). The flow is only diastolic in the case of a communication with the left ventricle.

Angiography, CT angiography and magnetic resonance imaging (MRI)

Clinically silent sinus of Valsalva aneurysm may be occasionally missed on echocardiography, but demonstrated by aortography (Figure 9.42) or a CT angiogram or MRI.

Risks

- Rupture of sinus of Valsalva aneurysm in up to 87% of cases.

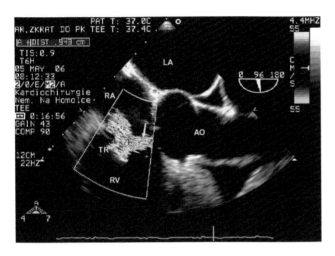

Figure 9.40
Transesophageal echo, 96 degrees. Rupture of the aneurysm of right Valsalva sinus into the right atrium (RA) with the shunt from aorta to the right atrium (arrow), concomitant tricuspid regurgitation (TR); the same patient as in Figure 9.35, 9.39 and 9.41. LA, Left atrium; AO, aorta; RV, right ventricle.

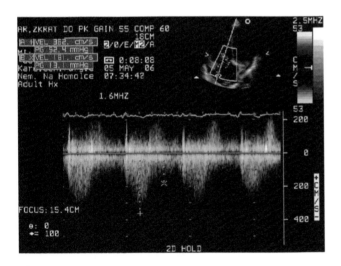

Figure 9.41
Continuous Doppler examination of the shunt flow from aorta to right atrium with systolic–diastolic flow due to the rupture of the aneurysm of Valsalva sinus; the same patient as in Figures 9.35, 9.39 and 9.40.

- IE (in 5–10% of patients with congenital sinus of Valsalva aneurysm).
- Oppression of adjacent structures.

Management

Surgical treatment in the presence of rupture or oppression of adjacent structures. Surgery for documented rupture of a sinus of Valsalva aneurysm should not be postponed. The procedure involves aneurysm resection and closure of its

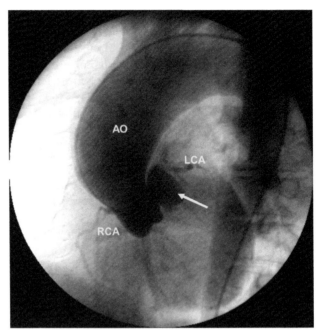

Figure 9.42
Aortogram with a large aneurysm of the left sinus of Valsalva (arrow) without rupture, accidental finding in a patient with congenital aortic stenosis. LCA, Left coronary artery; RCA, right coronary artery; AO, dilated ascending aorta.

orifice using a Dacron patch. Preventive surgical procedure in small aneurysms without rupture and oppression of adjacent structures is controversial.

Prognosis

A sinus of Valsalva aneurysm without rupture is asymptomatic and may manifest itself by mere oppression of adjacent structures. Rupture of a sinus of Valsalva aneurysm has occurred in 87% of reported cases.[1] Rupture will usually occur between 20 and 30 years of age; however, it may well occur later.[32] A case of rupture of a sinus of Valsalva aneurysm in pregnancy has also been reported.[33] Rupture may result in sudden death if there is perforation into the pericardium or if arrhythmia develops. Death from heart failure is more frequent, usually within 1 year of untreated rupture, while long-term survival is possible with minor perforations.[3]

MARFAN'S SYNDROME

Etiology and prevalence

Marfan's syndrome is one of the most frequent connective tissue disorders. There is autosomal dominant inheritance with complete penetrance, but variable clinical expression. The incidence is 1 per 5000 individuals, with men and women affected equally. Marfan's syndrome is caused by mutation of the fibrillin 1 gene on chromosome 15, or fibrillin 2 gene on chromosome 5, or the gene for transforming growth factor beta receptor type 2. More than 100 mutations for fibrillin 1 have been described. Approximately 25% of patients with Marfan's syndrome represent sporadic cases due to a new mutation with no family history.

Pathophysiology

Fibrillin abnormalities reduce the structural integrity of connective tissue, for example, deficient fibrillin in the aortic wall may trigger progressive aortic ectasia with cystic medionecrosis of the aortic wall. The walls of the aorta and the pulmonary artery become progressively weakened and dilate over the patient's life, and may result in aortic dissection or rupture (Figures 9.43–9.46). The changes appear mainly in the ascending aorta, where fibrillin 1 is primarily expressed (Figure 9.47). The wall stress increases with increased diameter and progression of media degeneration. The prevalence of aortic dilatation in Marfan's syndrome is 70–80%. Apart from cardiovascular manifestations (aortoannular ectasia, mitral valve prolapse), it has ocular, bone and articular manifestations.

Clinical manifestation

Tall statue with disproportionally long, thin limbs and digits (arachnodactylia), and spinal or chest wall deformities. The dilated aorta does not usually cause any symptoms. Acute aortic dissection presents with sudden severe retrosternal pain, which may irradiate to the back. The pain, however, may be atypical and misdiagnosed.

Diagnosis

Clinical assessment is essential. Molecular genetic testing for fibrillin 1 mutations may be provided, even though it is neither sensitive nor specific. Clinical signs vary from mild to severe, and none are pathognomonic.[34]

In 1996, revised Ghent criteria were offered as an international standard for the diagnosis of Marfan's syndrome.[35]

Major criteria

- *Skeletal:* Pectus excavatum requiring surgery, pectus carinatum, distance from head to symphysis divided by distance from symphysis to sole <0.85; arm span-to-height ratio >1.05; positive thumb sign (Figure 9.48); positive wrist sign (Figure 9.49); scoliosis of more than 20 degrees or spondylolisthesis; reduced extension of the elbows (<170 degrees); protrusio acetabula, pes planus.

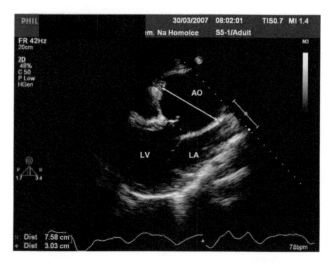

Figure 9.43
Transthoracic echo, parasternal long-axis view. Severely dilated aortic bulbus (arrow, 76mm) in a patient with Marfan's syndrome. It was possible to perform valve-sparing operation (reimplantation of aortic valve into the prosthesis). AO, Aorta; LV, left ventricle; LA, left atrium.

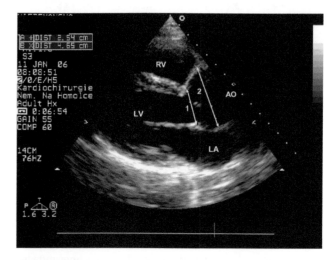

Figure 9.44
Transthoracic echo, long-axis parasternal view. Normal size of the aortic annulus (1), dilatation of the aortic bulbus (2). LV, Left ventricle; LA, left atrium; RV, right ventricle; AO, aorta.

- *Ocular:* Ectopia lentis.
- *Cardiovascular:* Dilatation of ascending aorta with or without aortic regurgitation, involving sinuses of Valsalva, dissection of the ascending aorta.
- *Dura mater:* Lumbosacral dural ectasia (by CT or MRI).
- *Family history/genetic:* A first-degree relative with diagnosed Marfan's syndrome, presence of fibrillin 1 mutation known to cause Marfan's syndrome.

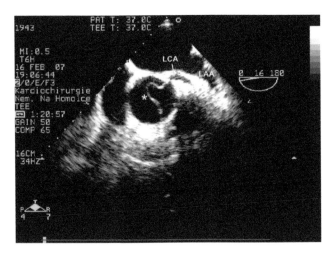

Figure 9.45
Transesophageal echo, 16 degrees. Aortic dissection type A, intimal flap (*) adjacent to left coronary artery (LCA). LAA, Left atrial auricle.

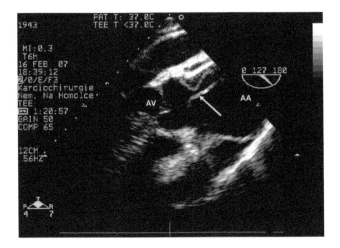

Figure 9.46
Transesophageal echo, 127 degrees, aortic dissection type A with intimal flap in the ascending aorta (arrow). AV, Aortic valve; AA, dilated ascending aorta.

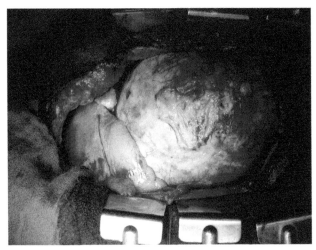

Figure 9.47
Aneurysm of the ascending aorta in Marfan's syndrome, surgical view. (Courtesy of Dr P Pavel, Dept of Cardiac Surgery, University Hospital Motol, Prague, Czech Republic.)

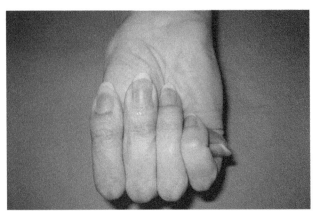

Figure 9.48
Positive thumb sign in a patient with Marfan's syndrome.

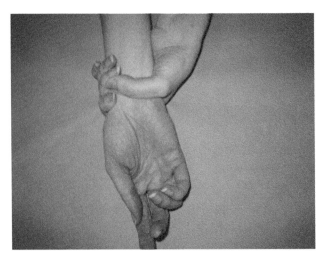

Figure 9.49
Positive wrist sign in a patient with Marfan's syndrome.

Minor criteria

- *Skeletal*: Pectus excavatum of moderate severity; scoliosis less than 20 degrees; thoracic lordosis; joint hypermobility; highly arched palate; typical appearance with dolichocephaly; malar hypoplasia; enophtalmus; retrognathia.
- *Ocular*: Abnormally flat cornea; hypoplastic iris; miotic pupil with reduced response to mydriatic drugs; hypoplastic ciliary muscle causing myopia.
- *Cardiovascular*: Mitral valve prolapse; calcification of mitral annulus in patients younger than 40 years of age; dilatation of proximal main pulmonary artery in the absence of pulmonary stenosis, or other cause in patients younger than 40 years of age; dilatation or

dissection of abdominal aorta in patients younger than 50 years of age.

- *Pulmonary*: Spontaneous pneumothorax: apical blebs (chest X-ray).
- *Skin*: Striae atrophicae not associated with pregnancy, recurrent or incisional hernia.

Requirements for systemic involvement: Skeletal criteria: one or two major plus two minor; ocular: at least two minor; cardiovascular: one major or one minor; pulmonary: one minor; skin: one minor; dura mater: one major; family history/genetic: one major.

Involvement of the cardiovascular system has a very high diagnostic strength.[34]

Echocardiography

Echocardiography is the main method for evaluation of cardiovascular involvement in patients with suspected Marfan's syndrome. It is used for their long-term follow-up, including indication of timely surgery and postoperative follow-up.

Aortic enlargement begins in Marfan's syndrome at the level of sinuses of Valsalva (Figures 9.43 and 9.44), in contrast to BAV, where the dilatation is distal to sino-tubular junction (Figures 9.3 and 9.25). The dilatation in Marfan's syndrome affects aortic sinuses near the sino-tubular junction; in later stages, also aortic annulus, bulbus (sinuses), ascending aorta. In normal adults the aortic root is usually <37mm, the upper limit of the normal size is 21mm/m^2, aneurysm is considered in dimensions >50% the upper normal limit, usually >50mm.[34,36–38]

For the diagnosis of aortic dissection, transesophageal echocardiography is often necessary (Figures 9.45 and 9.46). Acute aortic regurgitation may be caused by cusp prolapse after dissection. Chronic aortic regurgitation is caused by dilatation of the aortic annulus and root. Mitral valve prolapse is more frequent in females and younger patients with Marfan's syndrome.

CT angiography and MRI

These are valuable methods for imaging the whole aorta with the arch, great arteries and descending aorta, and should always be performed before surgery. Aneurysms of the descending aorta usually extend into the abdominal aorta.

Catheterization

This is usually not necessary if the aforementioned methods are used. Coronary angiogram should be performed on patients over 40 years of age.

Management

Lifestyle

Patients should be informed about potential complications and modify their lifestyle to reduce the risk of dissection if aortic dilatation is present. Physical activity depends on the severity of the disease. Recreational activities are possible for most patients, with the exclusion of strenuous exercise, isometric exercise, contact sports, weightlifting, jumping into water or any hits of the chest, rapid decompression and flying in unpressurized airplanes.[34] For adults with Marfan's syndrome and dilated aorta who want to be physically active, earlier surgery may be considered.

Medical treatment

Beta blockers have been shown to delay the onset of aortic dilatation, reduce the rate of aortic dilatation, reduce the risk of aortic dissection, and improve the survival rate in all age groups.[39,40] The long-term use of beta blockers is recommended for all adult patients with Marfan's syndrome who do not have contraindications for this treatment. For patients who cannot take beta blockers, ACE inhibitors or calcium channel blockers (verapamil) are recommended. ACE inhibitors may play a role in the prevention and treatment of aortic wall degeneration and disproportionate growth rate.[34]

Surgery

Elective surgery is performed to prevent fatal aortic dissection or rupture, and to treat aortic or mitral regurgitation. Inevitably, well-timed cardiovascular surgery considerably improves the prognosis.[41,42] The indication for elective surgery is based on aortic size, rate of growth and family history. Prophylactic aortic root replacement is usually recommended when the diameter of the aortic root reaches 50mm. However, in experienced institutions the ascending aorta may be replaced as soon as the diameter reaches 45mm.[15,34] Preventive surgery may be indicated even earlier in experienced centers with good results, when the aortic root is >40mm, for patients with a family history of sudden death or dissection, or for women before planned pregnancy. Early aortic root surgery is also recommended if the aortic root diameter is enlarging rapidly (>2–5mm per year), or in the presence of moderate aortic regurgitation. Early surgery (with an aortic root diameter 45–50mm) is recommended if the surgeon believes that the aortic valve can be spared.

Surgery is performed as composite valve graft repair or a valve-sparing procedure. Composite graft repair (modified Bentall procedure) consists of a mechanical aortic valve attached to synthetic prosthesis tube, the coronary ostia are reimplanted into the aortic graft (Figure 9.50).[43a] In the valve-sparing procedure, the patient's own aortic valve is spared and the ascending aorta is replaced by a synthetic

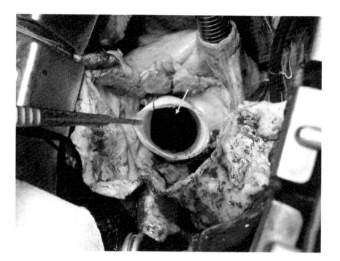

Figure 9.50
Bentall procedure in patient with aneurysm of ascending aorta, surgical view, composite conduit with mechanical aortic valve prosthesis (arrow), (Courtesy of Dr P Pavel, Chief, Dept of Cardiac Surgery, University Hospital Motol, Prague, Czech Republic.)

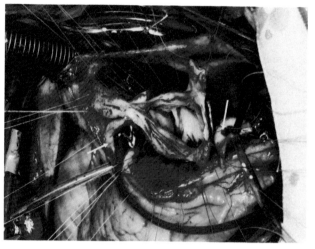

Figure 9.52
The same patient as in Figure 9.51, valve-sparing aortic valve surgery, reimplantation according David. Stitches are placed subannulary, coronary arteries with buttons will be reimplanted into the prosthesis (arrows). (Courtesy of Dr Stepan Cerny, Chief, Dept of Cardiac Surgery, Hospital Na Homolce, Prague, Czech Republic.)

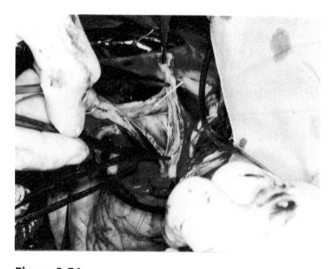

Figure 9.51
Valve-sparing surgery of the aortic valve in a patient with Marfan's syndrome, reimplantation according David; surgical view. Aortic valve has three pliable cusps without degenerative changes (arrow). Dilated aortic root with sinuses is completely excised. (Courtesy of Dr Stepan Cerny, Chief, Dept of Cardiac Surgery, Hospital Na Homolce, Prague, Czech Republic.)

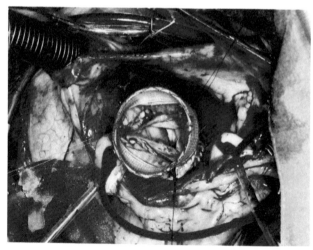

Figure 9.53
The same patient as in Figures 9.51 and 9.52; surgical view, aortic valve-sparing surgery, reimplantation according David. Native aortic valve is implanted inside the tubular Dacron aortic root prosthesis. (Courtesy of Dr Stepan Cerny, Chief, Dept of Cardiac Surgery, Hospital Na Homolce, Prague, Czech Republic.)

prosthesis. It is advantageous for patients with a structurally normal aortic valve and a dilated aorta. Better results are achieved if aortic root dilatation is <50mm. Two approaches exist: reimplantation of the patient's own valve into the prosthetic tube according David (Figures 9.51–9.55), or the remodeling technique according Yacoub.[43–45] The operative mortality of the valve-sparing procedure is low, and valve-related 5–10 year morbidity and mortality are superior to those of composite graft repair.[46,47] The great advantage of the valve-sparing procedure is a lower risk of IE and thromboembolism, and avoidance of lifelong anticoagulation therapy.

Emergency surgery is indicated for patients with aortic dissection type A (in ascending aorta) or intramural hemorrhage. The descending aorta should be replaced if the aortic diameter is >55–60mm, or the diameter increases rapidly (5–10mm per year), or if complications occur (pain, organ ischemia). Dissection type B (in the descending aorta) can be treated by an aortic stent graft.[48,49]

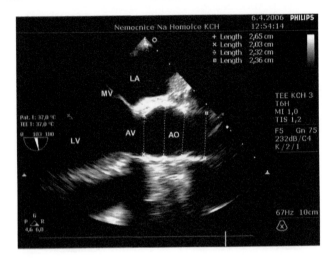

Figure 9.54

Transesophageal echo, 103 degrees. The same patient with Marfan's syndrome as in Figure 9.44 after valve-sparing surgery, reimplantation of own aortic valve into prosthesis according David. The aortic valve is competent, the prosthesis (Valsalva Gelweave) keeps the physiological shape of the aortic root. LV, Left ventricle; LA, left atrium; AV, aortic valve; MV, mitral valve; AO, prosthesis of the aortic root and ascending aorta.

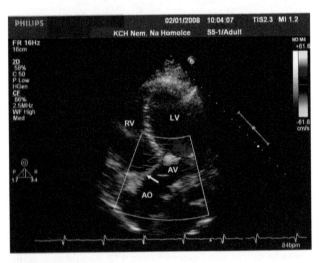

Figure 9.55

Transthoracic echo, with color Doppler mapping, apical view with aorta. Patient with Marfan's syndrome after valve-sparing surgery with reimplantation of native aortic valve (AV) into the prosthesis (arrow), normal function of the aortic valve without regurgitation. LV, Left ventricle; AO, aorta; RV, right ventricle.

Pregnancy

Women with Marfan's syndrome must have a detailed cardiovascular evaluation and genetic counseling prior to pregnancy because of the high risk of cardiovascular complications. The risk of dissection during pregnancy and after delivery is unpredictable, the highest risk is in the third trimester.[50] Enlargement of the aortic root >40mm identifies

a particularly high-risk group, even though the smaller dimensions do not prevent serious complications such as aortic dissection or rupture. During the whole pregnancy it is necessary to carefully monitor the blood pressure, and to monitor monthly the aortic root dimensions by echocardiography. Beta blocker use is advisable in all patients with Marfan's syndrome in pregnancy, not only with dilated aorta, but also with an aortic root width <40mm.[14,15] ACE inhibitors are contraindicated due to fetal risk. Bed rest is recommended in the case of progressive aortic dilatation or severe aortic regurgitation. In women with Marfan's syndrome and aortic root dilatation >40–45mm, elective surgery is strongly recommended before pregnancy.[15] A valve-sparing operation may be performed with good results, and without the necessity of lifelong anticoagulation therapy. Delivery by cesarean section is recommended for pregnant patients with Marfan's syndrome with aortic root dilatation >40–45mm because of the risk of dissection or rupture.[15,27] For vaginal delivery, adequate analgesia and shortening of the second stage of labor is recommended. Epidural and spinal anesthesia should be performed only after exclusion of dural ectasia or arachnoic cyst, which may cause a dilution of anesthetics. Careful monitoring of blood pressure and clinical status during and after delivery is imperative for all pregnant patients with Marfan's syndrome.

Infectious endocarditis

Antibiotic prophylaxis of IE is recommended prior to procedures that are associated with bacteremia.

Follow up

Patients with Marfan's syndrome require lifelong serial and systematic follow-up by a cardiologist, even after successful surgery. The disease may progress with aneurysm formation in the aortic arch and the descending aorta. Follow-up intervals depend on the severity of involvement, usually 12 months for unoperated patients with aortic root diameter <40mm or successfully operated patients. Ophthalmologic and orthopedic examination and the treatment may be necessary. First-degree relatives should be evaluated for Marfan's syndrome.

Prognosis

Prognosis depends mainly on the severity of cardiovascular involvement. Reduced life expectancy is caused predominantly by aortic dissection and rupture, or aortic (and mitral) regurgitation. Dissection typically occurs after the second decade of life and only infrequently during childhood and adolescence. The risk of aortic dissection increases with aortic diameter, and is especially high in patients with an aortic root diameter >55mm or in those with a positive family history.[51] Dissection may, however, also appear in nondilated aorta. The earlier diagnosis, adequate pharmacological treatment, and timely surgery improve the prognosis and life expectancy of patients with Marfan's syndrome. The average lifespan has increased from approximately 40 years of age in untreated patients to 70 years of age.[52–54] Nevertheless, cardiovascular complications are still the most common causes of patient loss, often due to sudden death or dissection in previously undiagnosed Marfan's syndrome. The 5- and 10-year survival rates of patients with Marfan's syndrome undergoing combined aortic valve and root replacement are 80 and 60%, respectively.[55]

References

1. Valdes-Cruz Lm, Cayre LO. Echocardiographic Diagnosis of Congenital Heart Disease. An Embryologic and Anatomic Approach, 1st edn. Philadelphia, PA: Lippicott-Raven Publishers, 1999.

2. Redington A, Shore D, Oldershaw P. Congenital heart disease in adults. 1st edn. London: WB Saunders Company, 1994.

3. Perloff JK. The clinical recognition of congenital heart disease, 4th edn. Philadelphia, PA: WB Saunders Company, 1994.

4. Niwa K, Perloff JK, Bhuta SM et al. Structural abnormalities of great arterial walls in congenital heart disease: Light and electron microscopic analysis. Circulation 2001; 103: 393–400.

5. Roberts CS, Roberts WC. Dissection of the aorta associated with congenital malformation of the aortic valve. J Am Coll Cardiol 1991; 17: 712.

6. Hahn R, Roman M, Mogtader AH, Devereux RB. Association of aortic dilatation with regurgitant, stenotic and functionally normal bicuspid aortic valves. J Am Coll Cardiol 1992; 19: 283–8.

7. Keane MG, Wiegers SE, Plappert T et al. Bicuspid aortic valves are associated with aortic dilatation out of proportion to coexistent valvular lesions. Circulation 2000; 102: 35–9.

8. Nistri S, Sorbo MD, Martin M et al. Aortic root dilatation in young men with normally functioning bicuspid aortic valves. Heart 1999; 82: 19–22.

9. Nkomo VT, Enriquez-Sarano M, Ammash NM et al. Bicuspid aortic valve associated with aortic dilatation. A community based study. Arterioscler Thromb Vasc Biol 2003; 23: 351–6.

10. Cecconi M, Manfrin M, Moraca A et al. Aortic dimensions in patients with bicuspid aortic valve without significant valve dysfunction. Am J Cardiol 2005; 95: 292–4.

11. Williams JCP, Barrett-Boyes BG, Lowe JB. Supravalvular aortic stenosis. Circulation 1961; 24: 1311–18.

12. Roberts WC. The congenitally bicuspid aortic valve. Am J Cardiol 1970; 26: 72–83.

13. DeFilippi CR, DuWayne MD, Willett L et al. Usefulness of Dobutamine echocardiography in distinguishing severe from nonsevere valvular aortic stenosis in patients with depressed left ventricular function and low transvalvular gradients. Am J Cardiol 1995; 75: 191–4.

14. Iung B, Gohlke-Bärwolf C, Tornos P et al. Recommendations on the management of the asymptomatic patients with valvular heart disease. Working group report. Eur Heart J 2002; 23(16): 1253–66.

15. Bonow RO, Carabello BA, Chatterjee K et al. ACC/AHA 2006 Guidelines for the management of patients with valvular heart disease. J Am Coll Cardiol 2006; 48(3): e1–148.

16. Vahanian A, Baumgartner H, Bax J et al. Guidelines on the management of valvular heart disease. The task force on the management of valvular heart disease of the European Society of Cardiology. European Heart J 2007; 28: 230–68.

17. Cribier A, Eitchaninoff H, Tron C et al. Treatment of calcific aortic stenosis with the percutaneous heart valve: Mid-term follow-up from the initial feasibility studies: The French experience. J Am Coll Cardiol 2006; 47(6): 1214–23.

18. Walker F. Subvalvar and supravalvar aortic stenosis. In: Gatzoulis MA, Webb GD, Daubeney PEF, eds. Diagnosis and Management of Adult Congenital Heart Disease. Edinburgh: Churchill Livingstone, 2003.

19. Connelly MS, Webb GD, Somerville J et al. Canadian consensus conference on adult congenital heart disease 1996. Can J Cardiol 1998; 14(3): 395–452.

20. Bonow RO, Carabello B, De Leon AC et al. ACC/AHA guidelines for the management of patients with valvular heart disease. J Am Coll Cardiol 1998; 32(5): 1486–588.

21. Otto CM. Valvular Heart Disease. Philadelphia, PA: WB Saunders Company, 1999.

22. Reich O, Tax P, Marek J et al. Long term results of percutaneous balloon valvoplasty of congenital aortic stenosis: Independent predictors of outcome. Heart 2004; 90(1): 70–6.

23. Keane JF, Driscoll DJ, Gersony WM et al. Second natural history study of congenital heart defects: Results of treatment of patients with aortic valve stenosis. Circulation 1993; 87(Suppl I): I-16–I-27.

24. Serraf A, Zoghby J, Lacour-Gayet F et al. Surgical treatment of subaortic stenosis: A seventeen-year experience. J Thorac Cardiovasc Surg 1999; 117(4): 669–78.

25. Erentug V, Bozbuga N, Kirall K et al. Surgical treatment of subaortic obstruction in adolescence and adults: Long-term follow up. J Card Surg 2005; 20(1): 16–21.

26. Paulus WJ. Chronic aortic regurgitation. In: Crawford MH, Di Marco JP, Cardiology, 1st edn. London: Mosby, 2001: 6.11.1–6.11.10.

27. Oakley C. Heart Disease in Pregnancy, 1st edn. London: BMJ Publishing Group, 1997.

28. David TE, Feindel CM, Webb GD et al. Aortic valve preservation in patients with aortic root aneurysm: Results of the reimplantation technique. Ann Thorac Surg 2007; 83(2): S732–5.

29. Wernly JA. Thoracic aorta disease. In: Crawford MH, Di Marco JP, eds. Cardiology, 1st edn. London: Mosby, 2001: 1.12.1–1.12.13.

30. Matherne GP. Aneurysms of the sinus of Valsalva. In: Allen HD, Gutgesell HP, Clark EB, Driscoll DJ, eds. Moss and Adams' Heart Disease in Infants, Children and Adolescents, 6th edn. Philadelphia, PA: Lippincott, Williams and Wilkins, 2001: 686–8.

31. Shah RP, Ding ZP, Quek SS. A ten-year review of ruptured sinus of Valsalva: Clinico-pathological and echo-Doppler features. Singapore Med J 2001; 42(10): 473–6.

32. Sakakibara S, Konno S. Congenital aneurysm of the sinus of Valsalva: A clinical study. Am Heart J 1962; 63: 708.

33. Cripps T, Pumphrey CW, Parker DJ. Rupture of the sinus of Valsalva during pregnancy. Br Heart J 1987; 57: 490.

34. Kaemmerer H, Oechslin E, Seidel H et al. Marfan syndrome: What internists and pediatric or adult cardiologists need to know. Expert Rev Cardiovasc Ther 2005; 3(5): 891–909.

35. DePaepe A, Devereux RB, Dietz HC et al. Revised diagnostic criteria for the Marfan syndrome. Am J Med Genet 1996; 62(4): 417–26.

36. Erbel R, Alfonso F, Boileau C et al. Diagnosis and management of aortic dissection. Recommendations of the Task Force on Aortic Dissection, European Society of Cardiology. Eur Heart J 2001; 22: 1642–81.

37. Johnston KW, Rutherford RB, Tilson MD et al. Suggested standards for reporting on arterial aneurysms: Subcommittee on reporting standards for arterial aneurysms. J Vasc Surg 1991; 13: 452–8.

38. Meijboom LJ, Timmermans J, Zwinderman A et al. Aortic root growth in men and women with the Marfan's syndrome. Am J Cardiol 2005; 96: 1441–4.

39. Halpern BL, Char F, Murdoch JL et al. A prospectus on the prevention of aortic rupture in the Marfan syndrome with data on survivorship without treatment. John Hopkins Med J 1971; 129(3): 123–9.

40. Shores J, Berger KR, Murphy EA et al. Progression of aortic dilatation and the benefit of long-term beta-adrenergic blockade in Marfan syndrome. N Engl J Med 1994; 330(19): 1335–41.

41. Svensson LG, Crawford ES, Coselli JS et al. Impact of cardiovascular operation on survival in the Marfan patient. Circulation 1989; 80: I233–42.

42. Gott VL, Cameron DE, Pyeritz RE et al. Composite graft repair of Marfan aneurysm of the ascending aorta: Results in 150 patients. J Card Surg 1994; 9(5): 482–9.

43a. Bentall H, De Bono A. A technique for complete replacement of the ascending aorta. Thorax 1968; 23(4): 338–9.

43. David TE, Feindel CM. An aortic valve-sparing operation for patients with aortic incompetence and aneurysm of the ascending aorta. J Thorac Cardiovasc Surg 1992; 103(4): 617–21.

44. David TE. Current practice in Marfan's aortic root surgery: Reconstruction with aortic valve preservation or replacement? What to do with the mitral valve? J Card Surg 1997; 12(Suppl 2): 147–50.

45. Sarsam MA, Yacoub M. Remodeling of the aortic valve annulus. J Thorac Cardiovasc Surg 1993; 105(3): 435–8.

46. Birks EJ, Webb C, Child A et al. Early and long-term results of a valve-sparing operation for Marfan syndrome. Circulation 1999; 100(Suppl 19): II-29–II-35.

47. DeOliveira NC, David TE, Ivanov J et al. Results of surgery for aortic root aneurysm in patients with Marfan syndrome. J Thorac Cardiovasc Surg 2003; 125(4): 789–96.

48. Nienaber CA, Fattori R, Lund G et al. Nonsurgical reconstruction of thoracic aortic dissection by stent-graft placement. N Engl J Med 1999; 340(20): 1539–45.

49. Fleck TM, Hutschala D, Tschernich H et al. Stent graft placement of the thoracoabdominal aorta in a patient with Marfan syndrome. J Thorac Cardiovasc Surg 2003; 125(6): 1541–3.

50. Pyeritz RE. Maternal and fetal complications of pregnancy in the Marfan syndrome. Am J Med 1981; (5): 784–90.

51. Groenink M, Lohuis TAJ, Tijssen JPG et al. Survival and complication-free survival in Marfan's syndrome: implications of current guidelines. Heart 1999; 82: 499–504.

52. Murdoch JL, Walker BA, Halpern BL et al. Life expectancy and causes of death in the Marfan syndrome. N Engl J Med 1972; 286(15): 804–8.

53. Silverman DI, Burton KJ, Gray J et al. Life expectancy in the Marfan syndrome. Am J Cardiol 1995; 75(2): 157–60.

54. Gott VL, Greene PS, Alejo DE et al. Replacement of the aortic root in patients with Marfan's syndrome. N Engl J Med 1999; 340(17): 1307–13.

55. Gott VL, Pyeritz RE, Cameron DE, Greene PS, Mckusick VA. Composite graft repair of Marfan aneurysms of the ascending aorta: Results in 100 patients. Ann Thorac Surg 1991; 52: 38–45.

10

Pulmonary stenosis

Division and anatomical notes

Right ventricular outflow tract obstruction (RVOTO) may be present at various levels: valvular, subvalvular (infundibular), supravalvular, or within the peripheral pulmonary artery branches. Pulmonary stenosis (PS) may be isolated or associated with other congenital heart diseases (CHD), e.g. atrial or ventricular septal defects (ASD and VSD, respectively). However, it is also part of more complex defects such as tetralogy of Fallot, double-outlet right ventricle, some forms of univentricular hearts, etc. PS may be part of Noonan's syndrome, where a dysplastic (thickened and rigid) pulmonary valve occurs, in some 60% of patients. However, this chapter deals only with isolated pulmonary stenosis (PS).

- *Valvular PS* is, in general, congenital. In most (80–90% of cases) pulmonary valvular stenoses, the valve is compliant, with fused commissures, bulging cusps and with a small aperture at the top (Figure 10.1). In some 10–20% of cases, the valve is dysplastic, with thickened, myxomatous, immobile cusps, with no commissural fusions. Often the annulus is hypoplastic.

- *Subvalvular PS* (Figure 10.2) results from muscular hyperplasia of the right ventricular infundibulum, which narrows dynamically or remains constantly narrowed, usually with a thickened, fibrotic endocardium. It may also be secondary in significant valvular PS. Subvalvular PS is part of tetralogy of Fallot (see Chapter 7); however, it may also occur isolated or in combination with other CHD, e.g. a VSD.

- '*Double-chambered right ventricle*' (subinfundibular stenosis) is a separate entity with midventricular obstruction of the right ventricle owing to hypertrophic muscle bundles ('moderator band') at the interface of the right ventricular inlet and outlet tract, often associated with VSD.

- *Supravalvular PS* is frequent in tetralogy of Fallot, Williams' syndrome, Noonan's syndrome, or congenital rubella syndrome (Figure 10.3). Artificial supravalvular PS may be the consequence of pulmonary artery banding in childhood.

- *Peripheral stenoses of pulmonary artery branches* may be present in tetralogy of Fallot and other CHD. They may be uni- or bilateral, isolated or multiple.

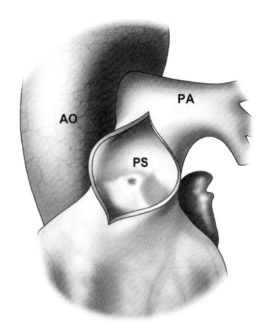

Figure 10.1
Valvar pulmonary stenosis. Pliable valve fused in commissures with small central orifice. AO, Aorta; PA, pulmonary artery; PS, pulmonary stenosis.

Prevalence

As an isolated defect, PS accounts for about 6–10% of all CHD. The male-to-female ratio is equal.

Pathophysiology

Obstruction in the RVOT leads to right ventricular pressure overload and right ventricular hypertrophy. The right ventricular chamber usually remains small, with reduced compliance. Systolic right ventricular function is maintained in compensated PS. With significant PS, there is an increase in systolic ventricular pressure and also, because of diastolic dysfunction, an increase in end-diastolic right ventricular and right atrial pressure. Right ventricular failure results in dilatation and systolic dysfunction of the right ventricle, and tricuspid regurgitation secondary to tricuspid annular dilatation. Chronic pressure overload may be associated with diastolic

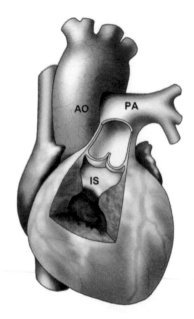

Figure 10.2
Subvalvular (infundibular) pulmonary stenosis.
AO, Aorta; PA, pulmonary artery; IS, infundibular stenosis.

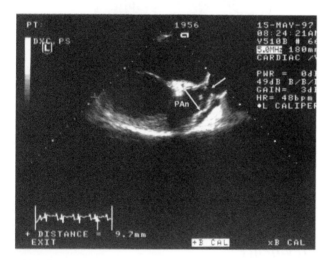

Figure 10.3
Supravalvular pulmonary stenosis (arrow), with narrowing to 9.7mm between the white crosses, normal size of the pulmonary annulus (PAn). Transesophageal echo, longitudinal view.

and systolic left ventricular dysfunction due to hypertrophy and dislocation of the interventricular septum.[1,2]

Necropsy in patients with severe PS will reveal multiple subendocardial infarctions involving the right ventricle and papillary muscles.

Clinical findings and diagnosis

Significant PS which has not been treated in childhood is a rare finding in adult patients. However, there may be a

progression in the severity of originally less significant lesions, restenosis, or infundibular PS over the years.

Symptoms

- Signs and symptoms depend on the severity of the stenosis.
- Patients are often asymptomatic.
- Fatigability and exertional dyspnea due to a low cardiac output.
- Presyncope, syncope, chest pain in severe stenoses.
- Palpitations.
- Signs of right-heart decompensation.
- Central cyanosis, if associated with a right-to-left shunt due to an associated shunt lesion (e.g. patent foramen ovale, ASD, VSD).
- Peripheral cyanosis if the cardiac output is reduced.

Clinical manifestation

Right ventricular heave, with or without a systolic thrill at the upper left sternal border.

Auscultatory findings

- A systolic click due to an abrupt bulging of the cusps of a compliant valve fused in commissures. It is not present in a dysplastic valve.
- Split second pulmonary heart sound, diminished in intensity.
- Ejection systolic murmur in the second left intercostal space, propagating to the neck. The murmur is transmitted into the back and to the posterior lung field. The louder and longer the murmer is, the more severe is the obstruction. With infundibular stenosis, the systolic murmur is in the third to fourth left intercostal space. In peripheral pulmonary artery stenosis, the murmur radiates into the posterior lung fields and the axilla.

Electrocardiogram (ECG)

- With mild PS, the ECG recordings may be normal.
- Right axis deviation of the axis QRS complex.
- In dysplastic pulmonary valve and Noonan's syndrome, left axis deviation.
- With advanced PS, a P-dextroatriale may be present.
- With significant PS, right ventricular hypertrophy.
- Incomplete or complete right bundle branch block.
- Atrial flutter, atrial fibrillation in the presence of right atrial dilatation.

Chest X-ray

- Normal with mild PS.
- Pulmonary vascular markings are normal or decreased.

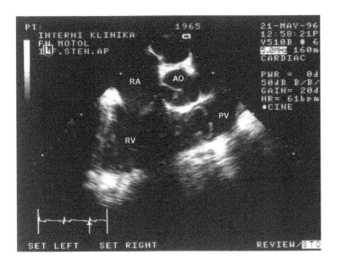

Figure 10.4
Valvar pulmonary artery stenosis with doming of the pulmonary valve, fused in commissures. AO, Aorta; PV, pulmonary valve; RA, right atrium; RV, right ventricle. Transesophageal echo, longitudinal view.

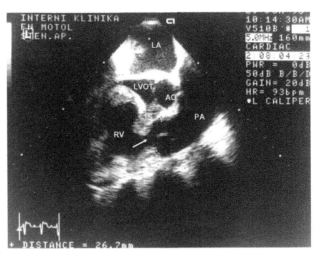

Figure 10.6
Infundibular pulmonary artery stenosis (arrow). PA, Pulmonary artery; RV, right ventricle; IS, infundibular septum; LVOT, left ventricular outflow tract; AO, aorta; LA, left artrium. Transesophageal echo, longitudinal view.

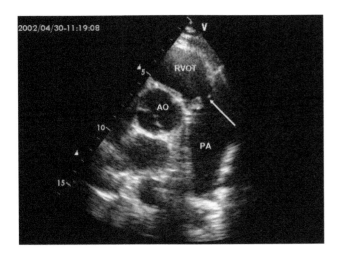

Figure 10.5
Valvar pulmonary stenosis, thickened dysplastic valve (arrow). RVOT, Right ventricular outflow tract; PA, pulmonary artery with mild poststenotic dilatation; AO, aorta. Transthoracic echo.

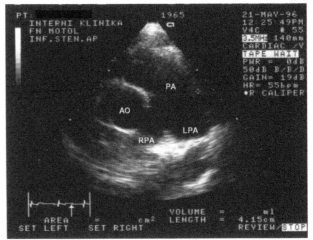

Figure 10.7
Poststenotic dilatation of the pulmonary artery (PA) to 41mm and dilatation of the left pulmonary artery, where the stenotic jet is preferentially directed. LPA, Left pulmonary artery; RPA, right pulmonary artery; AO, aorta. Trasthoracic echo, short-axis view on the level of the great arteries.

- Poststenotic dilatation of the pulmonary artery trunk or, alternatively, a dilatation of the left pulmonary artery branch, where the stenotic flow is preferentially directed to. The degree of dilatation must not be consistent with the degree of stenosis.
- The pulmonary valve may be calcified.

Echocardiography

- Determination of the location and significance of obstruction, which may be present at several levels (Figures 10.3–10.6).

- Determination of valve morphology (compliant valve with commissural fusion, or thickened and dysplastic valve) and function (Figures 10.4 and 10.5).
- Width of the pulmonary annulus, pulmonary artery trunk and branches (Figures 10.6 and 10.7).
- Right ventricular size, its systolic and diastolic function, right ventricular wall thickness.
- Diastolic and systolic left ventricular function.
- Tricuspid annular size and function.
- Association with other CHD (Figure 10.8).

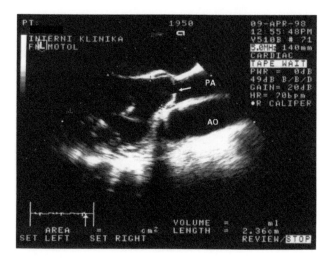

Figure 10.8
Valvar pulmonary stenosis (arrow) with the doming
of pulmonary valve in congenitally corrected transposition
of the great arteries. Aorta (AO) is in the front, pulmonary
artery (PA) behind, parallel course of the great
arteries without crossing.

In difficult-to-examine patients, transesophageal echocardiography may be of advantage, particularly to assess pulmonary valve morphology, width of the pulmonary trunk and the central segments of the pulmonary artery branches, and for better visualization of residual pulmonary regurgitation (Figure 10.9).

Spiroergometry

To assess physical fitness and oxygen consumption during exercise; measuring the saturation with pulsed oxymeter during exercise helps to rule out a potential right-to-left shunt.

Catheterization

- Catheterization is performed for diagnostic purposes only if the hemodynamic significance of the lesion is unclear, and in order to exclude peripheral pulmonary artery branch stenoses.
- Catheter-based intervention is performed as a therapeutic procedure (see 'Management' on page 91).
- Coronary arteriography is indicated prior to an elective cardiac surgical procedure in patients over 40 years of age, or in younger patients at risk for coronary artery disease or with suspected coronary artery anomalies.

Magnetic resonance imaging (MRI)

To quantify pulmonary regurgitation and to determine right ventricular function. It can be also used for noninvasive visualization of pulmonary artery branches.

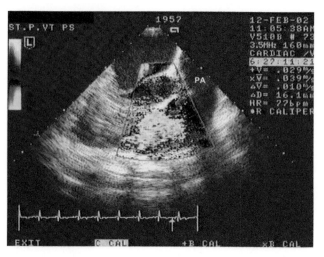

Figure 10.9
Severe pulmonary regurgitation after the surgical valvulotomy of the pulmonary stenosis in childhood in a 45-year-old female. Transesophageal echo, longitudinal view, color flow mapping. PA, Pulmonary artery.

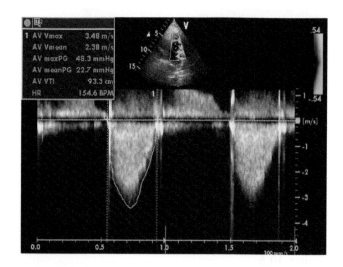

Figure 10.10
Mild pulmonary stenosis with maximal Doppler gradient <50mmHg. CW Doppler measurement under 2D control.

Computerized tomography (CT) angiography

Noninvasive visualization of pulmonary artery and its branches, and mediastinal structures including postoperative changes, adhesions, etc.

Assessing the significance of pulmonary stenosis

When assessing the significance of PS, account has to be taken to flow rate, heart rate, and right ventricular function. The

Table 10.1	*Hemodynamic severity of pulmonary stenosis (PS)*		
Pulmonary stenosis	Pulmonary valve orifice indexed to body surface area (cm²/m²)	Maximal Doppler or peak catheterization gradient (mmHg)	Mean Doppler echocardiographic gradient (mmHg)
Trivial		<25	
Mild	>0.8	25–49	<20
Moderate	0.8–0.5	50–79	20–40
Severe	<0.5	>80	>40

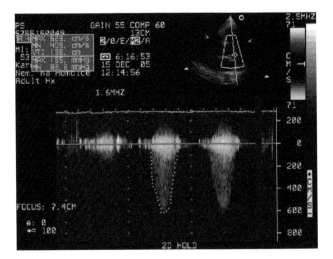

Figure 10.11
Severe unoperated pulmonary stenosis in 50-year-old female with maximal Doppler gradient on pulmonary valve 155mmHg. CW Doppler measurement under 2D control.

gradient depends on the flow across the valve, and on the ventricular function, which may decrease in the presence of systolic dysfunction (Figures 10.10 and 10.11). A grading of the hemodynamic severity of the PS is given in Table 10.1.

Management

The method of choice for the management of valvular PS in adulthood is catheter-based balloon valvuloplasty.[3] This procedure should be performed in centers experienced in the management of CHD. Balloon valvuloplasty may be unsuccessful in dysplastic and calcified valves, subsequently indicated for surgical management: valvulotomy or pulmonary valve replacement. For valve replacement, a human pulmonary homograft, less often a biological or mechanical prosthesis, is used.

Supravalvular and subvalvular PS should be managed at departments of cardiac surgery specializing in CHD. Peripheral pulmonary artery stenosis can occasionally be managed by balloon angioplasty with stenting.

Indications for balloon valvuloplasty or surgical intervention/reintervention4–6

- Total catheter gradient in RVOT at pullback >30–50mmHg at rest.
- Intervention in lower gradients on PS (30–40mmHg) is undertaken, especially in symptomatic patients, before pregnancy, or in active sportsmen and -women.
- Presence of symptoms (exertional dyspnea, angina, presyncope, syncope).
- Significant arrhythmia (often atrial flutter).
- Concomitant right-to-left shunt (e.g. ASD, VSD).
- Surgery is indicated in double-chambered right ventricle with a mid-ventricular obstruction in the right ventricle >50mmHg.
- A status after infectious endocarditis (IE) may be an indication for intervention.
- After valvuloplasty, surgery is indicated for severe residual pulmonary regurgitation with reduced exercise capacity for cardiac causes, deteriorating right ventricular function or deteriorating tricuspid valve regurgitation.

Residual findings

- Residual obstruction following catheter-based valvuloplasty or surgical valvulotomy; the obstruction may be progressive.
- Residual pulmonary regurgitation, which is initially tolerated. Pulmonary regurgitation may, however, result in right ventricular dilatation and dysfunction, dilatation of the tricuspid annulus with tricuspid regurgitation, reduced cardiac output and symptoms over decades (Figures 10.9, 10.12 and 10.13). This requires pulmonary valve replacement.
- Any form of pulmonary hypertension will augment pulmonary regurgitation.
- Residual stenosis of pulmonary artery peripheral branches reduces the hemodynamic significance of residual pulmonary regurgitation.

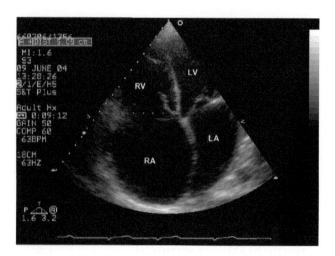

Figure 10.12
Persisting dilatation of the tricuspid annulus (51mm) in an adult patient after a successful balloon valvuloplasty of severe pulmonary stenosis. RV, Right ventricle; RA, right atrium; LV, left ventricle; LA, left atrium. Transthoracic echo, apical four-champer view.

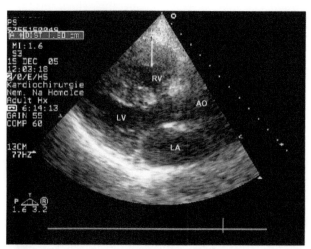

Figure 10.14
Extremely severe hypertrophy of the right ventricular anterior wall, the thickness is 18mm (arrow); the same patient as in Figure 10.11, this lady was successfully operated on. RV, Right ventricle; LV, left ventricle; LA, left atrium; AO, aorta. Transthoracic echo, long-axis parasternal view.

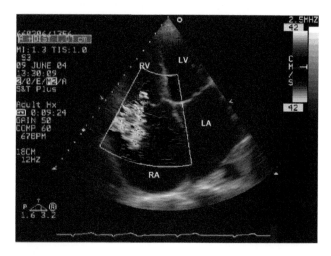

Figure 10.13
Moderate tricuspid regurgitation in the same patient as in Figure 10.12. Color flow mapping, transthoracic echo, four-chamber apical view. RV, Right ventricle; RA, right atrium; LV, left ventricle; LA, left atrium.

Risks

- Progression of PS, particularly of subvalvular PS.
- Underestimation of the hemodynamic consequences of protracted residual pulmonary regurgitation.
- Balloon valvuloplasty may result in acute pulmonary or tricuspid regurgitation, RVOT perforation, arrhythmia, venous thrombosis, etc.
- Surgical valvulotomy or balloon valvuloplasty of a significant PS may be followed by dynamic RVOT obstruction due to the hypertrophy of the infundibulum (Figure 10.14).

Pregnancy and delivery

Mild RVOTO is usually tolerated without problems.[7] During pregnancy and delivery, women with moderate and severe PS may develop right-heart decompensation, progressive tricuspid regurgitation, and supraventricular arrhythmias, even if they were asymptomatic before pregnancy. Therefore, more than mild PS should be removed before pregnancy. During pregnancy, balloon valvuloplasty of PS can be performed in critical cases, preferably after completion of organogenesis.

Infectious endocarditis

PS is associated with a relatively small risk of IE; however, IE prevention should be permanent even after surgical or balloon-based intervention.

Follow-up

Asymptomatic patients with mild PS may be followed-up by a general practitioner or an internist. Patients with moderate and severe PS require follow-up by a cardiologist, bearing in mind the potential of progressive valvular and subvalvular stenosis, residual pulmonary regurgitation, right ventricular size and function, tricuspid regurgitation and arrhythmias.

Prognosis

- Mild valvar PS does not usually progress, while moderate-to-severe stenosis does.

- Compared with aortic stenosis, PS usually has a less serious course and may be tolerated for years. Valve degeneration in the low-pressure pulmonary bed is slower compared to aortic valve stenoses.
- In some children with *mild* PS, the significance of PS may diminish as a result of growth. However, with *significant* PS, the severity rather tends to increase.
- Even severe PS may be asymptomatic for a prolonged period of time.
- Patients with syncope or angina are at risk of sudden death.
- Asymptomatic patients with mild to moderate PS and a peak gradient <60mmHg do not have a significantly limited prognosis.[5]
- The long-term survival of pediatric patients with isolated PS after surgical or catheter-based management is close to that in a healthy population. However, mortality on long-term follow-up is higher when a significant PS has not been eliminated until adulthood.[4]
- The short- and mid-term outcome of *balloon pulmonary valvuloplasty* in children and adults are excellent;[8,9] long-term data are currently unavailable.
- A favorable outcome of pulmonary valvuloplasty (with a decrease in Doppler-determined gradient <36mmHg without a need for reintervention) has been reported in 85% of patients with valvular PS not associated with dysplasia. By contrast, the outcome of valvuloplasty was suboptimal in 65% of patients with a dysplastic valve.[10]
- The long-term outcome of *surgical valvulotomy* is likewise excellent, with 96% of patients not requiring reoperation for 10 years; the 25-year survival rate is 97%, and 97% of surviving patients are in functional NYHA Class I.[7] Although overall survival after surgical treatment of isolated valvular PS remains excellent, many patients undergo late reintervention after 30 years of follow-up.[11]
- Some *secondary pulmonary regurgitation* is almost invariably present after balloon valvuloplasty, as well as after surgical valvulotomy. Its significance varies, usually being lower after a catheter-based procedure compared to surgery. Moderate to significant pulmonary regurgitation was seen in 28% of patients undergoing surgical valvulotomy.[7] Even severe residual pulmonary regurgitation is frequently well tolerated in the long run. Therefore, it is often regarded as an insignificant finding. However, even moderate residual pulmonary regurgitation has been associated with a reduced functional exercise capacity and an abnormal hemodynamic exercise response.[12] Prolonged volume overload results in right ventricular dilatation, systolic right ventricular dysfunction, and progressive tricuspid regurgitation. Right ventricle with a reduced compliance will develop diastolic dysfunction. The severity of residual pulmonary regurgitation increases in the presence of residual peripheral PS or pulmonary hypertension. If severe residual pulmonary regurgitation is present, valve replacement is required. In the case of secondary tricuspid regurgitation due to annulus dilatation the tricuspid annuloplasty is also performed.

References

1. Kelly DT, Spotnitz HM, Beiser GD, Pierce JE, Epstein SE. Effects of chronic right ventricular volume and pressure loading on left ventricular performance. Circulation 1971; 44: 403.
2. Stenberg RG, Fixler DE, Taylor AL, Corbett JR, Firth BG. Left ventricular dysfunction due to chronic right ventricular pressure overload. Resolution following percutaneous balloon valvuloplasty for pulmonary stenosis. Am J Med 1988; 84: 157.
3. Almeda FQ, Kavinsky CJ, Pophal SG, Klein LW. Pulmonic valvular stenosis in adults: Diagnosis and treatment. Catheter Cardiovasc Interv 2003; 60(4): 546–57.
4. Connelly MS, Webb GD, Somerville J et al. Canadian consensus conference on adult congenital heart disease 1996. Can J Cardiol 1998; 14(3): 395–452.
5. Redington A, Shore D, Oldershaw P. Congenital Heart Disease in Adults, 1st edn. London: WB Saunders Company, 1994.
6. Deanfield J, Thaulow E, Warnes C et al. Management of Grown up Congenital Heart Disease, The task force on the management of grown up congenital heart disease of the European Society of Cardiology. European Heart J 2003; 24: 1035–84.
7. Hayes CJ, Gersony WM, Driscoll DJ et al. Second natural history study of congenital heart defects. Results of treatment of patients with pulmonary valvar stenosis. Circulation 1993; 87(Suppl 2): I28–37.
8. Jarrar M, Betbout F, Farhat MB et al. Long-term invasive and noninvasive results of percutaneous balloon pulmonary valvuloplasty in children, adolescents, and adults. Am Heart J 1999; 138(5 Pt 1): 950–4.
9. Sharieff S, Shah-e-Zaman K, Faruqui AM. Short- and intermediate-term follow-up results of percutaneous transluminal balloon valvuloplasty in adolescents and young adults with congenital pulmonary valve stenosis. J Invasive Cardiol 2003; 15(9): 484–7.
10. McCrindle BW. Independent predictors of long-term results after balloon pulmonary valvuloplasty. Circulation 1994; 89: 1751–9.
11. Earing MG, Connolly HM, Dearani JA et al. Long-term follow-up of patients after surgical treatment for isolated pulmonary valve stenosis. Mayo Clin Proc 2005; 80(7): 871–6.
12. Marx GR, Hicks RW, Allen HD et al. Noninvasive assessment of hemodynamic responses to exercise in pulmonary regurgitation after operations to correct pulmonary outflow obstruction. Am J Cardiol 1988; 1: 595–601.

11

Transposition of the great arteries

Definition and anatomical notes

Transposition of the great arteries (TGA) refers to a condition where the position of the aorta and the pulmonary artery is reversed. In (complete) TGA, atrial and ventricular cardiac chambers are in atrioventricular concordance. The aorta arises from the morphologic right ventricle instead of the morphologic left, and the pulmonary artery arises from the morphologic left ventricle instead of the morphologic right ventricle (ventriculo-arterial discordance). The aorta is situated anterior and rightward from the pulmonary artery (d = dextroposition of the aorta). The pulmonary artery is localized posterior and leftward (Figures 11.1 and 11.2). The great vessels do not cross, and run in parallel (Figure 11.3). The coronary arteries arise from the aorta.

- *Simple transposition* (about 2 out of 3 cases) refers to TGA without associated defects.
- *Complex transposition* is associated with other defects, most often with ventricular septal defect and left ventricular outflow tract obstruction (LVOTO).

In TGA, the two circulations are separated, i.e. both circuits are parallel rather than in series. Desaturated blood from the body returns to the right atrium, the tricuspid valve, the morphologic right ventricle and to the aorta, so bypassing the lung. The aorta originates from the morphologic right ventricle, and is located anterior and rightward from the pulmonary artery. Oxygenated blood returns from the lungs via the left atrium, the mitral valve, and the morphologic left ventricle to the pulmonary artery, and is recirculated to the lungs.

The clinical manifestation depends on the presence of associated anatomic lesions. The *typical constellation* is:

1. *TGA with intact ventricular septum*
   Progressive cyanosis within the first days of life.
2. *TGA with large ventricular septal defect*
   Mild cyanosis; signs of congestive heart failure over the first weeks as pulmonary blood flow increases.
3. *TGA with ventricular septal defect (VSD) and LVOTO*
   Severe cyanosis at birth, depending on the degree of LVOTO (similar to tetralogy of Fallot).

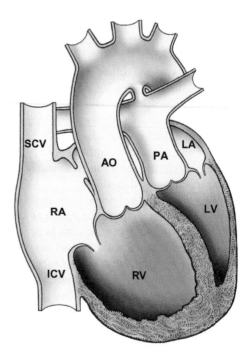

Figure 11.1
Transposition of the great arteries. ICV, Inferior caval vein; SCV, superior caval vein; RA, right atrium; RV, right ventricle; AO, aorta; PA, pulmonary artery; LA, left atrium; LV, left ventricle.

4. *TGA with VSD and pulmonary vascular obstructive disease*
   Progressive pulmonary vascular obstructive disease can prevent development of congestive heart failure, despite a large VSD.

TGA is incompatible with life, except accompanied by a communication between the two circuits (mostly an atrial septal defect (ASD) or a VSD, or a patent ductus arteriosus) which allows mixing of oxygenated and deoxygenated blood. In the first days after birth, mixing is taken over by a patent ductus arteriosus and a patent foramen ovale (PFO). In the presence of a VSD in complex TGA, blood mixes at ventricular level. At the same time, this is accompanied by rapid development of pulmonary vascular obstructive disease. Initial treatment in the newborn before surgery is continuous prostaglandin E_1 infusion to (re)open the duct and

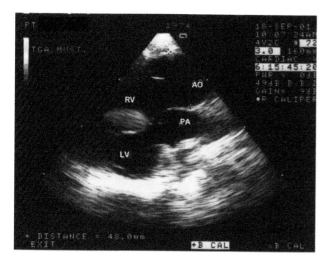

Figure 11.2
Transposition of the great arteries, long-axis parasternal view; transthoracic echo. AO, Aorta, dilated in front; LV, left ventricle; RV, right ventricle; PA, pulmonary artery arising from the left ventricle, behind aorta.

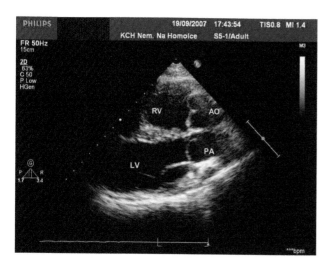

Figure 11.3
Transthoracic echo, parasternal long-axis view, d-transposition of the great arteries after Mustard correction. Aorta is in the front from the right ventricle, pulmonary artery is behind from the left ventricle, both great arteries run in parallel. AO, Aorta; PA, pulmonary artery; RV, right ventricle; LV, left ventricle.

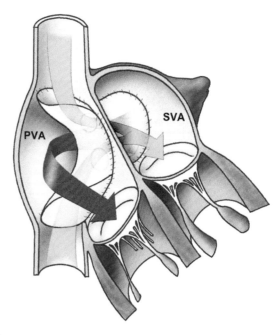

Figure 11.4
Mustard correction of transposition of the great arteries. Blue arrow shows the venous flow from superior and inferior caval veins through intra-atrial baffles to systemic venous atrium (SVA) and mitral valve orifice. Red arrow shows pulmonary venous flow redirected into pulmonary venous atrium (PVA) to tricuspid valve.

- Arterial switch procedure.
- Rastelli operation (in TGA with VSD and severe pulmonary stenosis).
- Atrial switch procedure (Mustard or Senning operation).
- Palliative Mustard or Senning operation (in TGA, VSD and pulmonary vascular obstructive disease).

Transposition of the great arteries after Mustard or Senning operation

Until the development of surgical atrial septectomy in the 1950s, no treatment was available for TGA. Since 1958, patients with TGA have been repaired at atrial level using the technique developed by Ake Senning, or, since 1963, the technique developed by William Mustard. The Mustard or Senning procedures (atrial 'switch') consist of retouring the systemic and pulmonary venous return at the atrial level.

In the Mustard modification, intra-atrial channels are created using a baffle from the patient's own pericardium, Dacron or Goretex (Figure 11.4). In the Senning modification, the patient's right atrial and atrial septal tissue is used (Figure 11.5). The venous blood flow is redirected by the baffle from the superior and inferior caval veins to the

to improve arterial oxygen saturation. In critical, severely hypoxemic patients with an inadequate interatrial communication and insufficient mixing, balloon atrial septostomy increases the shunt and mixing of blood at atrial level. This procedure is followed by corrective surgery (see the following sections in this chapter).

Associated cardiac anomalies define not only the clinical presentation but also the surgical management of TGA. Repair for TGA can be performed as:

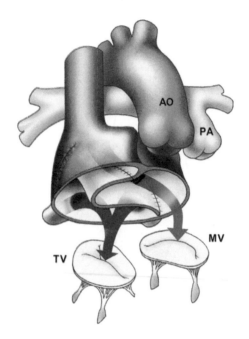

Figure 11.5
Sennings' correction of transposition of the great arteries. Blue arrow shows redirection of the systemic venous flow to mitral valve (MV), red arrow shows redirection of pulmonary venous flow to tricuspid valve (TV). AO, Aorta from right ventricle; PA, pulmonary artery from left ventricle.

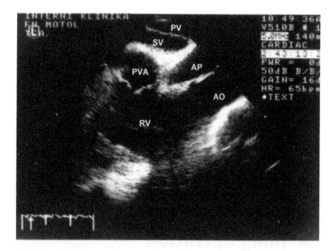

Figure 11.6
Transposition of the great arteries after Mustard correction; transesophageal echo, longitudinal view. Dilated aorta (AO) in front, arising from systemic right ventricle (RV). Behind aorta there is pulmonary artery (PA) coming from left ventricle. Pulmonary venous baffle (PV) is directed to pulmonary venous atrium (PVA). The baffle of systemic veins (SV) is directed to systemic venous atrium and mitral valve.

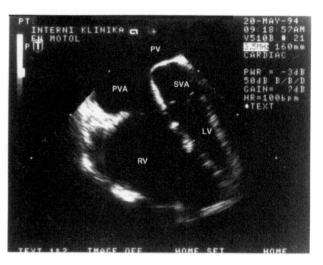

Figure 11.7
Transposition of the great arteries after Mustard correction; transesophageal echo, transversal view. PV, Pulmonary venous baffle; PVA, pulmonary venous atrium; SVA, systemic venous atrium; LV, small, subpulmonary left ventricle; RV, large subaortic right ventricle.

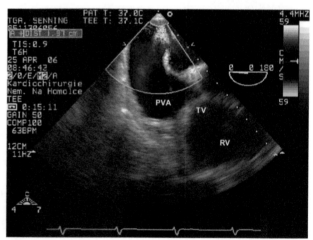

Figure 11.8
Transposition of the great arteries, Senning correction; transesophageal echo, 0 degrees. Red color shows laminar nonobstructive flow from the pulmonary veins baffle to the pulmonary veins atrium (PVA) and tricuspid valve (TV); RV, systemic right ventricle. Normal finding after Sennings' correction.

mitral valve and the morphologic left ventricle. Blood from the pulmonary veins is redirected to the tricuspid valve and the morphologic right ventricle. The atria are referred to as pulmonary venous atrium and systemic venous atrium. The morphologic left ventricle is referred to as subpulmonic ventricle, and the morphologic right ventricle as systemic or subarterial ventricle (Figure 11.6–11.9).

After the atrial switch operation, the morphologically right ventricle remains in the high-pressure systemic circulation, whereas the anatomically left ventricle remains in

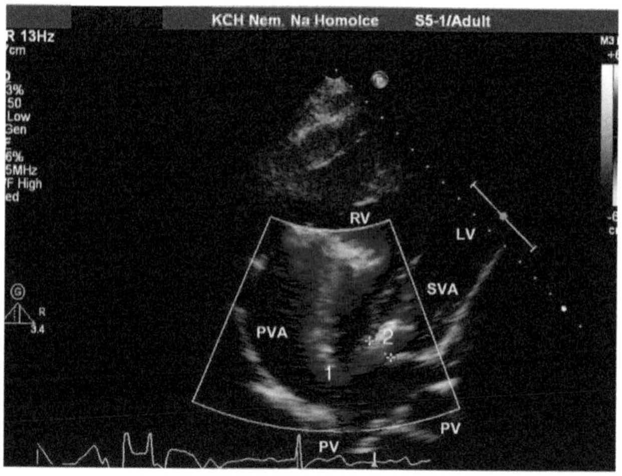

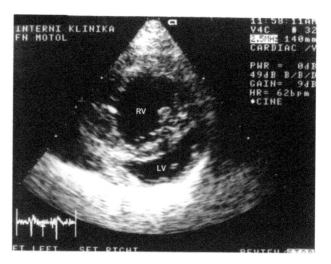

Figure 11.9

Transposition of the great arteries after Mustard correction; transthoracic echo, apical four-chamber view. 1, Pulmonary venous flow; 2, systemic venous flow; PVA, pulmonary venous atrium; RV, systemic high-pressure right ventricle; LV, subpulmonary low-pressure left ventricle; SVA, systemic venous atrium; PV, pulmonary veins.

Figure 11.11

Transposition of the great arteries after Mustard correction; transthoracic echo short axis. Circular shape of the systemic right ventricle (RV) and semilunar shape of the low-pressure subpulmonary left ventricle (LV).

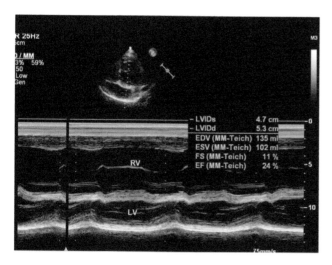

Figure 11.10

Transposition of the great arteries after Senning correction, M-mode, parasternal long-axis view. RV, Dilated, systemic right ventricle, with systolic dysfunction; LV, subpulmonary small left ventricle with normal ejection fraction (EF). Paradoxical septal motion.

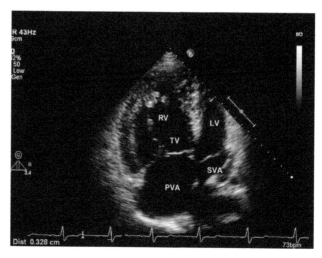

Figure 11.12

Transposition of the great arteries, Mustard correction; transthoracic echo. Systemic right ventricle (RV) is dilated with systolic dysfunction. Annulus of the tricuspid valve (TV) is dilated, motion of the leaflets is restrictive with mal-coaptation. Pulmonary veins atrium (PVA) is dilated; subpulmonary left ventricle (LV) is small. SVA, systemic veins atrium.

the low-pressure pulmonary circulation. The right ventricle becomes hypertrophied, dilated, featuring a circular cross-section, with the septum bulging leftward and contracting in favor of the right ventricle in systole (Figures 11.10 and 11.11). This adaptation mechanism to systemic pressures is usually effective during the first postoperative decades.

Later on, a proportion of patients will develop dysfunction and failure of the systemic right ventricle. This process is associated with the development of progressive tricuspid valve regurgitation (Figures 11.12 and 11.13). By contrast, the morphologic left ventricle is in a low-pressure circulation; consequently, its musculature does not tend to grow.

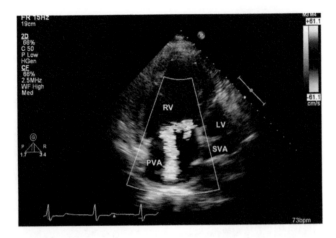

Figure 11.13
Transposition of the great arteries, Mustard correction; transthoracic echo, apical four-chamber view. The same patient as in Figure 11.18. Color flow shows massive regurgitation on the systemic AV valve, morphologically tricuspid. RV, Systemic right ventricle; LV, low-pressure left ventricle; PVA, pulmonary venous atrium; SVA, systemic venous atrium.

Risks and residual findings

- Without cardiac surgery, 90% of children with TGA die before 1 year of age. Almost only patients with TGA and a concomitant large VSD survive to adulthood without surgery.
- With improved diagnostic, medical, and surgical techniques, the overall survival rate is >90%.
- Today, most adult patients with TGA have had a Mustard or Senning operation, which has significantly improved long-term prognosis of children born with complete TGA. This type of correction was mainly used in the 1960s–1980s to treat TGA, but is now only rarely performed.
- Late survival after atrial switch procedure is ≤80% at 25–30 years.[1–5]
- Many patients feel well and lead a normal life.[6–8]
- However, progressive worsening of the systolic function of the systemic right ventricle, severe regurgitation on the morphologically tricuspid valve and heart failure may occur in a relatively short time, especially after 30 years of age.
- After the atrial switch procedure many patients have subnormal exercise capacities due to chronotropic incompetence, peripheral deconditioning, and impaired lung function.[9]

Long-term follow-up after intra-atrial repair for complete transposition shows that postoperative morphological and hemodynamic abnormalities exist in many patients. They may cause clinical deterioration in the long term, often necessitating therapeutic intervention. In order to detect anatomic and functional residuals and sequels, regular follow-up is necessary. The most important *residua and sequelae* are:

- failure of the right ventricle to sustain its function as the systemic pump;
- tricuspid regurgitation (from systemic high-pressure ventricle);
- obstruction of the LVOTO;
- obstructions of the systemic or the pulmonary venous blood flow;
- baffle leaks;
- arrhythmias;
- sudden death.

- The ability of the morphologic right systemic ventricle to support systemic circulation adequately in the long term is not known. Quantification of systolic and/or diastolic ventricular function under resting and/or stress conditions can be gained by Doppler echocardiogram, magnetic resonance imaging (MRI), computed tomography (CT), and radionuclide ventriculography.
- Significant systemic *right ventricular dysfunction* occurs in some 10% or more of cases. Severe systemic right ventricular dysfunction is a common cause of late death.[10,11] The incidence of right ventricular dysfunction rises with the duration of follow-up, particularly in the third to fifth decades of life. In addition, with increasing age, diastolic dysfunction also occurs.

The etiology of systemic ventricular dysfunction is multifactorial. Under discussion are duration and intensity of cyanosis and hypoxemia pre- and perioperatively, preexisting right ventricular dysfunction, abnormal geometry of the right ventricle, coronary perfusion – mainly from the right coronary artery, impaired myocardial flow reserve, myocardial perfusion defects, excessive right ventricular hypertrophy, higher age at operation, coexisting VSD.

- It is currently unknown how long the *tricuspid valve* (right-sided, systemic atrioventricular valve) can tolerate high systemic pressures. As after Mustard or Senning operation, the tricuspid valve is part of the high-pressure circulation, valve geometry, size and position of the papillary muscles in the morphologically right ventricle are not ideal for a high-pressure chamber. Dilatation of the tricuspid annulus, degenerative changes of the tricuspid valve and tricuspid regurgitation develop (Figures 11.12 and 11.13). Hemodynamically important *tricuspid regurgitation* can be found in up to 10% of patients following the atrial switch procedure. Tricuspid regurgitation is often progressive and is particularly observed in complex TGA. Tricuspid regurgitation is of outstanding importance when it results from systemic ventricular failure. In the presence of significant tricuspid regurgitation, systolic ventricular dysfunction is often underestimated.

- *Obstruction of the LVOTO* occurs in up to 33% of patients with complete transposition. The obstruction in cases with an intact ventricular septum predominantly represents dynamic stenosis, rarely being due to fibrosis or anomalous insertion of the mitral valve cords. In contrast, in the presence of a VSD, obstruction is often caused by a fibrotic tunnel. Some degree of LVOTO is mostly very well tolerated, and can even be protective against systemic ventricular failure.

- *Obstructions of the systemic or the pulmonary venous blood flow* represent an important complication. Obstructions can be incomplete or complete, isolated or combined in the systemic venous and pulmonary venous baffle leg.

- Baffle obstructions develop usually due to fibrosis, re-endothelialization or shrinkage of the baffle, and can worsen with time.

- Baffle obstruction can be a risk factor for cardiac death and contribute to exercise intolerance.[12]

- *Systemic venous obstructions* are present in 5–10% (up to 40%) of patients, and are typically located at the veno-atrial junctions or within the corresponding atrium. They can be seen predominantly in children who have undergone surgery in the first year of life, or in the early evolution of the atrial switch procedure.

- Some authors relate the development of obstructions to the location of sutures, to the extent of excision of the atrial septum, and to the size, form and material used for the baffle. Obstruction occurs more frequently with Dacron than with pericardial tissue (Figures 11.14 and 11.15).

- The dilation of the upstream caval veins, and/or a diameter of the azygos/hemiazygos vein >5mm, are signs of systemic venous obstruction. S*uperior* vena cava obstruction may develop without symptoms due to the decompression via the vena azygos system. Such collaterals may work as an overflow, and are mainly responsible for the development of the clinical symptoms, which occur in only 25–50% of the cases. Clinical examination alone, therefore, is not reliable in detecting and quantifying caval venous obstructions.

- Systemic venous obstruction can be of outstanding importance if it impedes ventricular filling, causing fixed stroke volume.

- *Pulmonary venous obstruction* is a severe complication encountered in 10% (up to 27%) of patients after atrial redirection. This complication is also associated with the surgical procedure, reflecting an unfavorable size or location of the baffle, age at time of surgery, or use of Dacron as the patch material. Obstruction of the pulmonary venous baffle manifests itself by dyspnea and pulmonary congestion, but there is no enlargement of the heart.

- Important *baffle leaks*, with a large shunt at atrial level, represent a rare complication, whereas small leaks are frequent (Figures 11.16–11.18). Baffle leaks may cause

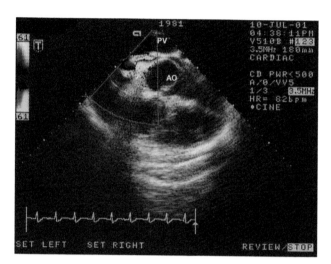

Figure 11.14
Transesophageal echo, transversal projection in a patient with transposition of the great arteries after Mustard correction with turbulent flow (color) in the narrowed and obstructed upper limb of the systemic venous baffle. PV, Pulmonary venous baffle; AO, aorta.

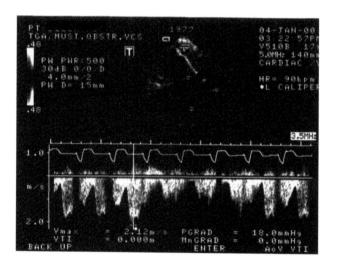

Figure 11.15
Pulse Doppler signal from narrowed and obstructed lower limb of the systemic venous baffle in a patient with transposition of the great arteries after Mustard correction. Transesophageal echo + pulse Doppler. Maximal velocity is >2m/s, whereas without obstruction there are much lower velocities in the atrial baffles.

right-to-left, left-to-right or bidirectional shunts, dependent on the ventricular compliance. A right-to-left or bidirectional shunt can be associated with cyanosis and paradoxical embolism.[13] Only 1–2% of patients have shunts requiring reoperation.

- Following the Mustard procedure, *sinus rhythm* is present in 77% of cases at 5 years and in only 40% at 20 years.[14] *Progressive sinus node dysfunction* and *supraventricular*

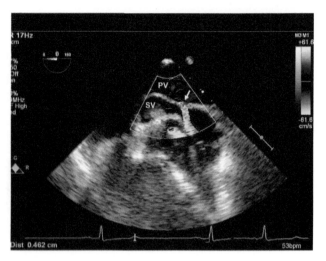

Figure 11.16
Transposition of the great arteries, Mustard correction; transesophageal echo, 0 degree. Color Doppler flow shows small leak (arrow) between pulmonary veins baffle (PV) and upper limb of the systemic vein baffle (SV) with small left-to-right shunt.

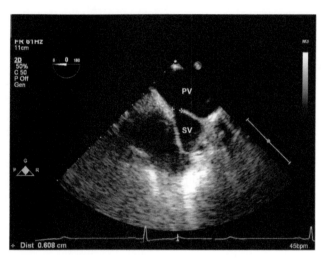

Figure 11.18
Transposition of the great arteries, Mustard; transesophageal echo. The same patient as in Figures 11.16 and 11.17. Small leak in the patch between pulmonary veins baffle (PV) and upper limb of the systemic veins baffle (SV).

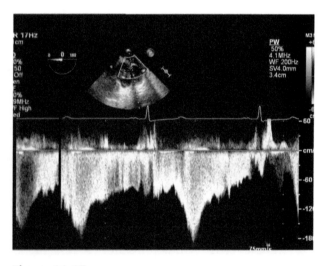

Figure 11.17
Transposition of the great arteries, Mustard correction; transesophageal echo. The same patient as in Figure 11.16. Continuous flow from left (pulmonary veins baffle) to right (systemic veins baffle).

tachycardia are common, increase with age and are often poorly tolerated. Sinus node dysfunction may develop due to fibrosis of the sinus node and the adjacent tissue as a result of atrial surgery.

- *Intra-atrial reentrant tachycardia* is the most common arrythmia.
- Supraventricular tachycardia and sinus node dysfunction can coexist.
- Atrial flutter occurs in about 20% of patients while atrial fibrillation and ventricular arrhythmia are less frequent. Inadequate sinus node acceleration during exercise

contributes to inadequate cardiac output and reduced exercise tolerance, as well as to the loss of atrial contraction.

- *Bradyarrhythmia* occurs frequently after intra-atrial correction.
- *Sudden death* seems to occur due to atrial arrythmia and loss of sinus rhythm in 6–17 % of patients, often during exercise.[5,15,16]

In rare cases, patients with TGA, VSD and pulmonary vascular obstructive disease have had a *'palliative' Mustard or Senning operation*, where an atrial switch procedure has been performed, while the VSD remains open. This operation improves systemic arterial oxygen saturation and quality of life in selected patients with TGA, VSD, and severe pulmonary vascular obstructive disease. Late survival for early survivors at 15 years is 54%.[17]

Clinical findings and diagnosis

Symptoms

- Following intra-atrial TGA repair, many patients are asymptomatic or show only slightly reduced exercise tolerance. Exertional dyspnea and paroxysmal nocturnal dyspnea already herald severe dysfunction and failure of the systemic right ventricle or, less often, obstruction of the pulmonary venous baffle.

Clinical findings

- Increased jugular vein filling without pulsation is only sometimes present in *superior* vena cava obstruction.

Significant *inferior* systemic venous obstruction can be associated with hepatomegaly without pulsation. Obstruction of both systemic venous baffle legs results in morning swelling of the face, leg edema and, possibly, even ascites.

- Patients with a low cardiac output state that they feel tired and dyspneic.
- Syncope occurs more often due to tachyarrhythmia than because of bradyarrhythmia. In particular, atrial flutter with fast conduction is very poorly tolerated. Another rare cause of syncope may be central nervous embolism.

Auscultatory findings

- As the aorta is situated anterior, close to the chest wall, the second sound is usually single and loud.
- A systolic ejection murmur along the left upper sternal border reflects LVOTO.
- A systolic regurgitant murmur at the left lower sternal border and at the apex is usually indicative of tricuspid regurgitation.
- An early diastolic murmur resembles baffle obstruction or significant tricuspid regurgitation.

Electrocardiogram (ECG)

- There is usually a rightward tilt of the cardiac axis and right ventricular hypertrophy.
- Sinus rhythm is infrequent; there is usually a supraventricular escape rhythm originating from the lower part of the atrium or a junctional rhythm.
- Exercise may result in resumption of sinus rhythm, which is not evident at rest.

Holter ECG monitoring and exercise tests

- Holter ECG monitoring and exercise tests should be performed at least once a year, even in asymptomatic patients, after the Mustard or Senning operation.
- Repeated Holter monitoring is particularly indicated in presyncopal and syncopal states.

Chest X-ray

- The upper mediastinum is usually narrow relative to the apposition of the great vessels in TGA; however, it may become broad by a dilated superior vena cava and the vena azygos system in case of superior systemic venous baffle obstruction.
- A small heart with pulmonary congestion or pulmonary edema is pathognomonic for pulmonary venous baffle obstruction.
- Mild cardiomegaly is a rule following atrial switch operation.

Echocardiography

- A transthoracic examination (TTE) may be difficult to perform in some adults. In particular, proper assessment of the baffle can be problematic. TTE is mostly sufficient to evaluate ventricular size and function, as well as atrio-ventricular valve function (Figures 11.9–11.13).
- Casually, TTE allows us to visualize the intra-atrial baffle in four-chamber apical projection (Figure 11.9), long-axis parasternal view or, alternatively, in subcostal projection.
- Exact assessment of the intra-atrial baffle in adults will often require transesophageal echocardiography (TEE) (Figures 11.6–11.8).
- The systemic venous baffle is situated anterior and medial, whereas the pulmonary venous baffle is located posterior and lateral (Figure 11.8).
- Moreover, attention is focused on LVOTO (Figures 11.14 and 11.15), and on the presence of baffle leaks (Figures 11.16–11.18).
- Transtricuspid and transmitral diastolic flow may be difficult to assess.
- A cross-section of the right ventricle is circular, while that of the left ventricle is crescent-shaped (Figure 11.11).

Catheterization

- Invasive diagnostic procedures should be performed in specialized centers only.
- Catheterization and angiography are carried out prior to catheter-based or surgical procedures, or in the case of inconclusive diagnosis.
- If systemic venous baffle obstruction is suspected, selective angiography of the vena cava superior and inferior is undertaken. The gradient may be small in the case of decompression of the obstruction via the venous azygos system.
- Pulmonary venous baffle obstruction, which may be unilateral, requires bilateral simultaneous assessment of capillary wedge pressure and diastolic right ventricular pressure.
- Selective angiography of the right and left pulmonary artery branches may identify the site of obstruction.
- Right ventricular end-diastolic pressure after the atrial switch operation is usually higher than the end-diastolic pressure in a normal systemic left ventricle.
- Complete catheterization, including coronary angiography, is recommended in patients older than 40 years of age and/or prior to a reintervention.

Radionuclide angiography/MRI

- Radionucide angiography is mainly used to assess systemic ventricular function.
- MRI particularly provides exact assessment of biventricular function and evaluation of baffle obstruction.

Management of residual findings

- *Systemic right ventricular dysfunction* is often treated empirically by afterload reduction, beta blockers, diuretics and/or by cardiotonic agents. Currently, these strategies have not been evaluated in clinical randomized trials, and only scarce data are available from small trials demonstrating a beneficial effect of ACE inhibitors, angiotensin-II antagonists or beta blockers on systemic right ventricular function and exercise capacity at best in a subset of patients.[18–21]
- Some patients with a systemic right ventricular and electromechanical dyssynchrony may benefit from cardiac resynchronization therapy.[22]
- Patients with severe symptomatic right ventricular dysfunction should be listed for heart transplantation.
- In adults, 'late arterial switch' is still considered experimental. This type of reoperation necessitates a prior left (subpulmonary) ventricular reconditioning to systemic pressures, using pulmonary artery banding and conversion as a second step months later. Operative mortality is high and this type of operation is currently performed only in a few centers worldwide.
- *Tricuspid regurgitation* may necessitate tricuspid valve replacement or tricuspid valve repair, provided the tricuspid regurgitation does not result from systemic ventricular failure. If so, tricuspid surgery will usually not be able to secure long-standing improvement. The procedure is associated, in adults, with higher mortality rates compared with standard mitral valve replacement.
- Transcatheter device closure of atrial *baffle leaks*, e.g. using the Amplatzer septal occluder, is a suitable alternative to surgical closure.[13]
- *Superior and inferior systemic venous baffle obstruction* is managed by catheter-based angioplasty, possibly with stent implantation, or surgically.[23]
- Management of *pulmonary venous baffle obstruction* is difficult and surgery is often required in significant obstruction.
- *Atrial flutter, atrial and nodal reentry tachycardia* may require ablation therapy under control of electroanatomical mapping using three-dimensional mapping and navigating system (e.g. CARTO).[24] The procedure should only be performed in a specialized center with experience in CHD.
- *A modified Maze procedure* can be performed in patients who require cardiac surgery.
- Permanent stimulation for sino-atrial (*SA*) *nodal dysfunction* has often been performed, particularly in former times (in up to 25% of patients).[25,26] The pacemaker lead is inserted, via the superior systemic venous baffle leg, into the morphologic left ventricle, where it should be actively fixed. Before a transvenous stimulation lead is inserted, a residual shunt (baffle leak) should be ruled out using transesophageal echocardiography to exclude the risk for paradoxical embolism, and to assess the diameter of the baffle leg because of the risk of obstruction. An alternative approach is epicardial stimulation.

Pregnancy

Pregnancy is often well tolerated, particularly if the patient is in a low functional class and has good systemic ventricular function. However, the long-term effect of pregnancy on the systemic ventricle is not known. Moreover, a high incidence of obstetric complications and mortality in the offspring occurs.[27] Deterioration of systemic right ventricular function may occur during pregnancy or after delivery – in about 10% of patients – and is sometimes irreversible.[28] Moreover, arrythmia, stroke and death tend to occur.[29] It is appropriate to plan pregnancy after an atrial switch operation, together with experienced cardiologists and obstetricians. ACE inhibitor therapy should be discontinued before a planned pregnancy.

Infectious endocarditis

The risk of infectious endocarditis (IE) is high, especially in patients with valvular dysfunction and if foreign material has been used during the operation.

Transposition of the great arteries after Rastelli operation

Patients with TGA, VSD, and severe fixed valvular or subvalvular pulmonary stenosis may undergo anatomical correction according to Rastelli (Figures 11.19–11.27). This operation has the advantage of incorporating the left ventricle as the systemic ventricle. A large intraventricular baffle is sutured into place, closing the VSD and redirecting the left ventricular outflow to the more anterior placed aortic valve. The connection between the left ventricle and the pulmonary artery is closed and a valved conduit (a valved Hancock Dacron conduit, a porcine xenograft or a human homograft) is placed between the right ventricle and the pulmonary artery (Figures 11.23 and 11.24).

Risks and residual findings

- Despite excellent early results, late follow-up indicates a high prevalence of pulmonary conduit obstruction, LVOTO, arrhythmia, and death.[30]
- A typical late finding is conduit degeneration with *valvular stenosis* and/or *regurgitation*. *Stenosis* of the *extracardiac conduit* is usually located at the proximal or

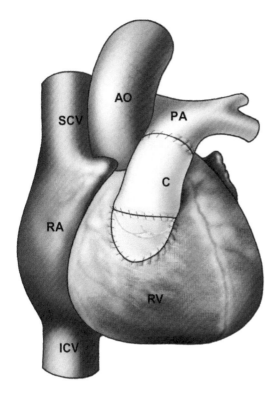

Figure 11.19
Rastelli correction of transposition of the great arteries.
ICV, Inferior caval vein; SCV, superior caval vein; RA, right atrium;
RV, right ventricle; AO, aorta; PA, pulmonary artery;
LA, left atrium; LV, left ventricle; C, conduit from right
ventricle to pulmonary artery.

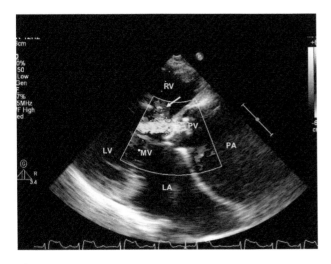

Figure 11.20
Unoperated 41-year-old lady with d-transposition of the great
arteries, ventricular septal defect (arrow), severe pulmonary
stenosis, moderate pulmonary regurgitation (color flow),
pulmonary hypertension and extremely large pulmonary artery
aneurysm (11cm in diameter). LV, Left ventricle; MV, mitral
valve; LA, left atrium; PV, pulmonary valve, severely calcified,
severely stenotic and moderately insufficient; PA, pulmonary
artery arising from the left ventricle with huge aneurysm.

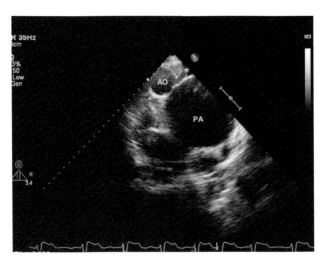

Figure 11.21
Transthoracic echo from higher intercostal space. Unoperated
d-transposition of the great arteries; the same patient as in
Figure 11.20. Aorta (AO) is in the front and right with
severely dilated coronary arteries (*), pulmonary artery
(PA) is behind, to the left, arising from the left ventricle and
severely dilated.

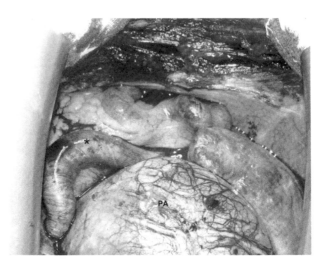

Figure 11.22
d-Transposition of the great arteries, unoperated until
adulthood; the same patient as in Figures 11.20 and 11.21.
Surgical view. Dilated and tortuous coronary arteries (*) and
aneurysm of the pulmonary artery (PA). (Courtesy of Dr Stepan
Cerny, Chief of the Dept of Cardiac Surgery, Hospital Na Homolce,
Prague, Czech Republic.)

distal conduit anastomosis. Valve degeneration and
calcification often occur some time after surgery.
Obstruction may also result from conduit kinking.
- Left ventricular dysfunction may be a sequel of preoperative hypoxemia and intraoperative injury.

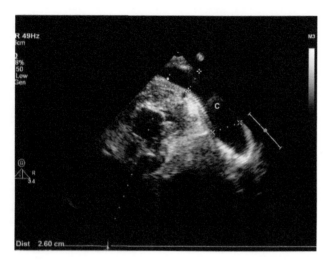

Figure 11.23
Transposition of the great arteries, Rastelli correction performed in adulthood; transthoracic echo. Conduit (C) with bioprothesis from the right ventricle to pulmonary trunk-bifurcation. See also Figure 11.24.

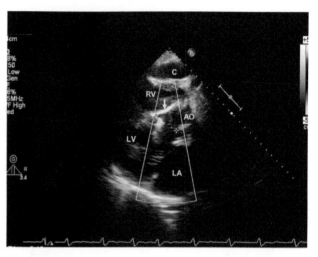

Figure 11.25
Transposition of the great arteries after Rastelli correction. Aorta is redirected over the left ventricle by patch (arrow); color flow shows laminar unobstructed flow from the left ventricle (LV) to aorta (AO) through original ventricular septal defect. LA, Left atrium; RV, hypertrophic right ventricle; C, conduit from the right ventricle to pulmonary artery branches.

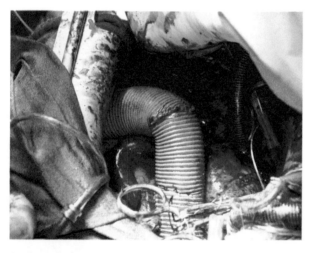

Figure 11.24
Transposition of the great arteries, Rastelli correction in adulthood. Surgical view. Conduit with bioprosthesis from the right ventricle to pulmonary trunk. (Courtesy of Dr Stepan Cerny, Chief of the Dept of Cardiac Surgery, Hospital Na Homolce, Prague, Czech Republic.)

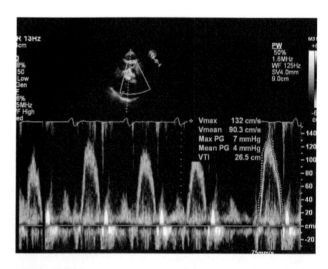

Figure 11.26
Transposition of the great arteries after Rastelli correction; transthoracic echo, pulsed Doppler flow in the left ventricular outflow tract shows laminar flow without obstruction from the left ventricle through original ventricular septal defeat now redirected to aorta. See also Figure 11.25.

- There may be atrioventricular valve regurgitation, with mitral regurgitation being a prognostic serious finding.
- *Subaortic obstruction* may occur in the area of the intracardiac patch (Figures 11.25–11.27).
- Aortic regurgitation may develop in the long run.
- At the site of the patch, there may be a residual interventricular shunt.
- Sustained ventricular and supraventricular tachycardia occur.

Clinical examination and diagnosis
Auscultatory findings

- An audible pulmonary component of the second sound is inconsistent with obstruction, whereas a nonsplit second sound will usually signal stenosis and fibrosis or calcification of the pulmonary conduit valve.

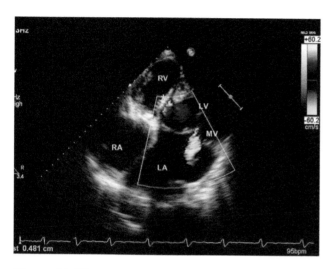

Figure 11.27
Transposition of the great arteries, after Rastelli correction; transthoracic echo, apical four-chamber view. The same patients as in Figures 11.20–11.26. Hypertrophic right ventricle (RV). RA, Right atrium; LV, left ventricle; MV, mitral valve with small residual regurgitation; LA, dilated left atrium; *, patch; red colored flow from left ventricle to outflow tract and aorta.

• A systolic ejection murmur is usually present at the left upper sternal border due to pulmonary stenosis and, in the presence of pulmonary regurgitation, also a diastolic murmur.

ECG

• Rightward deviation of the cardiac axis.
• Often complete right bundle branch block.

Chest X-ray

• Mild cardiomegaly is frequent.
• Calcification of the extracardiac pulmonary conduit may be found.
• A side difference in the pulmonary vasculature may suggest pulmonary artery branch stenosis.

Echocardiography

• The native pulmonary artery is usually closed during surgery.
• The conduit is visualized in the parasternal short axis from a higher intercostal space.
• Two-dimensional echocardiography will visualize calcifications, Doppler echocardiography will determine obstruction severity, color Doppler echocardiography will semiquantitatively determine the significance of pulmonary regurgitation.
• The significance of pulmonary stenosis can be assessed by determining the gradient in tricuspid regurgitation.

• A residual shunt at ventricular level, and aortic and mitral valve function are evaluated using routine techniques.
• Transesophageal echocardiography will be required in adults with poor-quality images.

Catheterization

Catheterization is performed only in the case of doubt regarding the presence and significance of pulmonary stenosis, residual VSD or if pulmonary artery branch stenosis is suspected.

Management

• After Rastelli operation, reintervention is indicated in significant graft stenosis (pullback cath-gradient >60mmHg), in significant regurgitation, in significant obstruction across the LVOT, in significant VSD.
• Balloon dilatation of the conduit is often not successful.
• Balloon angioplasty, possibly with stent implantation, is often successful in patients with pulmonary artery branch stenosis.

Pregnancy

Women can have successful pregnancies after Rastelli repair, provided significant residua are absent. In particular, pulmonary conduit degeneration and subaortic stenosis can become a problem and should ideally be eliminated before pregnancy. Careful cardiac evaluation before, during and after pregnancy is essential.[31]

Infectious endocarditis

The risk of IE is high when using foreign materials; however, the risk is also present with degenerated homografts.

Prognosis

• Rastelli repair can be performed with a low early mortality.[30]
• After 20 years, freedom from death and transplantation was 52%, freedom from death and reintervention after 15 years was 21%.[30]
• A considerable percentage of patients require repeated conduit changes because of conduit degeneration.[32]

Transposition of the great arteries after anatomical correction according to Jatene

Anatomical correction at the level of the great arteries (arterial 'switch') has been performed since the mid-70s (Figure

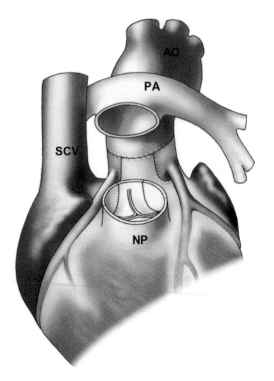

Figure 11.28
Arterial correction of transposition of the great arteries according to Jatene. NP, Neopulmonary valve, morphologically aortic; PA, pulmonary artery; AO, aorta; SCV, superior caval vein.

11.28). Anatomical operation should be undertaken in the early neonatal age, when the left ventricular mass is still adequate for the systemic circulation. Otherwise the left ventricular mass decreases rapidly if the left ventricle remains in the low-pressure pulmonary circulation.

The operation consists of dividing the aorta and pulmonary artery above the valvular level, connecting the aorta to the left ventricle, and the pulmonary artery to the right ventricle. The semilunar valves remain attached to their ventricle. The original pulmonary valve becomes the aortic valve and vice versa. The coronary arteries are removed from their attachment to the aorta and reimplanted with a cuff of aortic wall into the neoaorta. An intramural course of the coronary arteries occurs in some 3–7% of TGA patients, may cause intraoperative technical problems and contribute to a higher postoperative mortality rate. If present, a VSD or ASD is also closed as part of the operation.

There is a structural difference between the normal neonatal aorta and pulmonary artery. The neoaortic valve (morphological pulmonary valve) has thinner cusps, contains less collagen and elastin compared to the aortic valve, and is not designed for long-term function in a high-pressure circulation. It may degenerate and regurgitate early.

The great arteries in TGA differ from each other and from normal vessels. In the sinus of the pulmonary artery of untreated TGA, there is a dedifferentiation of smooth muscle cells, providing an explanation for the neoaortic root dilatation after the arterial switch operation.[33]

Risks and residual findings

- Supravalvular pulmonary artery stenosis, caused by scarring at the anastomosis, requires reintervention in about 5–30% of patients.
- Supravalvular aortic stenosis occurs less often, with reintervention required by some 2% of patients.
- Right ventricular outflow tract obstruction (RVOTO) arises in the presence of a hypertrophic infundibulum.
- Progressive dilatation of the neoaortic root occurs more often in complex TGA.
- Neoaortic valve regurgitation (anatomical pulmonary valve) occurs in up to 50% of patients.
- Coronary artery orifice stenoses may occur due to scarring in the area of anastomosis or impaired growth of the anastomosis, resulting in myocardial ischemia at rest or during exercise.

Management

- After the arterial switch operation there may be a need for interventional or surgical intervention on the supravalvular pulmonary stenosis.
- Progressive significant aortic regurgitation, possibly with dilatation of the neoaortic root, may require surgical reintervention.
- Treatment of coronary stenosis is still a matter of debate. Primary percutaneous transluminal coronary angioplasty (PTCA) of stenotic proximal coronary arteries after the arterial switch procedure seems to be effective.[34]

Infectious endocarditis

The risk of IE is dependent on the morphological finding and function of the semilunar valves, and/or other residual findings.

Follow-up

All TGA patients should be followed-up by a cardiologist with experience in managing CHD, working in close cooperation with a specialized center.

Prognosis

- Today, the arterial switch operation is the procedure of choice for all forms of TGA.
- Long-term outcome data are as yet unavailable.

- After up to 15 years of follow-up, the late outcome of TGA after the arterial switch operation is better than that of the atrial switch operation.[35–37]
- The late mortality is low.
- Reoperations are less frequent than after atrial switch operation.[37]
- Patients with complex TGA are more prone to reintervention.
- Pulmonary stenosis is a major cause for reoperation.[36]
- Supravalvular pulmonary stenoses are of concern.[38]
- Progressive neoaortic root dilation and neoaortic regurgitation have been reported, and some of these patients require neoaortic root or valve surgery.[33,40]
- Coronary stenosis is dependent of the prior coronary status; 3% to 11% of all survivors have proximal coronary stenosis or complete occlusion developing after arterial switch operations.[34]
- Left ventricular function is generally good. However, a significant proportion of asymptomatic children have impaired LV contractility and reversible myocardial perfusion defects and mild wall motion abnormalities on stress.[41]
- Sinus rhythm is maintained in almost all patients after arterial switch operation.
- The incidence of postoperative dysrhythmia is significantly lower compared to the *atrial* switch operation.
- Late postoperative infarction has been reported in 1–2%, asymptomatic collateralized coronary artery occlusion in 1–2%, respectively.
- The incidence of perfusion defects during exercise testing is high, yet their clinical relevance remains unclear.
- *On long-term follow-up, attention is focused on coronary artery function and neoaortic valve function.*

References

1. Dodge-Khatami A, Kadner A, Berger Md F et al. In the footsteps of Senning: Lessons learned from atrial repair of transposition of the great arteries. Ann Thorac Surg 2005; 79(4): 1433–44.
2. Moons P, Gewillig M, Sluysmans T et al. Long term outcome up to 30 years after the Mustard or Senning operation: A nationwide multicentre study in Belgium. Heart 2004; 90(3): 307–13.
3. Oechslin E, Jenni R. 40 years after the first atrial switch procedure in patients with transposition of the great arteries: Long-term results in Toronto and Zurich. Thorac Cardiovasc Surg 2000; 48(4): 233–7.
4. Roos-Hesselink JW, Meijboom FJ, Spitaels SE et al. Decline in ventricular function and clinical condition after Mustard repair for transposition of the great arteries (a prospective study of 22–29 years). Eur Heart J 2004; 25(14): 1264–70.
5. Wilson NJ, Clarkson PM, Barratt-Boyes BG et al. Long-term outcome after the Mustard repair for simple transposition of the great arteries. 28-year follow-up. J Am Coll Cardiol 1998; 32(3): 758–65.
6. Bolger AP, Gatzoulis MA. Towards defining heart failure in adults with congenital heart disease. Int J Cardiol 2004; 97 (Suppl 1): 15–23.
7. Ebenroth ES, Hurwitz RA. Functional outcome of patients operated for d-transposition of the great arteries with the Mustard procedure. Am J Cardiol 2002; 89(3): 353–6.
8. Moons P, De Bleser L, Budts W et al. Health status, function abilities, and quality of life after the Mustard or Senning operation. Ann Thorac Surg 2004; 77(4): 1359–65.
9. Hechter SJ, Webb G, Fredriksen PM et al. Cardiopulmonary exercise performance in adult survivors of the Mustard procedure. Cardiol Young 2001; 11(4): 407–14.
10. Carrel T, Pfammatter JP. Complete transposition of the great arteries: Surgical concepts for patients with systemic right ventricular failure following intraatrial repair. Thorac Cardiovasc Surg 2000; 48(4): 224–7.
11. Oechslin EN, Harrison DA, Connelly MS, Webb GD, Siu SC. Mode of death in adults with congenital heart disease. Am J Cardiol 2000; 86(10): 1111–16.
12. Gewillig M, Cullen S, Mertens B, Lesaffre E, Deanfield J. Risk factors for arrhythmia and death after Mustard operation for simple transposition of the great arteries. Circulation 1991; 84 (Suppl 5): III187–III92.
13. Balzer DT, Johnson M, Sharkey AM, Kort H. Transcatheter occlusion of baffle leaks following atrial switch procedures for transposition of the great vessels (d-TGV). Catheter Cardiovasc Interv 2004; 61(2): 259–63.
14. Gelatt M, Hamilton RM, McCrindle BW et al. Arrhythmia and mortality after the Mustard procedure: A 30-year single-center experience. J Am Coll Cardiol 1997; 29(1): 194–201.
15. Kammeraad JA, van Deurzen CH, Sreeram N et al. Predictors of sudden cardiac death after Mustard or Senning repair for transposition of the great arteries. J Am Coll Cardiol 2004; 44(5): 1095–102.
16. Sun ZH, Happonen JM, Bennhagen R et al. Increased QT dispersion and loss of sinus rhythm as risk factors for late sudden death after Mustard or Senning procedures for transposition of the great arteries. Am J Cardiol 2004; 94(1): 138–41.
17. Burkhart HM, Dearani JA, Williams WG et al. Late results of palliative atrial switch for transposition, ventricular septal defect, and pulmonary vascular obstructive disease. Ann Thorac Surg 2004; 77(2): 464–8; discussion 468–9.
18. Dore A, Houde C, Chan KL et al. Angiotensin receptor blockade and exercise capacity in adults with systemic right ventricles: A multicenter, randomized, placebo-controlled clinical trial. Circulation 2005; 112(16): 2411–16.
19. Hechter SJ, Fredriksen PM, Liu P et al. Angiotensin-converting enzyme inhibitors in adults after the Mustard procedure. Am J Cardiol 2001; 87(5): 660–3, A11.
20. Lester SJ, McElhinney DB, Viloria E et al. Effects of losartan in patients with a systemically functioning morphologic right ventricle after atrial repair of transposition of the great arteries. Am J Cardiol 2001; 88(11): 1314–16.
21. Robinson B, Heise CT, Moore JW et al. Afterload reduction therapy in patients following intraatrial baffle operation for transposition of the great arteries. Pediatr Cardiol 2002; 23(6): 618–23.
22. Janousek J, Tomek V, Chaloupecky VA et al. Cardiac resynchronization therapy: A novel adjunct to the treatment and prevention of systemic right ventricular failure. J Am Coll Cardiol 2004; 44(9): 1927–31.
23. Brown SC, Eyskens B, Mertens L et al. Self expandable stents for relief of venous baffle obstruction after the Mustard operation. Heart 1998; 79(3): 230–3.
24. Zrenner B, Dong J, Schreieck J et al. Delineation of intra-atrial reentrant tachycardia circuits after Mustard operation for transposition of the great arteries using biatrial electroanatomic mapping and entrainment mapping. J Cardiovasc Electrophysiol 2003; 14(12): 1302–10.
25. Hornung TS, Derrick GP, Deanfield JE, Redington AN. Transposition complexes in the adult: A changing perspective. Cardiol Clin 2002; 20(3): 405–20.
26. Kirjavainen M, Happonen JM, Louhimo I. Late results of Senning operation. J Thorac Cardiovasc Surg 1999; 117(3): 488–95.
27. Drenthen W, Pieper PG, Ploeg M et al; ZAHARA Investigators. Risk of complications during pregnancy after Senning or Mustard (atrial) repair of complete transposition of the great arteries. Eur Heart J 2005; 26(23): 2588–95. (Epub 2005 Aug 25).

28. Guedes A, Mercier LA, Leduc L et al. Impact of pregnancy on the systemic right ventricle after a Mustard operation for transposition of the great arteries J Am Coll Cardiol 2004; 44(2): 433–7.

29. Siu SC, Sermer M, Colman JM et al; Cardiac Disease in Pregnancy (CARPREG) Investigators. Prospective multicenter study of pregnancy outcomes in women with heart disease. Circulation 2001; 104(5): 515–21.

30. Kreutzer C, De Vive J, Oppido G et al. Twenty-five-year experience with Rastelli repair for transposition of the great arteries. J Thorac Cardiovasc Surg 2000; 120(2): 211–23.

31. Radford DJ, Stafford G. Pregnancy and the Rastelli operation. Aust NZ J Obstet Gynaecol 2005; 45(3): 243–7.

32. Dearani JA, Danielson GK, Puga FJ, Mair DD, Schleck CD. Late results of the Rastelli operation for transposition of the great arteries. Semin Thorac Cardiovasc Surg Pediatr Card Surg Annu 2001; 4: 3–15.

33. Lalezari S, Hazekamp MG, Bartelings MM, Schoof PH, Gittenberger-De Groot AC. Pulmonary artery remodeling in transposition of the great arteries: Relevance for neoaortic root dilatation. J Thorac Cardiovasc Surg 2003; 126(4): 1053–60.

34. Kampmann C, Kuroczynski W, Trubel H et al. Late results after PTCA for coronary stenosis after the arterial switch procedure for transposition of the great arteries. Ann Thorac Surg 2005; 80(5): 1641–6.

35. Hutter PA, Kreb DL, Mantel SF et al. Twenty-five years' experience with the arterial switch operation. J Thorac Cardiovasc Surg 2002; 124(4): 790–7.

36. Losay J, Touchot A, Serraf A et al. Late outcome after arterial switch operation for transposition of the great arteries. Circulation 2001; 104 (Suppl 12 1): I121–I126.

37. Williams WG, McCrindle BW, Ashburn DA et al; Congenital Heart Surgeon's Society. Outcomes of 829 neonates with complete transposition of the great arteries 12–17 years after repair. Eur J Cardiothorac Surg 2003; 24(1): 1–9; discussion 9–10.

38. Rehnstrom P, Gilljam T, Sudow G, Berggren H. Excellent survival and low complication rate in medium-term follow-up after arterial switch operation for complete transposition. Scand Cardiovasc J 2003; 37(2): 104–6.

39. Hovels-Gurich HH, Seghaye MC, Ma Q et al. Long-term results of cardiac and general health status in children after neonatal arterial switch operation. Ann Thorac Surg 2003; 75(3): 935–43.

40. Schwartz ML, Gauvreau K, del Nido P, Mayer JE, Colan SD. Long-term predictors of aortic root dilation and aortic regurgitation after arterial switch operation. Circulation 2004; 110 (11 Suppl 1): II128–II132.

41. Hui L, Chau AK, Leung MP, Chiu CS, Cheung YF. Assessment of left ventricular function long term after arterial switch operation for transposition of the great arteries by dobutamine stress echocardiography. Heart 2005; 91(1): 68–72.

12

Congenitally corrected transposition of the great arteries

Definition and anatomical notes

Congenitally corrected transposition of the great arteries (CCTGA) is a rare defect in which the ventricles are arranged in atrioventricular (AV) discordance and, at the same time, a ventriculo-arterial discordance exists (double discordance). Despite the natural disarrangement of the cardiac chambers and valves, the blood streams in normal sequence, and the flow is functionally correct. However, the morphologic *right* ventricle supports systemic circulation (Figure 12.1).

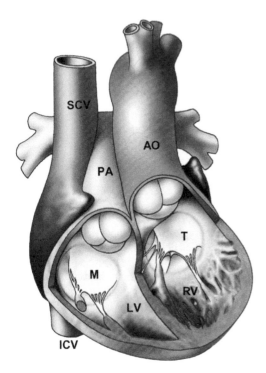

Figure 12.1
Congenitally corrected transposition of the great arteries.
AO, Aorta; PA, pulmonary artery; SCV, superior caval vein;
ICV, inferior caval vein; M, morphologically mitral valve;
T, morphologically tricuspid valve; LV, morphologically left
ventricle; RV, morphologically right ventricle, systemic, subaortic.

Congenitally corrected transposition evolves in embryonic development by erroneous rotation of the bulboventricular tube leftward instead of rightward. As a result, the structures derived from it (e.g. AV valves, ventricles) are inverted. The atria and the sinus venosus remain physiologically situated. The ventricles are localized more 'side-by-side', and the ventricular septum runs perpendicular to the frontal plane (normally, the ventricles are situated rather more one behind the other, with the ventricular septum running oblique). The aortopulmonary septation does not follow a spiral course, with the origin of the aorta being anteriorly to the left and the origin of the pulmonary artery posteriorly to the right. Aorto-mitral continuity is absent, whilst fibrotic continuity between the pulmonary artery and the right-side mitral valve is present.

Isolated CCTGA without an associated defect is rare. CCTGA often occurs in combination with a large ventricular septal defect (VSD; up to 75%) in any position (often subpulmonary), pulmonary stenosis (PS; up to 75%), systemic AV valve anomalies (in 30%) and congenital complete heart block (in 5%).[1] The atrial and ventricular septa show 'malalignment'.

Left ventricular outflow tract obstruction (LVOTO) can be valvular and/or subvalvular. Subvalvular pulmonary artery stenosis may be due to abundant tricuspid valve tissue – protruding via VSD into the subpulmonary area (Figure 12.2) – or by a fibrotic annulus or membrane, abundant fibrotic or myxomatous tissue, or a muscular tunnel in the LVOT.

Tricuspid valve abnormalities, most often dysplasia, have been reported in pathological studies in a high percentage of CCTGA. The tricuspid valve differs from the mitral valve, in addition to the number of cusps, in its more apical origin of the septal cusp and insertion of the chordae into the septum (Figure 12.3). Ebsteinoid tricuspid valve anomaly consist of abnormal apical shift of the septal and posterior cusps, and occurs in about one third of cases with CCTGA (Figure 12.4).

The right ventricle in CCTGA shows its typical trabeculization, including the septomarginal trabecule (Figures 12.4, 12.5). The right ventricle is located on the left side and is working under high systemic pressure, ejecting blood into

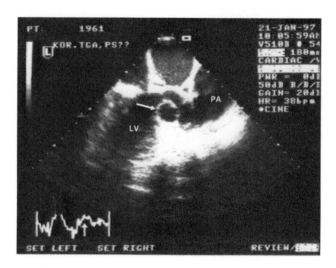

Figure 12.2

Transesophageal echo, longitudinal projection. Congenitally corrected transposition of the great arteries (CCTGA), subvalvar pulmonary stenosis (PS) (arrow) is caused by abundant tissue of the tricuspid valve, which is prolapsing through the ventricular septal defect (VSD) into the left ventricular outflow tract below pulmonary artery in adult patient with CCTGA, VSD and PS (valvar and subvalvar). PA, Pulmonary artery; LV, left ventricle.

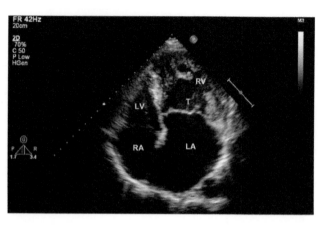

Figure 12.4

Transthoracic echo, apical four-chamber view. Isolated congenitally corrected transposition of the great arteries in adult patient with Ebsteinoid anomaly of the tricuspid valve (T), dilatation of the tricuspid annulus and lack of coaptation of the tricuspid cusps with severe tricuspid regurgitation. Dilatation and dysfunction of the systemic right ventricle (RV), which may be identified by coarse trabeculization, severely dilated left atrium (LA), normal size of the subpulmonic left ventricle (LV) and right atrium (RA).

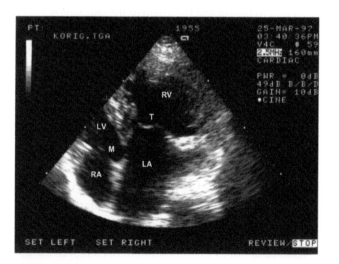

Figure 12.3

Transthoracic echo, apical four-chamber view. The left-sided artioventricular valve is located more apically, therefore it is tricuspid valve and the diagnosis is congenitally corrected transposition of the great arteries. LV, Morphologically left ventricle; RV, morphologically right ventricle; LA, left atrium; RA, right atrium; M, mitral valve; T, tricuspid valve.

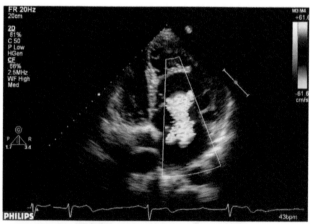

Figure 12.5

Transthoracic echo, apical four-chamber view, congenitally corrected transposition of the great arteries. The same patient as in Figure 12.4. Color flow shows severe tricuspid regurgitation, which begins deep in the right ventricle in the apically displaced orifice of the tricuspid valve. Functionally it is 'mitral' regurgitation.

aorta. The coronary sinuses of the aorta are situated posteriorly, with the noncoronary sinus situated anteriorly. The coronary arteries are inverted, with the morphologically left coronary artery running to the right and the morphologically right coronary artery running to the left in front of the subpulmonary outflow tract. A single coronary artery may also be present.

The position of the sinus node is normal.[2] The AV node is atypically situated, anteriorly and superiorly in the right atrium, between the auricle orifice and the lateral edge of the fibrotic continuity between mitral annulus and pulmonary valve. Many patients have an anomalous second AV node. The bundle of His runs anteriorly and cranially, superficially, in front of the pulmonary artery, by the pulmonary valve annulus, crossing – through the VSD – to the left side of the ventricular septum. The branches are inverted, with the left being on the right side and vice versa. The conduction system is elongated and readily vulnerable, not only during surgery but also during spontaneous degeneration and fibrosis. The incidence of complete AV block is reported to be 5–10% at birth, with an annual increase of 2%.

About 25% of CCTGA patients show dextrocardia or mesocardia, with 18% of patients having a right-side aortic arch.

Prevalence

In general, CCTGA is a rare congenital heart defect, accounting for <1% of all congenital heart defects. If excluding patients with univentricular AV connection (a functionally common ventricle), the incidence of CCTGA is about 0.5% of all congenital heart defects. Isolated CCTGA may be first diagnosed in adulthood.

Pathophysiology

The systemic venous return from the right atrium (on the right), passes across a morphological mitral valve to a morphological left ventricle (on the right) and to the pulmonary artery, originating posteriorly from the left ventricle. The pulmonary veins drain into the left atrium (on the left), and the blood passes across the morphologically tricuspid valve and the morphologically right ventricle (situated to the left and slightly anterior) from which the aorta arises. The morphologically right ventricle is the high-pressure, systemic ventricle. The aorta is situated anteriorly and to the left from the pulmonary artery, therefore, the older expression for the defect, l-TGA. The great arteries and the outflow tracts run in parallel (Figure 12.1).

Similar to the situation following Mustard's correction, a systemic right ventricle and tricuspid valve are situated on the systemic side of the circulation. A systemic right ventricle features a bigger end-diastolic volume than the left ventricle; as a result, it is capable of maintaining an adequate cardiac output in the presence of a lower ejection fraction.

Why some individuals develop systemic right ventricular failure while other patients live until old age without failure is not fully clear. Differences in genetic predisposition may play a role. Insufficient coronary supply to a hypertrophied myocardium of the systemic ventricle by the right coronary artery has also been incriminated.

In children with CCTGA, but not in adults, exercise results in an increase in right ventricular ejection fraction. In many adult patients, this systemic right ventricle runs out of its functional reserve, resulting in systolic dysfunction and failure over years. As the ventricle in the subpulmonary position is the morphologically left ventricle, in the presence of left ventricular hypertrophy this ventricle has a theoretical potential to tolerate pressure overload well.

Progressive tricuspid regurgitation (i.e. systemic AV valve) may be due to either a congenital or an acquired morphological abnormality, or to tricuspid annulus dilatation in the presence of right ventricular dilatation. On echocardiography, tricuspid regurgitation in CCTGA looks like mitral regurgitation with a dysfunctional spherical ventricle, and it indeed is a 'mitral' regurgitation in terms of function (Figure 12.5).

Isolated CCTGA is not associated with cyanosis. In the presence of significant PS *and* a VSD, CCTGA is associated with cyanosis due to a right-to-left shunt at ventricular level. In the presence of an equipoise magnitude of the VSD and subpulmonary obstruction, the defect is balanced. The pulmonary vessel bed is at that time protected against the development of pulmonary vascular obstructive disease. With balanced defect, cyanosis is not significant.

Clinical findings and diagnosis

Unless CCTGA manifests itself in childhood, it may be asymptomatic for decades, especially if isolated, i.e. without associated defects. In adulthood, most often from the third decade of life on, CCTGA may manifest itself by syncope or presyncope, and/or sudden exercise intolerance in the presence of a complete AV block. A complete AV block is characteristic of CCTGA and its incidence rises with age; it may even be intermittent.

CCTGA with VSD and PS is associated with cyanosis, which, however, may be mild and inconspicuous for a long time. The cyanosis may deteriorate if the PS progresses due to degenerative changes.

Mild systemic right ventricular dysfunction and tricuspid regurgitation are often tolerated by adults for some time, and clinically manifest themselves as mitral insufficiency. After a clinically silent period of different duration, heart failure develops; however, in young patients, this manifests differently and substantially less conspicuously compared with older patients. Shortness of breath may be only mild; clinical signs of congestion in the pulmonary circulation and swelling of legs are often absent. Hepatomegaly and signs of a low cardiac output are present in patients with severe dysfunction of the systemic ventricle and heart failure.

Symptoms

- The course may be minimally symptomatic for decades.
- Symptoms reflect the associated cardiac anomalies.
- A higher degree AV block with or without syncope.
- Decreased exercise tolerance.
- Mild cyanosis in the presence of a VSD or atrial septal defect (ASD) in combination with PS.
- Systemic ventricular or bilateral cardiac decompensation.

Clinical manifestations

- Palpable second heart sound left of the upper sternum.
- Hyperactive precordium in the case of VSD.

- Systolic thrill in case of VSD or PS.
- Cyanosis, if PS and VSD are present.

Auscultatory findings

- A single and loud second heart sound (A2) in the second left sternal border (due to the position of the aorta close under the chest wall).
- With complete AV block, the intensity of the first sound may vary.
- Systolic regurgitant murmur at the apex, or along the left lower sternal border with tricuspid regurgitation, propagating rather to the left lower sternum than to the axilla, as the regurgitation flow is often directed eccentrically medially into the left atrium.
- A noisy systolic murmur along the left lower sternal border in the presence of a VSD.
- A systolic ejection murmur in the upper left or right sternal border in the presence of LVOTO, with the subpulmonary component of obstruction being predominant in most cases.
- An early diastolic rumble at the apex in case of a significant tricuspid regurgitant, or a large VSD.

Electrocardiogram (ECG), (Figure 12.6.)

- Abnormal septal activation from the right to the left.
- Deep Q waves in II, III, aVF and V1–V3, V4R.
- As an exception, a QS pattern may be apparent in all precordial leads.
- Absent Q waves in I, aVL and V5–V6.
- The cardiac axis is usually deviated to the left; however, no left anterior hemiblock is involved as the left branch is on the right.
- Signs of atrial and/or ventricular hypertrophy. A 'mitral' P wave appears in the presence of morphologic left ventricular hypertrophy associated with a major left-to-right shunt or mitral valve regurgitation. High 'pulmonary' P waves occur in pulmonary hypertension or PS.
- In CCTGA, T waves tend to be high and positive in the precordial leads.
- Varying degree of (progressive) AV block.
- Atrial arrhythmias.
- Wolf-Parkinson-White syndrome.

Holter electrocardiogram monitoring

It is indicated, because of conduction disorders and pre-excitation syndrome (see previous section), also in asymptomatic adult patients with CCTGA. In symptomatic patients, Holter ECG monitoring is performed repeatedly.

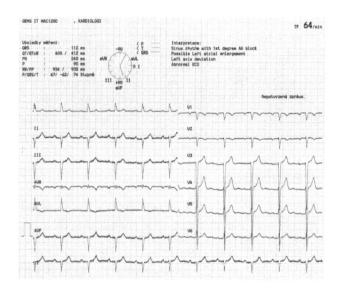

Figure 12.6
ECG in a patient with isolated congenitally transposistion of the great arteries.

Chest X-ray

- The anterior and leftward position of the aorta results in a straight left upper cardiac border without the pulmonary knob.
- A septal notch on the ventricular shadow is evident over the diaphragm.
- Cardiomegaly and pulmonary venous congestion, and left atrial enlargement, are evident in the case of systemic ventricular decompensation or 'tricuspid' regurgitation.
- Increased pulmonary vascular markings are evident in the presence of a major left-to-right shunt.
- The pulmonary vasculature is poor in the presence of a significant pulmonary artery stenosis.
- Abnormalities of the cardiac position (e.g. dextrocardia).

Echocardiography

- Adults with CCTGA are often difficult to examine along the parasternal long axis (Figure 12.7). Due to the abnormal anterior position of the aorta and the sagittal course of the ventricular septum, it may be impossible to obtain conventional projections. Of advantage are apical four-chamber projection and parasternal short-axis projection.
- In adulthood, isolated CCTGA may present in echocardiography as 'mitral' regurgitation associated with 'left ventricular' dysfunction (Figure 12.5).
- First and foremost, CCTGA is recognized by the more apical origin of the left-sided AV valve. Unlike the mitral valve, the tricuspid valve chords are inserted in the septum, whereas the mitral valve chords are inserted into the free-moving left ventricular wall.

- The left-sided tricuspid AV valve may be dysplastic with thickening and shortening of cusps, or may show Ebstein's anomaly with abnormal apical shift of the septal and posterior leaflets, and anterior leaflet elongation, etc.
- The degree and progression of regurgitation on the left-sided, systemic, tricuspid AV valve are of outstanding importance.
- The fibrotic continuity between the AV and semilunar valve with CCTGA is to the right; between the mitral and pulmonary valves.
- The ventricle situated to the left features trabeculization typical of the right ventricle. The quantification of the functional capability of the left-sided systemic, morphologically right ventricle is also of outstanding importance.
- The blood vessel situated anteriorly and to the left is the aorta.
- From the apical projection, the pulmonary artery is located at the site where usually the aorta is; the pulmonary artery can be visualized up to its bifurcation (Figure 12.8).
- The parallel course of the great arteries will be shown best in short-axis parasternal projection.
- The parallel course of blood vessels is also well visualized by transesophageal echocardiography in the longitudinal projection (Figures 12.9 and 12.10).
- In the presence of a VSD, shunt direction and significance should be assessed.
- Presence and relevance of pulmonary valvular and subvalvular stenosis, mechanism of subvalvular stenosis needs clarification, with the advantage of transesophageal echocardiography when the transthoracic image is not adequate (Figure 12.10).
- Also, any additional associated congenital anomaly, e.g. patent ductus arteriosus, mitral valve dysplasia, coarctation of the aorta etc., should be depicted.

Catheterization

Catheterization is no longer necessary to establish a diagnosis or to assess intracardiac morphology. Catheterization is indicated in the following cases:

- when there is a need to exactly determine pulmonary artery pressure and pulmonary vascular resistance, especially so in CCTGA with VSD, prior to elective surgery, and/or high-grade systemic AV valve regurgitation and/or systemic ventricular failure;
- to quantify the magnitude of a shunt;
- to determine the morphology of a subpulmonary outflow tract obstruction, the subpulmonary outflow tract gradient, and the pulmonary artery size;
- angiography may be required to exactly determine the morphology of a VSD;
- coronary angiography prior to cardiac surgery.

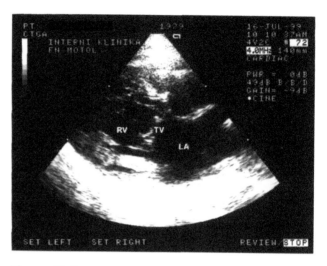

Figure 12.7
Transthoracic echo, parasternal long-axis view, congenitally corrected transposition of the great arteries due to abnormal anterior position of aorta, this view is often difficult to achieve. RV, Right ventricle; LA, left atrium; TV, tricuspid valve.

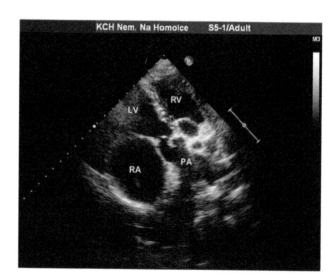

Figure 12.8
Transthoracic echo, congenitally corrected transposition of the great arteries, apical view with pulmonary artery (PA), which arises posteriorly from the morphologically left ventricle (LV). RA, Right atrium; RV, right ventricle.

Exercise testing with oximetry

On longitudinal follow-up, it will help to assess the course of physical fitness, exercise-induced arrhythmias, change in saturation etc.

Radionuclide angiography

This technique may help to specify and quantify the right ventricular function.[3]

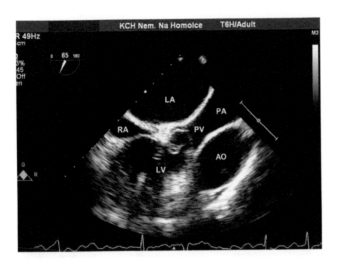

Figure 12.9
Transesophageal echo, congenitally corrected transposition of the great arteries, pulmonary stenosis is valvar with doming of the pulmonary valve (PV) as well as subvalvar. Pulmonary artery (PA) is behind aorta (AO), both great arteries have parallel course; LA, left atrium; RA, right atrium; LV, left ventricle.

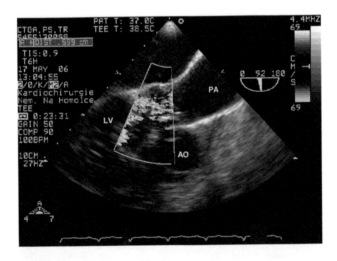

Figure 12.10
Transesophageal echo, 92 degrees, adult with congenitally corrected transposition of the great arteries, and subvalvar pulmonary stenosis and ventricular septal defect. Pulmonary artery (PA) lies behind aorta (AO). The color flow shows turbulent flow in the left ventricular outflow tract due to the subvalvar pulmonary stenosis. LV, Left ventricle.

Magnetic resonance imaging (MRI)

MRI is used to specify right ventricular anatomy or function in more detail.

Management

CCTGA as such does not require surgical correction as long as there is good systemic AV valve function. According to the

Canadian Consensus Conference, the following situations may warrant intervention or intervention re-intervention:[1]

- VSD or residual VSD;
- systemic AV valve regurgitation if moderate or worse;
- systemic AV valve regurgitation, if moderate or worse, following prior surgical repair;
- PS or subpulmonary stenosis with an invasive pullback gradient >60mmHg;
- stenosis across a prior left ventricle-to-pulmonary artery conduit with an invasive pullback gradient >60mmHg;
- complete AV block with symptoms, progressive or profound bradycardia, or poor exercise heart rate response;
- symptomatic deterioration;
- deteriorating systemic ventricular function.

In individuals experiencing minor symptoms, surgery is preferably postponed until symptoms have developed. However, the systolic dysfunction of the systemic ventricle may be the limiting factor, increasing the surgical risk especially in systemic AV valve regurgitation.

Surgical management is indicated for associated defects, if they are significant. Complete repair may involve:

- tricuspid valve replacement;
- VSD closure;
- relief of LVOTO;
- alternative approaches such as double-switch procedures (Senning with arterial switch), atrial switch, and Rastelli (RV-PA conduit with VSD closure);
- heart transplantation.

Tricuspid valve replacement with a mechanical prosthesis

This procedure is indicated in more than mild or moderate AV valve regurgitation associated with a fairly good systemic right ventricular function. Valvuloplasty of the malformed tricuspid valve is often not feasible or successful, and therefore is not generally recommended.

Tricuspid valve replacement associated with right ventricular dysfunction leads to systemic right ventricular failure, and shows high mortality rates. Considering the complexity of the anomaly, the procedure should only be performed in centers with a large body of experience.

Some authors have suggested timely cardiac surgery in isolated CCTGA with tricuspid regurgitation to prevent ventricular overload and injury to the systemic right ventricle. However, other authors tend to prefer, particularly in asymptomatic adults with pre-existing ventricular dysfunction, a conservative approach with subsequent heart transplantation, should cardiac decompensation develop.

Ventricular septal defect closure

VSD closure is performed if the shunt is significant, if symptoms of congestive heart failure occur, or when pulmonary vascular pressure is increasing. Special techniques for VSD closure have been developed to avoid injury to the conduction system.

Intracardiac removal of the pulmonary or subpulmonary obstruction

The procedure is only rarely possible because of the wedging position of the outflow tract and the close relationship with the conducting system and left coronary artery. Repair may comprise insertion of a *valved conduit* from the morphologic left, subpulmonary ventricle to the pulmonary artery. Closure of a VSD is indicated when the defect is associated.

Double-switch procedure

This term means atrial and arterial switch procedure. These methods require retraining of the left ventricle for systemic pressure, and the risk in adults is usually too high. Such complex surgery is performed in children with an approximate mortality rate of 10%. In adults, however, adequate data are not available.[4]

The Senning–Rastelli procedure[5]

This procedure can be performed if pulmonic stenosis and a large VSD are present. The procedure consists of switching the venous return at atrial level (Senning's or Mustard's operation) and performing a Rastelli procedure. During the Rastelli procedure, the morphologic left ventricle is directed to the aorta by a tunnel between the VSD and the aortic valve. A conduit is placed from the morphologic right ventricle to the bifurcation of the pulmonary artery. By this procedure, the morphologically left ventricle becomes the systemic ventricle.

Heart transplantation

Heart transplantation may be indicated in refractory heart failure secondary to severe systemic right ventricular dysfunction, or dysfunction of both ventricles, or in the presence of associated significant inoperable defects. Eligible for heart transplantation are patients with CCTGA and heart failure in functional Classes III and IV. A contraindication to transplantation is a high and fixed pulmonary vascular resistance.

Conservative therapy

Drug therapy should be timely and adequately effective. However, there are only limited data regarding the role of ACE inhibitors or beta blockers on maintaining systemic right ventricular function. Diuretics and digitalis may be indicated in symptomatic patients. The current guidelines do not make a single reference to spironolactone therapy, which, however, could in theory be effective in preventing the development of myocardial fibrosis. In the presence of atrial fibrillation, anticoagulation therapy is administered.

Permanent pacemaker

The risk for developing complete AV block is high both in the natural history and following surgery. An intermittent or permanent AV block results in permanent dual-chamber cardiac pacing. Considering the morphology of the subpulmonary ventricle, which is left-sided and features a smooth wall, active electrode fixation is recommended. Transvenous pacing increases the risk of paradoxical embolism associated with a shunt defect, in which case pacing with epicardial leads is preferred. There may be a benefit in biventricular pacing.

Catheter-based balloon dilatation of a PS is not recommended because of the risk of a complete AV block.

Residual findings and risks

- Progressive systemic ventricular dysfunction and progression of 'tricuspid' regurgitation. Given the long asymptomatic course of CCTGA, and the high operative risk in adulthood, the decision-making as to the timing of surgery is difficult.
- Valve replacement will not necessarily prevent further worsening of systolic systemic right ventricle function.
- Residual VSD.
- A complete AV block is frequent. Fibrosis of the conduction system is progressive in nature and may cause AV blocks of various degrees. The average incidence of any AV block is 75%, and that of complete AV block 30% in all CCTGA age groups.[6] The incidence of complete AV block is reported to be 5–10% at birth, with an annual increase of 2%.[7]
- Wolf-Parkinson-White with accessory bundles to the left and right is also frequent in CCTGA. In the case of Ebsteinoid tricuspid valve anomaly, the accessory conduit is to the left, with delta waves appearing in V1.
- Sudden death from arrhythmia.
- Residual pulmonary conduit (homograft) obstruction due to homograft degeneration may occur, often on the proximal anastomosis. Furthermore, conduit compression can go off the sternum, especially so in heart dilatation.

Pregnancy and delivery

- Pregnancy and delivery may be associated with appreciable deterioration of systemic right ventricular function, and/or the tricuspid (systemic) regurgitation.[8]

- In a series of 60 pregnancies of women with CCTGA, 88% of deliveries were vaginal, and 83% were live births.
- Women with CCTGA show increased morbidity rates and increased risk for abortion.
- Pregnancy is contraindicated with significant cyanosis, significant systemic ventricular dysfunction, or with significant pulmonary artery stenosis or high-grade systemic AV valve regurgitation.
- Patients require careful follow-up by a cardiologist during pregnancy, and monitoring during and immediately after childbirth. Infectious endocarditis (IE) prevention is advisable.

Infectious endocarditis

The risk of IE is increased because of valvular regurgitation, subpulmonary obstruction, and VSD. IE is reported to occur in 11% of cases of CCTGA, and may be the cause of death.

Follow-up

Even asymptomatic adults with CCTGA should be followed by a cardiologist experienced in congenital heart defects and closely collaborating with a specialized center.

Prognosis

- The median survival of operated or unoperated CCTGA patients is 40 years in historical studies.
- CCTGA patients without major associated anomalies may live long; however, these are usually single case reports.
- Isolated CCTGA without associated anomalies may stay asymptomatic for a long period of time, and therefore may be diagnosed for the first time in adulthood.
- The incidence of progressive systemic right ventricular dysfunction with significant tricuspid regurgitation increases with age. Between 20 and 40 years of age, the incidence of significant tricuspid regurgitation was about 20%. More than 20% of individuals developed heart failure after 40 years of age. In individuals older than 50 years of age, the incidence rates of significant tricuspid regurgitation and heart failure were >60%, with arrhythmia occurring in >80% of individuals in this age group.[4,9,10]
- The mortality of children undergoing VSD closure with pulmonary homograft implantation is <10%. However, the need for re-operation of a degenerated pulmonary conduit or homograft is up to 50% of patients at 10 years after the primary surgical procedure.
- The mortality of re-operation, particularly if involving tricuspid valve replacement, is high, some 30%.

- In a series of 111 CCTGA patients, out of which 51 had surgery prior to 1988, the overall early operative mortality was 20%, with overall mortality being 23%. Most patients with predominant cyanosis showed improvement of symptoms after surgery; with 14% of patients dying within 6 postoperative months. However, in patients with prevailing heart failure symptoms, the 6-month postoperative mortality rate was 37%, and 26% of survivors remained in Class III or IV, or their condition required reoperation.[11] Tricuspid valve replacement should thus be performed in time, before right ventricular dysfunction and symptomatic heart failure have set in.
- On long-term follow-up, in most series, adults with CCTGA have 10-year mortality rates of 25–36% and a mean age at death of 38.5 years.[7,10,12] The predominant cause of death (in >50% of cases) was heart failure with progressive systemic AV valve regurgitation, sudden death in documented supraventricular and ventricular arrhythmia, IE, or related to cardiac surgery or heart transplantation.
- The risk factors for death on long-term follow-up after operation are Ebstein malformation of the tricuspid valve and preoperative systemic (right) ventricular dysfunction.[12]

References

1. Therrien J, Gatzoulis M, Graham T et al. Canadian Cardiovascular Society Consensus Conference 2001 update: Recommendations for the Management of Adults with Congenital Heart Disease – Part II. Can J Cardiol 2001; 17(10): 1029–50.
2. Anderson RH. The conduction tissues in congenitally corrected transposition. Ann Thorac Surg 2004; 77(6): 1881–2.
3. Espinola-Zavaleta N, Alexanderson E, Attie F et al. Right ventricular function and ventricular perfusion defects in adults with congenitally corrected transposition: Correlation of echocardiography and nuclear medicine. Cardiol Young 2004; 14(2): 174–81.
4. Dyer K, Graham TP. Congenitally corrected transposition of the great arteries: current treatment options. Curr Treat Options Cardiovasc Med 2003; 5(5): 399–407.
5. Ilbawi MN, DeLeon SY, Backer CL et al. An alternative approach to the surgical management of physiologically corrected transposition with ventricular septal defect and pulmonary stenosis or atresia. J Thorac Cardiovasc Surg 1990; 100: 410.
6. Perloff JK. The Clinical Recognition of Congenital Heart Disease, 4th edn. Philadelphia, PA: WB Saunders Company, 1994.
7. Huhta JC, Danielson GK, Ritter DG et al. Survival in atrioventricular discordance. Pediatr Cardiol 1985; 6: 57–60.
8. Therrien J, Barnes I, Somerville J. Outcome of pregnancy in patients with congenitally corrected transposition of the great arteries. Am J Cardiol 1999; 84(7): 820–4.
9. Presbitero P, Somerville J, Rabajoli F, Stone S, Conte MR. Corrected transposition of the great arteries without associated defects in adult patients: Clinical profile and follow-up. Br Heart J 1995; 74: 57–9.
10. Connelly MS, Liu PP, Williams WG et al. Congenitally corrected transposition of the great arteries in the adult: Functional status and complications. J Am Coll Cardiol 1996; 27: 1238–43.
11. Lundstrom U, Bull C, Wyse RKH, Somerville J. The natural and 'unnatural' history of congenitally corrected transposition. Am J Cardiol 1990; 65: 1222–9.
12. Hraska V, Duncan BW, Mayer Jr JE et al. Long-term outcome of surgically treated patients with corrected transposition of the great arteries. J Thorac Cardiovasc Surg 2005; 129(1): 182–91.

13

Patent ductus arteriosus

Definition and anatomical notes

Patent ductus arteriosus (PDA) is an embryologic remnant, and connects the roof of the pulmonary artery to the proximal descending aorta. In the left-sided aortic arch, the duct's pulmonary orifice is located just leftward from the pulmonary artery bifurcation; the aortic orifice is on the medial side of the aorta, at the level or just distal to the origin of the left subclavian artery (Figure 13.1). The arterial duct can present in a variety of sizes and configurations: it may be short and wide, or narrow and long. Depending on its morphology and configuration, Krichenko classified five types of ducts:[1] type A ('conical' ductus) is the most frequent one, and is funnel-shaped with a wider aortic orifice (well-defined aortic ampulla) and a localized narrowing (constriction) near the pulmonary artery end. The narrowing at the pulmonary orifice is due to the fact that the duct begins to close spontaneously right from the pulmonary end. The duct's width is determined by its narrowest point and is no greater than 4mm in diameter in 78% of patients. Rarely, large ducts measuring ≥10mm in diameter can be seen, more often in adults. Also rarely, the arterial duct may be dilated in an aneurysm-like manner. In adulthood, atherosclerotic lesions develop in the duct wall, which is fragile and calcified.[2]

PDA in adulthood can be divided, by their size and clinical severity, into:

- *Clinically silent duct ('silent PDA')*: Detectable only by echocardiography.
- *Small duct*: Continuous murmur, negligible hemodynamic relevance, normal left ventricular size, no pulmonary hypertension.
- *Moderate duct*: Continuous murmur, wide pulse arterial pressure (as in aortic regurgitation), left ventricular dilatation, a degree of pulmonary hypertension, which is usually reversible.
- *Large ductus*: Usually not occurring in adults unless associated with Eisenmenger syndrome.
- *Eisenmenger syndrome*: No continuous murmur, severe, irreversible pulmonary hypertension, differentiated hypoxemia and cyanosis (see below).

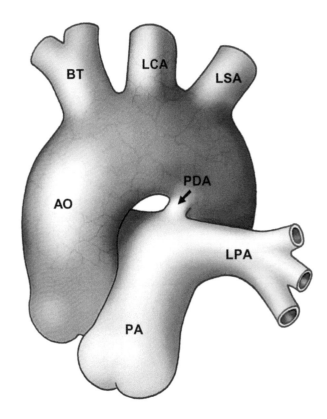

Figure 13.1
Patent ductus arteriosus. AO, Aorta; PA, pulmonary artery; LPA, left branch of pulmonary artery; BT, brachiocephalic trunk; LCA, left carotid artery; LSA, left subclavian artery.

Prevalence

PDA accounts for about 5–10% of all congenital heart disease (CHD), with girls affected about twice as often as boys.[3] The ductus arteriosus closes functionally during the first 48 hours after birth; a PDA is considered to be abnormal and a CHD if it remains widely patent beyond the second week of life. PDA occurs more often in pre-term infants, in children born at relatively high altitudes above sea level, in children born to mothers infected with rubella in the first trimester of pregnancy or, occasionally, with genetic predisposition reported.[4]

In adults, the prevalence of PDA has declined during the last few decades, and PDA is seen only very rarely as the duct has been closed surgically or using a catheter-based procedure in most children in their early childhood. In adulthood, one can find a small duct unrecognized in childhood, or a small residual shunt following catheter-based closure. Still, rarely, one can see a patient with Eisenmenger syndrome associated with PDA, a combination to be considered in the differential diagnosis of pulmonary hypertension, especially in young women.

Pathophysiology

In fetal life, when the lungs are not functional, only a small amount of blood passes through the lungs. The fetal ductus arteriosus is important to divert the right ventricular cardiac output away from the high-resistance pulmonary vascular bed to the systemic circulation. The majority of blood flows from the right ventricle and pulmonary artery via the ductus arteriosus to the descending aorta. The function ceases to exist after delivery when the infant begins to breathe and oxygen tension increases. The ductal wall contains a muscular layer contracting as the result of a decrease in prostaglandin levels after delivery because of elimination of the placental source and its metabolism in the now functioning lungs.[4] A functional closure begins several hours postpartum, with functional closure being complete within 24–48 hours postpartum in term neonates. Complete anatomical closure with fibrosis occurs during the next 2–3 weeks. A fibrous band without lumen results, and is called ligamentum arteriosum. A duct permanently patent after delivery is a CHD. A PDA is usually an isolated lesion. However, in some cases of critical CHD, maintenance of the duct patency is of vital importance for the infant to survive the first hours after birth (e.g. in pulmonary atresia with an intact ventricular septum, complete transposition of the great arteries in the absence of shunt at the atrial/ventricular level, aortic atresia, etc.).

A clinically silent and small ductus arteriosus does not create any hemodynamic overload, only an increased risk of infectious endarteritis in countries with limited health care resources and limited access to health care.[5] A moderate and a large ductus arteriosus with a left-to-right shunt pose a volume overload for the left ventricle. The direction and magnitude of the shunt via the duct are dependent on the pulmonary to systemic resistance ratio and duct size. A patent duct with severe, irreversible pulmonary hypertension in the presence of pulmonary vascular obstructive disease (Eisenmenger syndrome) indicates a right-to-left shunt at the level of the great arteries, and implies pressure overload for the right ventricle. As, in PDA with pulmonary hypertension and a right-to-left shunt, desaturated blood enters the aorta distal to the origin of the carotid arteries, hypoxic stimulation of respiratory centers does not occur, and differential cyanosis between the upper and lower limbs is present.

Clinical findings and diagnosis

The clinical findings depend on the size, amount of shunt and the presence or absence of pulmonary arterial hypertension or Eisenmenger syndrome. A small, incidentally detected PDA does not present with any symptoms or abnormal findings.

Inspection

PDA in adulthood is rare, with the most frequent finding being a clinically silent or small duct, which is unremarkable during inspection. However, one should consider the rare possibility of a PDA associated with Eisenmenger syndrome, whose diagnosis need not be obvious at first sight. In this case, the right-to-left shunt only occurs at the level or just distal to the origin of the left subclavian artery; as a result, central cyanosis is not evident in the upper part of the body. Drumstick fingers/clubbing and cyanosis are only evident in the lower limbs, and occasionally also in the left upper limb with a difference between the right and left upper limbs. Unlike peripheral cyanosis in vasoconstriction, which will resolve on warming up, this central cyanosis will increase in intensity, with the above differences becoming even more visible during exercise.

Symptoms

- A small PDA is asymptomatic in adulthood.
- Adults with moderate ducts were asymptomatic in about 25% of cases, while the remaining ones experienced dyspnea, palpitations or atypical chest pain.[6]
- PDA with a significant left-to-right shunt can result in left-heart failure; however, such cases are rare in clinical practice in developed countries as most ducts are surgically or interventionally closed during childhood.
- A PDA with Eisenmenger syndrome may remain undetected and the diagnosis inappropriately delayed. Patients may show relatively few symptoms, and are free of pronounced exertional dyspnea as the respiratory centers are not exposed to hypoxia. During exercise, patients may complain of lower limb fatigability or pain, with the latter associated with hypertrophic osteoarthropathy. Hoarseness may be due to laryngeal nerve compression by the severely dilated pulmonary artery secondary to pulmonary hypertension. In the end stage, the patient may show signs of right-heart decompensation. Inspection and the auscultatory findings may be inconspicuous on cursory examination.

Auscultatory findings

- A clinically silent duct is free of murmur.
- A small duct is typically associated with a continuous murmur (systolic–diastolic), reflecting systolic and

diastolic left-to-right shunt between the aorta and the pulmonary artery. The continuous murmur, or so called 'machinery' murmur, is the hallmark physical finding and is best heard in the first to second left intercostal space parasternally or below the left clavicula.

- A diastolic rumble can be heard at the apex in the presence of a moderate or large ductus arteriosus.
- A large ductus arteriosus shortens the duration of the murmur, and there may only be a systolic component in the presence of a severely increased pulmonary artery pressure.
- Eisenmenger syndrome is associated with balanced pressures in the great arteries; there may be no murmur, but the intensity of the pulmonary component of the second heart sound may be prominent. In addition, a high-frequency diastolic murmur of pulmonary regurgitation or a pansystolic murmur of tricuspid regurgitation can be audible.

Electrocardiogram (ECG)

The ECG is completely normal in the presence of a small duct. Moderate to severe ducts with a large left-to-right shunt present with left atrial overload and left ventricular hypertrophy; a prolonged PR interval can be seen in 10–20% of cases. P pulmonale and right ventricular hypertrophy are present in patients with Eisenmenger syndrome.

Chest X-ray

Pulmonary vasculature and heart size are dependent on the direction and magnitude of the shunt. A chest X-ray is completely normal in small ductus arteriosus. Pulmonary vascular markings (shunt vascularity) reflect increased left-to-right shunt in the presence of a moderate to large ductus arteriosus. The central pulmonary arteries are prominent, in particular in the presence of pulmonary arterial hypertension. Calcification of the duct between the aortic arch and the pulmonary artery may be evident in adulthood, in particular in older adults.

Echocardiography

Echocardiography is the mainstay diagnostic method, and the method of choice to confirm and to characterize the PDA. However, its visualization in the ductal area in adults is inferior to that in children. Using color Doppler echocardiography, the parasternal short-axis view and the suprasternal projection show, at a certain tilt of the probe, the duct directly as continuous flow from the aorta to the pulmonary artery bifurcation or to the left pulmonary artery. In the suprasternal view, a pulsed Doppler signal shows diastolic reverse flow in the descending aorta under the site of duct origin, and diastolic forward flow in the aortic arch above the duct origin. Right in the duct, continuous (systolic-diastolic) flow will be detected (Figure 13.2).

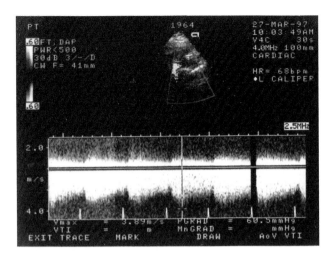

Figure 13.2
Continuous Doppler examination from suprasternal view, continuous systolic and diastolic flow of higher velocities, typical for smaller patent ductus arteriosus without pulmonary hypertension. The flow is directed from aorta to pulmonary artery, both in systole and diastole.

The velocity of the systolic–diastolic continuous flow will depend on the pressure difference between the pulmonary artery and the descending aorta. This typical finding is not present in patients with Eisenmenger syndrome. The duct may be identifiable morphologically; however, the shunt flow velocity is low in Eisenmenger syndrome due to the low pressure difference and the flow is directed from the pulmonary artery to the descending aorta (Figures 13.3 and 13.4). Transesophageal echocardiography and contrast echocardiography may be helpful in some cases (Figures 13.5 and 13.6). Echocardiography is the diagnostic method of choice to exclude associated congenital heart defects.

Catheterization

Diagnostic catheterization is limited to certain patients: (1) prior to elective closure of the PDA; or (2) in the presence of pulmonary hypertension and increased pulmonary vascular resistance to determine their reversibility using vasodilator agents (e.g. oxygen, nitric oxide, prostaglandins, sildenafil, etc.). Aortic angiography describes the morphology of the ductus arteriosus, which is essential before device closure. Prior to elective surgical closure, selective coronary angiography should be performed in patients over 40 years of age, as well as the assessment of the degree of duct calcification.

Magnetic resonance imaging (MRI) or computerized tomography (CT) scan

These techniques can be used for noninvasive anatomical assessment and to detect aneurysms. A CT scan can also

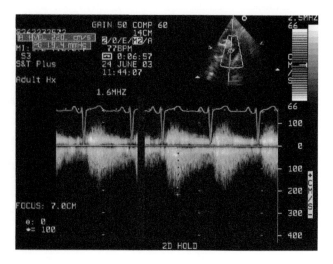

Figure 13.3

Doppler examination, suprasternal view, adult patient with patent ductus arteriosus and severe pulmonary hypertension – Eisenmenger syndrome. The flow is directed from pulmonary artery to aorta, predominantly in systole. The pulmonary artery pressure in this patient was suprasystemic: systolic pulmonary artery pressure was 160mmHg, mean pulmonary artery pressure was 110mmHg, diastolic pulmonary pressure was 70mmHg, the arterial pressure on brachial artery was 100/60mmHg.

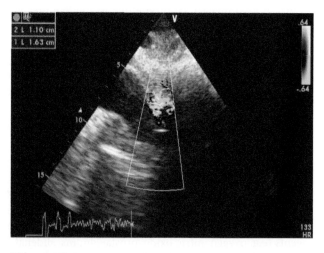

Figure 13.4

Patent arterial duct, 2D echocardiography, suprasternal view. The color flow indicates the systolic turbulent flow from pulmonary artery to descending aorta in a patient with patent ductus arteriosus and Eisenmenger syndrome with severe, suprasystemic pulmonary hypertension. The same patient as in Figure 13.3.

determine the degree of duct calcifications. MRI can be used to calculate Qp/Qs, a process which may be difficult to perform using catheterization.

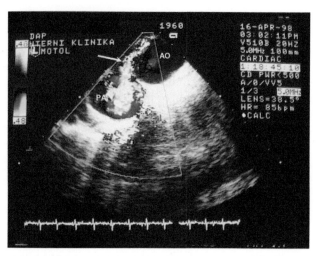

Figure 13.5

Transesophageal echo, modified longitudinal projection of descending aorta, color-flow mapping shows continuous flow from descending aorta to pulmonary artery via patent ductus arteriosus (arrow). AO, Descending aorta; PA, pulmonary artery.

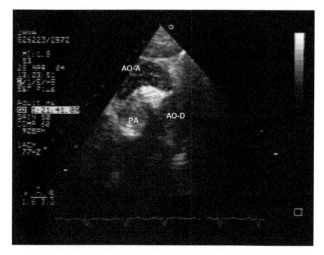

Figure 13.6

Suprasternal view, contrast echocardiography in patent ductus arteriosus with Eisenmenger syndrome. Contrast injected to peripheral vein can be seen as dense contrast in the pulmonary artery (PA) and passes through the duct to descending aorta (AO-D), but also partly retrograde to the aortic arch (AO-A).

Upper or lower limb oximetry

Oximetry obtained on both fingers and toes helps to confirm the diagnosis of PDA with Eisenmenger syndrome (differential cyanosis).

Open-lung biopsy

Open-lung biopsy may be considered if the reversibility of the pulmonary hypertension is uncertain from the

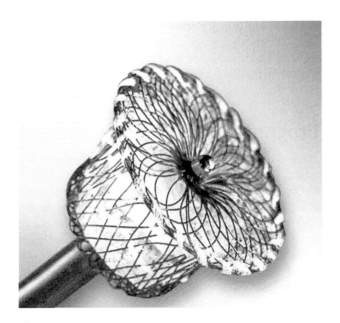

Figure 13.7
Amplatzer™ occluder for patent ductus arteriosus.

hemodynamic assessment.[2] It is performed very rarely to obtain a representative specimen of lung tissue to determine the reversibility of pulmonary vascular changes, but this may be clear from the hemodynamic investigation. Open-lung biopsy is a procedure associated with a high risk and should be performed only by a specialist in a tertiary care center with substantial experience in CHD. It may be hazardous and is almost never performed in adult patients.

Management

Catheter-based PDA closure has become the method of choice. Several systems for duct closure have been developed: the Rashkind occluder, featuring the shape of a twin umbrella; Sideris 'double-button' occluder; detachable spirals (Cook, Gianturco); and the ductal Amplatzer occluder (Figure 13.7). When comparing outcomes, the Rashkind and Sideris occluders have been found to show a higher incidence of residual shunts (12–25%); therefore, it is detachable spirals and the Amplatzer occluder which are currently in widespread use.[7,8]

Detachable spirals show reasonable outcomes with PDA below <4mm in diameter, while bigger PDA are associated with a higher incidence of distal embolism and fewer cases of complete closure.[9] With ducts >4mm (up to 10.6mm) in diameter, it is therefore more appropriate and safer to use the Amplatzer occluder.[10–13] With bigger ducts, 44–56% are completely closed immediately after the procedure; the number of complete closures rises to 66–76% within 24 hours, being 94.6–100% at 6 months, and 100% of completely closed ducts after 1 year.[10,13]

With particularly big ducts (10–16mm in diameter) associated with pulmonary hypertension, catheter-based closure was successfully performed using an Amplatzer occluder for muscular ventricular septal defects.[14,15] Hemodynamic testing is appropriate in patients with PDA and pulmonary hypertension prior to the closure. At 1 year after closure, there was a decrease in the systolic pulmonary artery pressure from 106mmHg to 37mmHg.[14]

Surgical closure is currently performed with those PDA which cannot be closed using a catheter-based technique, or in which a catheter-based closure failed. Surgical PDA closure carries a higher risk in adults compared with children. Ductal ligation is usually performed. In a very short and wide duct (window-like) or calcified duct, which does not permit ligation, the Dacron patch is used to close the PDA. Calcified duct usually occurs in adulthood and poses an increased risk if closed surgically.

Intervention is appropriate:

- In both symptomatic and asymptomatic patients with significant left-to-right shunting (subsequent enlargement of the left ventricle) through a moderate to large PDA in the absence of fairly significant pulmonary hypertension.
- After endarteritis.
- There has not been unanimity in terms of the indication for intervention in patients with a small PDA without volume load of the left ventricle; there is no hemodynamic reason to close the PDA and the risk for IE is low. A strategy for closure is usually advocated in children and young adults because of the low risk of device closure.
- In PDA with pulmonary hypertension, catheter-based closure (see 'Management') should be considered so long as the pulmonary hypertension is reversible. Careful hemodynamic assessment is required before closure in a tertiary care center with expertise in CHD; pulmonary vascular reactivity must be evaluated. The procedure carries a higher risk compared with PDA without pulmonary hypertension. Hemodynamic testing should be undertaken prior to the closure.

Intervention is not indicated/contraindicated:

- Clinically silent PDA (the risk of endarteritis is very low).
- PDA associated with severe pulmonary hypertension (systolic pulmonary artery pressure >2/3 systolic systemic arterial pressure, or pulmonary arteriolar resistance >2/3 systemic arteriolar resistance) or established Eisenmenger syndrome. Closure may be considered if there is a net left-to-right shunt of at least Qp:Qs >1.5:1, or evidence of pulmonary artery reactivity when challenged with vasodilators.[2]

Risks and residual findings

- Surgical closure carries a risk in the presence of a calcified duct (device closure is preferred).
- Catheter-based closure is not appropriate in patients after infectious endocarditis/endarteritis, and in some cases of ductal aneurysm.
- Residual shunts are usually small and tend to close spontaneously over time.
- The risk of distal occluder embolism is in the range of 0–4.7% in large trials using an Amplatzer occluder.[10,12,13] With detachable spirals, the risk of distal embolism is higher (36%) with PDA >4mm,[9] the risk of fatal embolism was 0.3%.[10]
- There have been occasional case reports of aortic or pulmonary obstruction in small children.[16]
- There have been occasional case reports of intravascular hemolysis using an Amplatzer occluder in PDA.[17,18]

Pregnancy

With small and clinically silent PDA in functional NYHA Class I–II, pregnancy and delivery are very well tolerated. With major symptomatic ducts, closure is more appropriate before pregnancy. Pregnancy is contraindicated in patients with Eisenmenger syndrome.

Infectious endocarditis/endarteritis

The risk of infectious endarteritis is low in the absence of Eisenmenger syndrome. According to the recently published guidelines of the American Heart Association, endocarditis prophylaxis is no longer recommended in patients with a PDA and absence of a history of infectious endocarditis and cyanosis.[19] In patients with a residual shunt after closure and Eisenmenger syndrome, the risk of infectious endocarditis/endarteritis is present and requires antibiotic prevention. Prevention of infectious endocarditis/endarteritis is to be maintained after catheter-based closure of PDA for a period of 6 months.[19,20]

Follow-up

The cardiologist follows patients after surgical or catheter-based closure, those with PDA and Eisenmenger syndrome and individuals with yet unclosed and not negligible patent duct. The cardiologist will also follow all patients not undergoing duct closure until adulthood. Regular echocardiographic follow-up is scheduled depending on the clinical status.

The general practitioner will follow a clinically silent duct and patients after surgical closure in childhood without residual shunt or other residual findings, without pulmonary hypertension and clinical complaints.

Prognosis

Surgical duct closure in full-term infants is associated with mortality rates <1% and a good long-term prognosis; recanalization is rare. Surgical closure carries a significantly higher risk in adults with atherosclerotic lesions involving the duct wall. Occasionally, a patch closure on cardiopulmonary bypass instead of ligation will be used to close calcified ducts.[4]

Currently, catheter-based duct closure is clearly preferred to surgical closure; its outcome is good, with mortality rates at about 0.3%. Complete closure at 2 years, in a series of adult patients when using the twin-umbrella technique, was reported in 86% of cases;[6] the figure was 93% in adolescents and adults when using the detachable spiral, but a mere 84% when closing ducts >4mm in diameter.[9] With the Amplatzer occluder, complete closure at 1 year (even with bigger ducts) is reported in 100% of cases; however, the groups included a smaller proportion of adult patients.[12,13]

Symptom remission (dyspnea, palpitations, atypical chest pain) has been reported in some 60–75% of patients after closure.[6] These symptoms are nonspecific in adulthood.

References

1. Krichenko A, Benson LN, Burrows P et al. Angiographic classification of the isolated, persistently patent ductus arteriosus and implications for percutaneous catheter occlusion. Am J Cardiol 1989; 63: 877–80.
2. Therrien J, Dore A, Gersonz W et al. Canadian Cardiovascular Society Consensus Conference 2001 update: Recommendations for the management of adults with congenital heart disease. Part I. Can J Cardiol 2001; 17(9): 940–59.
3. Perloff JK. The Clinical Recognition of Congenital Heart Disease, 4th edn. Philadelphia, PA: WB Saunders Company, 1994.
4. Schneider DJ, Moore JW. Patent ductus arteriosus. Circulation 2006; 114: 1873–82.
5. Sadiq M, Latif F, Ur-Rehman A. Analysis of infective endarteritis in patent ductus arteriosus. Am J Cardiol 2004; 93: 513–15.
6. Harrison DA, Benson LN, Lazzam C et al. Percutaneous catheter closure of the persistently patent ductus arteriosus in the adult. Am J Cardiol 1996; 77: 1094–7.
7. O'Donnel C, Neutze JM, Skinner JR, Wilson NJ. Transcatheter patent ductus arteriosus occlusion: Evolution of techniques and results from the 1990s. J Paediatr Child Health 2001; 37(5): 451–5.
8. Donti A, Formigari R, Bonvicini M et al. Transcatheter closure of the patent ductus arteriosus with new-generation devices: Comparative data and follow-up results. Ital Heart J 2002; 3(2): 122–7.
9. Wang JK, Liau CS, Huang JJ et al. Transcatheter closure of patent ductus arteriosus using Gianturco coils in adolescents and adults. Catheter Cardiovasc Interv 2002; 55(4): 513–18.
10. Faella HJ, Hijazi ZM. Closure of the patent ductus arteriosus with the Amplatzer PDA device: Immediate results of the international clinical trial. Catheter Cardiovasc Interv 2000; 51(1): 50–4.

11. Podnar T, Gavora P, Masura J. Percutaneous closure of patent ductus arteriosus: Complementary use of detachable Cook patent ductus arteriosus coils and Amplatzer duct occluders. Eur J Pediatr 2000; 159(4): 293–6.

12. Thanapoulos BD, Hakim FA, Hiari A et al. Patent ductus arteriosus equipment and technique. Amplatzer duct occluder: intermediate-term follow up and technical considerations. J Interv Cardiol 2001; 14(2): 247–54.

13. Bilkis AA, Alwi M, Hasri S et al. The Amplatzer duct occluder: experience in 209 patients. J Am Coll Cardiol 2001; 37(1): 258–61.

14. Thanapoulos BD, Tsaousis GS, Djukic M et al. Transcatheter closure of high pulmonary artery pressure persistent ductus arteriosus with the Amplatzer muscular ventricular septal occluder. Heart 2002; 87(3): 260–3.

15. Demkow M, Ruzyllo W, Siudalska H, Kepka C. Transcatheter closure of a 16mm hypertensive patent ductus arteriosus with the Amplatzer muscular VSD occluder. Cathater Cardiovasc Interv 2001; 52(3): 359–62.

16. Duke C, Chan KC. Aortic obstruction caused by device occlusion of patent arterial duct. Heart 1999; 82(1): 109–11.

17. Joseph G, Mandalay A, Zacharias TU, George B. Severe intravascular hemolysis after transcatheter closure of a large patent ductus arteriosus using the Amplatzer duct occluder: Successful resolution by intradevice coil deployment. Catheter Cardiovasc Interv 2002; 55(2): 245–9.

18. Godart F, Rodes J, Rey C. Severe haemolysis after transcatheter closure of a patent arterial duct with the new Amplatzer duct occluder. Cardiol Young 2000; 10(3): 265–7.

19. Wilson W, Taubert KA, Gewitz M et al. Prevention of infective endocarditis; guidelines from the American Heart Association. Circulation 2007; 116(15): 1736–54.

20. Horstkotte D, Follath F, Gutschik E et al. Guidelines on prevention, diagnosis and treatment of infective endocarditis, executive summary; the task force on infective endocarditis of the European society of cardiology. Eur Heart J 2004; 25(3): 267–76.

14

Ebstein's anomaly of the tricuspid valve

Definition and anatomical notes

Ebstein's anomaly is a rare congenital heart anomaly of the tricuspid valve and right ventricle. It is characterized by abnormal adherence of the tricuspid valve leaflets (usually septal and posterior) to the underlying myocardium, and displacement of the functional tricuspid valve orifice more apically and anteriorly into the right ventricle and towards the right ventricular outflow tract (Figures 14.1–14.4). The right ventricle is divided into a dilated atrialized portion and a muscular portion, which represents the true apical right ventricle. The adherence of tricuspid valve leaflets to the myocardium is caused by a failure of delamination during development. These abnormalities usually cause severe tricuspid regurgitation, with extreme dilatation of the right atrium and an atrialized portion of right ventricle. Arrhythmias are frequent. Cyanosis may be present due to right-to-left shunt via frequently present atrial septal defect or patent foramen ovale. There is a great variability among patients with Ebstein's anomaly.[1,2]

Typical features of Ebstein's anomaly include:

- The septal and posterior leaflets are displaced towards the right ventricular apex and adhere to the right ventricular endomyocardium. The posterior cusp may be missing. Physiologically, in healthy adults the tricuspid valve is attached more apically than the mitral valve. However, a shift of >2cm from the level mitral attachment in adults is considered abnormal.[3,4]
- The anterior leaflet originates appropriately at the annular level, and is redundant and enlarged in a sail-like manner. It usually has many attachments to the right ventricular free wall, causing tethering of the leaflet, and may show multiple fenestrations. The chordal attachments are abnormally numbered and placed.
- The original anatomical tricuspid valve annulus is severely dilated in adults and the shape of the functional tricuspid valve orifice is eccentric, with a lack of coaptation of the leaflets and severe tricuspid regurgitation.
- The right ventricle is divided into an atrialized and a muscular portion. The 'atrialized' right ventricle extends from the true tricuspid annulus to the displaced attachment of the septal and posterior leaflets. It is a

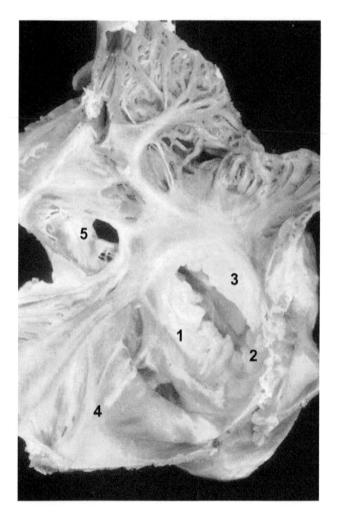

Figure 14.1
Ebstein's anomaly of the tricuspid valve. 1, Septal cusp; 2, posterior (mural) cusp; 3, anterior cusp; 4, atrialized part of the right ventricle; 5, fossa ovalis with atrial septal defect; view from right atrium. (Courtesy of Dr SY Ho, PhD, Royal Brompton Hospital, London.)

thin-walled, low-pressure chamber containing right ventricular myocytes. The right atrium, together with the atrialized part of the right ventricle is usually very large, often >10cm in diameter in adults.

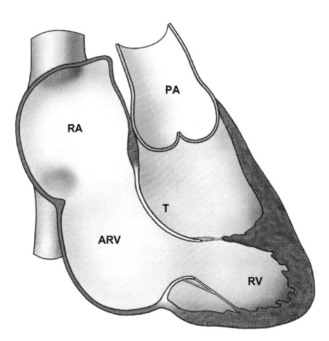

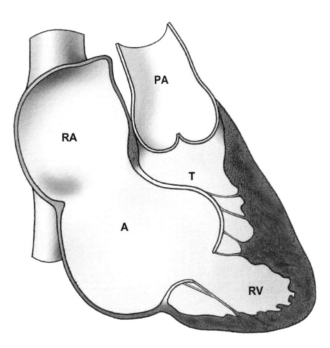

Figure 14.2
Ebstein's anomaly of tricupid valve, type A (according Carpentier). Free movement of tricuspid leaflets, mild septal and posterior leaflet displacement, mild dilatation of the atrialized right ventricle (ARV). T, Anterior leaflet of the tricuspid valve; RA, right atrium;
PA, pulmonary artery; RV, true apical functional right ventricle.

Figure 14.3
Ebstein's anomaly of tricupid valve, type B (according Carpentier). Restricted motion of the anterior cusp of the tricuspid valve (T) due to its fixation to the right ventricular wall by multiple short cords and papillary muscles, or by muscular bands, causing tethering of the leaflet. Important septal and posterior leaflet apical displacement, large dilatation of the atrialized right ventricle (ARV). T, Anterior leaflet of the tricuspid valve; RA, right atrium;
PA, pulmonary artery; RV, true apical functional right ventricle.

- The functional right ventricle is small, usually with lack of an inlet component and with a small trabecular component.
- The right ventricle infundibulum can be obstructed by the redundant anterior leaflet or by its chordal attachments.
- Many patients with Ebstein's anomaly (50–93%) have an interatrial communication – patent foramen ovale or atrial septal defect, mostly with a right-to-left or bidirectional shunt. Pulmonary stenosis or atresia occurs in 20–25% of cases. An accessory pathway (Wolff-Parkinson-White (WPW) syndrome) is present in about 4–26% of cases.
- Ebstein's anomaly of the tricuspid valve also occurs in corrected transposition of the great arteries. In this defect, the tricuspid valve is localized in the systemic position (see Figure 12.4).

Carpentier classifies Ebstein's anomaly into four types, with types A and B (Figures 14.2 and 14.3) being the most common in adults, surviving without operation:

- *Type A*: Freely moving leaflets; the shift of the septal leaflet is not big, the right ventricular atrialized part is small, and the volume of the functional right ventricle is adequate (Figure 14.2).

- *Type B*: The enlarged anterior leaflet is partly mobile (Figure 14.3). The atrialized portion of the right ventricle is large, sometimes akinetic or dyskinetic; the volume of the right ventricle is small.
- *Type C*: The movement of the anterior leaflet is restricted; the volume of the right ventricle is small, and the right ventricular outflow tract can be obstructed (Figure 14.4).
- *Type D*: With the exception of a small infundibular component, there is nearly a complete atrialization of the right ventricle. The functional right ventricle is virtually absent.

Prevalence

- Ebstein's anomaly is an infrequent defect with prevalence <1% of all congenital cardiac anomalies; mild forms may not be diagnosed until adulthood.
- The anomaly occurs with equal frequency in both sexes.
- Most cases are sporadic, but familial cases have been reported.

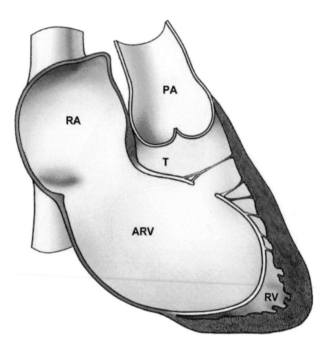

Figure 14.4
Ebstein's anomaly of tricupid valve, type C (according Carpentier). Immobile cusps, fixed to the underlying myocardium of the right ventricle and infundibulum, restrictive tricuspid valve orifice below pulmonary valve in the right ventricular outflow tract, extreme dilatation of the atrialized right ventricle (ARV). T, Anterior leaflet of the tricuspid valve; RA, right atrium; PA, pulmonary artery; RV, true apical functional right ventricle.

- Maternal exposure to lithium and benzodiazepine have been implicated as a potential cause.

Pathophysiology

- The tricuspid valve is usually significantly regurgitant due to a lack of leaflet coaptation (annulus dilatation), restricted movement of the septal and posterior leaflets (adhesion to the right ventricular endomyocardium), and abnormal morphology and tethering by tendinous cords of the anterior tricuspid valve leaflet.
- The thin-walled atrialized segment of the right ventricle may bulge in an aneurysm-like manner in systole.
- The interatrial communication leads to the shunt, which is dependent on the left and right atrial pressures. In severe tricuspid regurgitation and elevated right atrial pressure, the shunt is predominantly right-to-left and causes cyanosis. If the pressures in both atria are balanced, the shunt is bidirectional and cyanosis is mild or there is none. Right-to-left shunt may be only intermittent (during exercise or pregnancy). If the right atrial pressure is low in rare mild cases, the shunt may be even be predominantly left-to-right.

- Pulmonary artery pressure and pulmonary vascular resistance are usually low; the pulmonary flow can be severely reduced.
- The atrialized segment of the right ventricle contains right ventricular myocytes, which may cause ventricular tachycardia or ventricular fibrillation on mechanical irritation (e.g. during cardiac catheterization).
- Interestingly, the functional part of the right ventricle has an absolutely lower count of myocytes and a bigger proportion of connective tissue, which may be the reason for dilatation (particular in the infundibular part) and reduced function.
- Patients with Ebstein's anomaly have also been shown to have impaired right ventricular diastolic function and reduced right atrial compliance.
- There is often a mitral valve prolapse with regurgitation.
- Ebstein's anomaly should not be regarded as a disease confined to the right side of the heart.[5,6] Because of the massive dilatation of the right-heart chambers, the banana-shaped left ventricle has an impaired geometry and a reduced end-diastolic volume. Leftward bulging of the interventricular septum may impair the left ventricular function. In older adults, there is often a left ventricular diastolic dysfunction with an elevated pulmonary wedge pressure.
- An increased quantity of connective tissue has also been reported in the left ventricular wall.[7] The paradoxical septal movement reduces the left ventricular systolic function.
- Patients with Ebstein's malformation are prone to arrhythmias. Stretching and fibrosis of the dilated right atrium causes: atrial flutter and fibrillation; associated accessory muscular pathways for atrioventricular conduction, and abnormal fibrous encasement of the atrioventricular node and bundle of His; or fibrotic and dysplastic right ventricular tissue provide substrate for developing supraventricular and ventricular tachyarrhythmias, which are usually poorly tolerated.[1,8]
- Sudden death is encountered in 3–10% of patients, secondary to supraventricular or ventricular tachycardia.

Clinical findings and diagnosis
Clinical manifestations

- Asymptomatic course in many middle-aged patients with mild Ebstein's anomaly.
- Fatigue, diminished exercise tolerance.
- Palpitations and shortness of breath, particularly on exertion.
- Tachycardia.
- Chest pain resembling angina pectoris.
- Right-heart decompensation.

Physical examination

- Cyanosis (ruddy facial coloring = violaceous hue), intermittent or permanent, indicating significant right-to-left shunting or low cardiac output.
- Usually normal jugular venous and arterial pulse forms.
- Precordium often normally active (silent chest).
- Hepatomegaly.

Auscultatory findings

- The first sound is widely split and its second component is very loud due to the delayed closure of the large anterior leaflet of the tricuspid valve.
- The second sound may be widely split in the presence of delayed pulmonary valve closure; yet the split cannot always be heard because of the low pulmonary artery pressure.
- Serial clicks.
- Third and fourth sounds are usually present.
- Triple or quadruple rhythm (S4, split S1, split S2, S3).
- Systolic murmur from tricuspid regurgitation at the lower left sternal border, radiating toward the apex (right ventricular dislocation). The intensity of the murmur does not usually increase during inspirium, providing the functionally insufficient right ventricle is unable to raise stroke volume.
- Short mid-diastolic murmurs.

Electrocardiogram (ECG)

- Right atrial hypertrophy.
- The PR interval may be prolonged in the presence of intra-atrial or atrioventricular conduction disturbance.
- Right bundle branch block.
- Second QRS complex attached to the normal QRS.
- Deep Q waves in II, III, aVF, V1–V4 reflect the dislocated right ventricle; however, they may be mistaken for a myocardial infarction, especially if associated with chest pain.
- A preexcitation syndrome occurs in 10–25% of cases; usually WPW syndrome type B, with a right-side accessory pathway and delta wave in V5–V6. The accessory pathways may even be multiple.
- Intermittent left bundle branch block or tachycardia with aberrant conduction, resembling left bundle branch block, raises suspicion of the presence of Mahaim fibers.
- Supraventricular tachycardia develops in 25–30% of patients: atrial fibrillation, atrioventricular nodal reentry tachycardia, focal atrial tachycardia, atrial flutter.
- Ventricular tachycardia may develop in 1% of cases.
- Low voltage is possible in all leads.

Echocardiography

In adults with Ebstein's anomaly, echocardiography is difficult to perform because of the heart dislocation and dilatation. Adequate depth of the examination has to be selected.

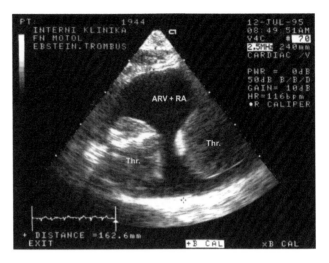

Figure 14.5
Ebstein's anomaly of the tricuspid valve. Transthoracic echo, parasternal long axis. Only the extremely dilated atrialized right ventricle (ARV) and right atrium (RA) can be visualized, its diameter in short axis is >160mm. There are two huge thrombi (Thr.) in this cavity, each >80mm in diameter. Unoperated lady with Ebstein anomaly, 61 years of age, only mildly symptomatic, NYHA Functional Class II.

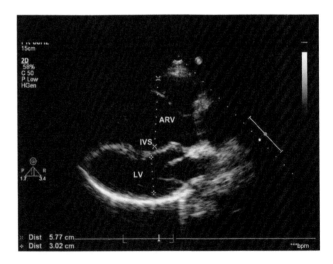

Figure 14.6
Ebstein's anomaly of the tricuspid valve. Transthoracic echo, long-axis parasternal view. Small left ventricle (LV) of 30mm in diastole, large right ventricle with large atrialized part (ARV), 58mm in diastole; the interventricular septum (IVS) is bulging into the left ventricle in diastole due to the right ventricular volume overload.

Standard projections will primarily show the dilated atrialized part of the right ventricle (Figures 14.5 and 14.6). The most informative approach for proper diagnosis is an apical four-chamber projection, often from as far back as the posterior axillary line (Figures 14.7 and 14.8).

Transesophageal echocardiography may be very useful, but the examination is not simple or easy to read. This is

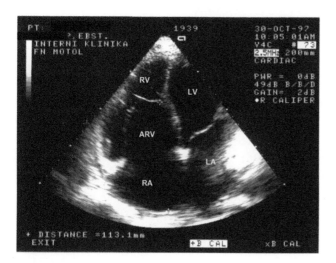

Figure 14.7

Ebstein's anomaly, type B. Transthoracic echo, apical four-chamber view from the lateral–back approach. Severely dilated right atrium (RA) with atrialized right ventricle (ARV), dilated true apical right ventricle (RV) mobile anterior leaflet. This 58-year-old man also had a dilated left ventricle (LV) and left atrium (LA), with severe systolic dysfunction of both ventricles, and died whilst on the waiting list for heart transplantation.

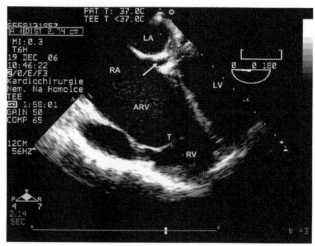

Figure 14.9

Ebstein's anomaly of the tricuspid valve. Transesophageal echo, 0 degrees, four-chamber view. T, Anterior cusp of the tricuspid valve, fixed to the lateral wall of the right ventricle; RV, true functional right ventricle; ARV, large atrialized part of the right ventricle; RA, right atrium; LA, left atrium; LV, left ventricle; arrow, coronary sinus.

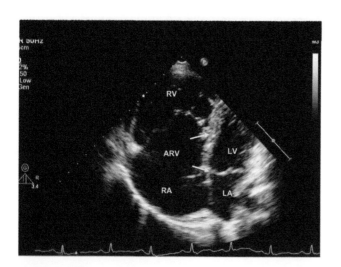

Figure 14.8

Ebstein's anomaly, type B. Transthoracic echo, apical four-chamber view from the lateral–back approach. Apical displacement of the septal cusp of the tricuspid valve is 40mm (arrows), right atrium (RA) with atrialized right ventricle (ARV), dilated true apical right ventricle (RV). LV, Left ventricle; LA, left atrium.

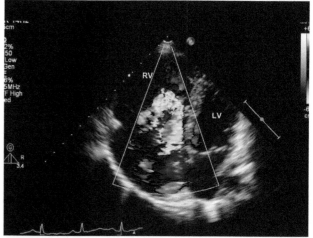

Figure 14.10

Ebstein's anomaly of the tricuspid valve. Transthoracic echo with color Doppler, apical four-chamber view. Color flow indicates severe tricuspid regurgitation from the apically displaced tricuspid orifice. RV, Right ventricle; LV, left ventricle.

because of the dislocation of the heart, which is caused by the extreme dilatation of the right atrium and the atrialized right ventricle (Figure 14.9).

The critical feature for establishing a diagnosis of Ebstein's anomaly is the apical shift of the tricuspid leaflet coaptation site, which is ideally verified using color Doppler

mapping in the presence of tricuspid regurgitation (Figures 14.10 and 14.11).

Echocardiographic examination is focused on:

• Size of the right atrium and the atrialized segment of the right ventricle.

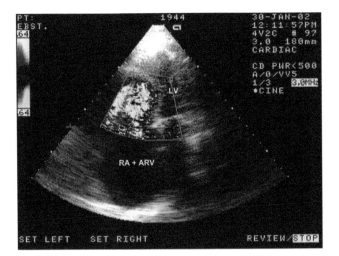

Figure 14.11
Ebstein's anomaly of the tricuspid valve, type C. Transthoracic echo with color Doppler, apical four-chamber view. Color flow indicates severe tricuspid regurgitation from the extremely apically displaced tricuspid orifice. Due to its unusual location, tricuspid regurgitation could be underestimated or even missed. RA + ARV, right atrium and dilated atrialized right ventricle; LV, left ventricle.

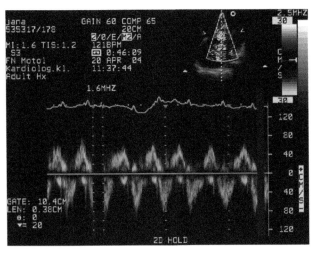

Figure 14.13
Pulsed Doppler echocardiography. Severe tricuspid regurgitation in a patient with Ebstein's anomaly of the tricuspid valve. Due to a large unrestrictive regurgitant orifice and low pulmonary artery pressure, the regurgitant flow is low velocity and laminar ('free-flow').

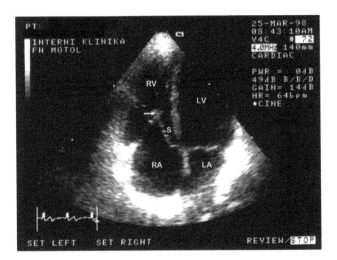

Figure 14.12
Ebstein's anomaly of the tricuspid valve, type A. Transthoracic echo, apical four-chamber view. Septal leaflet of the tricuspid valve is attached normally, without displacement in this view; however, the tricuspid orifice is dislocated apically. The anterior leaflet is moving freely, ARV and tricuspid regurgitation are small. RV, Right ventricle; RA, right atrium; arrow, tricuspid orifice; S, septal leaflet of the tricuspid valve; LV, left ventricle of normal size; LA, left atrium.

- Tricuspid valve:
  - morphology, degree of dysplasia, size and mobility of the anterior leaflet, length and origin of the tendons;
  - apical dislocation of the tricuspid valve orifice;
  - amount of apical shift of the posterior and septal tricuspid valve leaflets (*note*: in some projections, the septal leaflet may look quite normal, adhering to the septum only partly in the posterior part; Figure 14.12);
  - tricuspid regurgitation: the jet may be directed atypically from the apex across the dilated atrialized right ventricular segment (Figure 14.11); several regurgitation jets may be evident; tricuspid regurgitation usually has a low gradient, and may be unrestricted and laminar (free-flow) in the case of very large regurgitant orifice (Figure 14.13);
  - tricuspid annulus size.
- Size and function of the 'functional' apical right ventricle.
- Size and function of the left ventricle.
- Interatrial communication: presence and size; shunt amount and direction (transesophageal and contrast echocardiography) (Figure 14.14).
- Associated cardiac anomalies.
- Presence of mitral valve prolapse and mitral regurgitation.
- Presence of thrombi in the dilated cardiac chambers (Figures 14.5, 14.15 and 14.16).

Chest X-ray

- Varying size of the heart from normal to an extreme cardiomegaly (balloon-shaped heart) (Figure 14.17).
- The enlarged right atrium can produce a rightward curvature, and make up the entire cardiac silhouette.
- The left-heart border is straightened in its upper segment because of bulging of the infundibulum, overlapping the silhouettes of the aortic root and pulmonary artery.

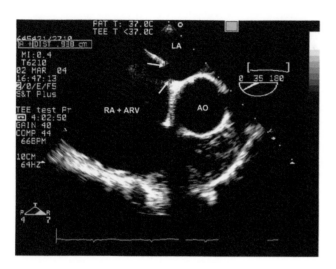

Figure 14.14
Transesophageal echo, transversal plane. Ebstein's anomaly of the tricuspid valve with small atrial septal defect type II (arrows) with bidirectional shunt. AO, Aorta; LA, left atrium; RA, right atrium; ARV, atrialized right ventricle.

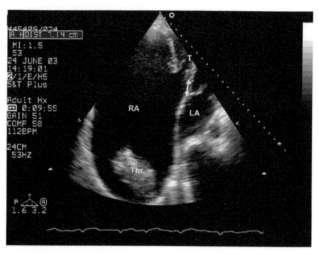

Figure 14.16
Transthoracic echo of the same patient as in Figure 14.15. Displacement of the septal cusp of the tricuspid valve is 22mm (arrow); large right atrium with thrombus (Thr.). LA, Left atrium; T, tricuspid valve.

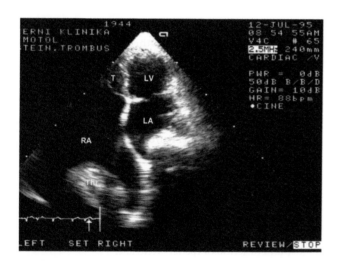

Figure 14.15
Ebstein's anomaly of the tricuspid valve. Transthoracic echo, apical four-chamber view. There is a huge thrombus (Thr.) in the extremely dilated right atrium (RA). LV, Left ventricle; LA, left atrium; T, septal cusp of the tricuspid valve, in this projection without displacement.

- Pulmonary vascular markings are normal or diminished.
- The cardiac stem is narrow, the pulmonary artery and aorta show no dilatation (Figure 14.17).

Holter monitoring

Holter monitoring should be performed repeatedly, especially in symptomatic patients.

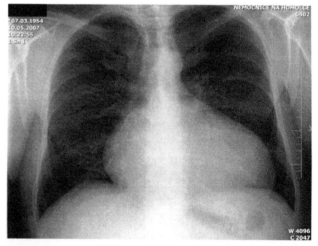

Figure 14.17
X-ray with the typical shape of the heart with Ebstein's anomaly.

Exercise testing with pulse oximetry

- Arterial saturation may deteriorate during exercise.
- Longitudinal follow-up of performance in mildly symptomatic patients is helpful in indicating surgery.

Electrophysiological studies

- Electrophysiological studies are indicated in the presence of symptomatic arrhythmia.

- May be indicated in asymptomatic patients with preexcitation syndrome, especially those who carry out professions associated with risk or a family history of sudden death.

Catheterization

- Diagnostic catheterization is not routinely performed. Particularly in former times, it was associated with morbidity and mortality secondary to catheterization-induced arrhythmia.
- Selective coronary angiogram is performed prior to surgery in patients over 40 years of age or in those with a high risk of coronary artery disease.
- Right-heart catheterization, with evaluation of pulmonary artery pressure, pulmonary arterial resistance, pulmonary wedge pressure and transpulmonary gradient, is important to assess in older patients with a severe form of Ebstein's anomaly before a planned bidirectional Glenn procedure.

Management

Indications for intervention:

- Deterioration of functional exercise capacity, Functional Class >II.
- Increasing heart size on chest X-ray with a cardiothoracic index >60%.
- Significant cyanosis with saturation at rest <90%.
- Severe symptomatic tricuspid regurgitation.
- Transient ischemic attack or cerebrovascular events.
- Atrial flutter, atrial fibrillation, supraventricular arrhythmia in the presence of accessory pathways.

Surgical management should only be undertaken in a department of cardiac surgery which is experienced with CHD surgery.

Operative aims:
- Tricuspid valve repair is preferred.
- Valve replacement if repair is impossible.
- Plication or no-plication of the atrialized right ventricle (optional).
- Closure of any associated atrial septal defect or patent foramen ovale.
- Interruption of accessory conduction pathways.
- Maze procedure as additional procedure in atrial fibrillation or flutter and volume-reduction of the right atrium.

Currently adopted surgical techniques
Repair of the tricuspid valve

- *Danielson (Mayo Clinic) annuloplasty*: Construction of a monocuspid valve with the use of the enlarged anterior

tricuspid leaflet; transverse plication of the free wall of the 'atrialized' right ventricular portion, posterior tricuspid annuloplasty, and excision of redundant right wall.[9]
- *Carpentier repair*: Mobilization of the anterosuperior leaflet, longitudinal plication of the 'atrialized' portion of the right ventricle, plication of the tricuspid valve annulus with rotation and reattachment of the anterosuperior leaflet on the right atrioventricular groove.[10] Using this technique, with the annuloplastic ring when necessary, it was possible to perform valvuloplasty in 98% of patients.[11]
- *Dearani-Danielson technique*: The base of the papillary muscles is brought, with sutures, toward the ventricular septum. The posterior angle of the tricuspid orifice is closed by plication. Posterior annuloplasty and anterior purse-string annuloplasty.[1,12]
- *Sebening technique* (Deutsches Herzzentrum München): Monocusp-plasty by 'single-stitch technique' with anterolateral shifting of the valvular plane. Relocation of the anterior leaflet is achieved by stitching the papillary muscle(s) to the septum in the direction of the 'true' valvular annulus as a primary procedure. This operation is performed without plication of the 'atrialized' portion. In the Augustin/Sebening technique an additional stabilization of the valvular plane is performed by placement of additional stitches at the right-lateral aspect of the anterior leaflet towards the septal leaflet.[13]

Tricuspid valve replacement

Biological prosthesis in the tricuspid position, when valvuloplasty is not possible, has better long-term results and is preferred to *mechanical prosthesis*.[1,14] The prosthesis is usually implanted in the right atrium above coronary sinus, which is left in the right ventricle. Leaving coronary sinus in the right atrium poses a high risk of complete atrioventricular block.

Bidirectional Glenn procedure

One-and-half ventricular repair (bidirectional Glenn procedure) is usually performed in high-risk patients with a severely reduced size of the right ventricle, or a severely dysfunctional and enlarged right ventricle, extended atrialized right ventricle and long-standing atrial fibrillation.[1,15] End-to-side anastomosis of the superior vena cava to the right pulmonary artery is performed in addition to the intracardiac repair (see Figure 15.2).[16] It reduces venous return to the dysfunctional right ventricle by almost half, and optimizes preload to the left ventricle. Construction of the shunt in patients with left ventricular dysfunction is possible if left ventricular end-diastolic pressure is <15mmHg, the transpulmonary gradient is <10mmHg and the mean pulmonary artery pressure is <18–20mmHg.[1]

Fontan procedure

Fontan procedure (total cavopulmonary connection) in the presence of tricuspid valve stenosis and/or right ventricular hypoplasia.

Intraoperative radiofrequency ablation or cryoablation

This technique represents an important adjunctive treatment for intractable arrhythmias. Concomitant procedures include right-sided Maze procedure, ablation of accessory pathways, and ablation of atrioventricular nodal reentry tachycardia.[1,17]

Heart transplantation

This may be recommended in patients with failed repair, or in severe biventricular dysfunction.

Catheter ablation

Catheter ablation of the accessory pathway after previous mapping can be performed with a high success rate. It is appropriate to use three-dimensional electroanatomical mapping (CARTO); there may be several accessory pathways.

Anticoagulation therapy

Anticoagulation therapy may be indicated in chronic atrial fibrillation, documented thrombi or spontaneous echocontrast in the dilated right atrium, and on suspicion of pulmonary or systemic embolism, unless causal surgical and catheter-based management is possible.

Risks and residual findings

- Those surviving *unoperated* to adulthood usually have milder forms of the anomaly; however, it does become symptomatic at the age of 40–50.
- A major risk in Ebstein's anomaly in adulthood is arrhythmia: supraventricular tachycardia in the WPW syndrome, atrial fibrillation and flutter, sinus node dysfunction, ventricular arrhythmia.
- Sudden death, most likely secondary to arrhythmia.
- Progression of tricuspid regurgitation, right ventricular dysfunction and right-heart decompensation.
- Progression of cyanosis due to right-to-left shunt on the atrial level.
- Paradoxical embolism into the central nervous system, transient ischemic attacks, cerebral abscess in patients with severe hypoxemia.
- Thrombus formation in a dilated right atrium and atrialized part of the right ventricle.
- A late sequel of surgery may be a complete atrioventricular block, whose risk is particularly high when suturing

a valvular prosthesis under the coronary sinus, with potential recurrent atrial and ventricular arrhythmia. A permanent pacemaker is needed in 11% of adults after operation.[18] Epicardial leads may be of benefit.

- Progression of tricuspid regurgitation and right-heart failure may be seen even after surgical tricuspid valvuloplasty. Patients with bidirectional cavo-pulmonary anastomosis have better tolerance of the residual tricuspid valve dysfunction.
- Bioprosthesis degeneration, thrombosis or infection of mechanical tricuspid valve prosthesis.
- There is a high operative risk in adults with very severe tricuspid regurgitation lasting for a long time, NYHA Functional Class IV and atrial fibrillation. The most common cause of early postoperative death in adults is right ventricular failure with low cardiac output and anuria, not reacting to inotropic support and volume expansion.[11]

Pregnancy

In asymptomatic females with good ventricular function, pregnancy may be well tolerated. There is a certain risk of right ventricular decompensation and arrhythmias in the presence of pregnancy-induced right ventricular volume overload. Atrioventricular nodal reentry tachycardia or atrial flutter may develop. A right-to-left shunt poses the patient at risk for paradoxical embolism. Hypoxemia poses a risk to the fetus. Pregnancy is contraindicated in significant cyanosis, serious arrhythmia and right-heart failure.

Infective endocarditis

Prophylaxis is advised given the malformed valve; however, the rise of infective endocarditis is not very high because of the slow flow rates at the tricuspid valve.

Follow-up

Follow-up should be undertaken by a cardiologist with expertise in CHD, in cooperation with a specialized department of arrhythmology.

Prognosis

- The severest forms of Ebstein's anomaly result in intrauterine death or death at a neonatal age.
- Conversely, survival until older age without operation, with only insignificant symptoms, has been reported in patients with mild forms of the anomaly.
- Most patients are somewhere in between these first two extremes.

- The mean age of death in patients with Ebstein's anomaly in historical studies is about 20 years of age, with one-third dying before reaching 10 years of age.[7,19]
- Adverse prognostic factors include progression of cyanosis, X-ray heart enlargement, newly occurring arrhythmia, progression of dyspnea and fatigability.
- Ebstein's repair has good functional outcomes in children, despite residual tricuspid regurgitation.[17]
- Surgical early mortality in patients with Ebstein's anomaly of the tricuspid valve depends on the experince of the surgeon, ranging between 1.8 and 54%. In experienced centers, the early mortality is between 5 and 7%.[1,11]
- The combination of bidirectional cavo-pulmonary anastomosis and intracardiac repair decreased operative mortality in high-risk groups (massive tricuspid regurgitation, extended atrialized right ventricle, poor right ventricle contractility, longstanding atrial fibrillation) from 24 to 0%.[15] Bidirectional Glenn is indicated in patients at very high risk with a small functional right ventricle or severe dysfunction of the right ventricle.
- The mid-term prognosis after repair is good, with the 10- and 20-year survival rates between 86 and 82%, respectively.[11,18]
- Freedom from reoperation was similar in patients with tricuspid valve repair (83%) and replacement (82%) at 10 years.[1]
- The most frequent cause of death from Ebstein's anomaly in adulthood is arrhythmia and, less often, heart failure.
- Sudden death occurs regardless of the severity of disease, especially in patients over 50 years of age.[20]
- Predictor of death is a cardiothoracic index >60–65%, or development of chronic atrial fibrillation, which predicts death within 5 years.[21]

Conditions to be distinguished from Ebstein's anomaly

Uhl anomaly of the right ventricle

With Uhl anomaly, the parietal right ventricular myocardium is complete or partially absent.[22] The right ventricular wall is paper-thin, thinner than the right atrial wall, and the right ventricle and right atrium are dilated. The absence of the myocardium results in impaired right ventricular kinetics, akinesis of the lateral and anterior right ventricular wall, and in paradoxical septal movement. The tricuspid valve is structurally normal; it may regurgitate. It differs from the tricuspid valve in Ebstein's anomaly by the completely normal origin of leaflets at the site of the tricuspid annulus and orifice.

Uhl anomaly often manifests by cardiac failure and is not dominated by arrhythmias, which mostly occur in older patients. Most patients die in childhood. Uhl anomaly is often confused with arrhythmogenic cardiomyopathy of the right ventricle.

Arrhythmogenic cardiomyopathy of the right ventricle

Arrhythmogenic cardiomyopathy (previously dysplasia) is characterized by a patchy and localized replacement of the right (and left) ventricular musculature by fibro-fatty tissue, separating the endocardial and epicardial layers. This finding may progress. More extensive involvement may be associated with generalized and segmental myocardial kinetic impairment with areas of localized sac-like dilatation. Echocardiography may fail to demonstrate dysplasia; MRI is a more sensitive method. Arrhythmogenic cardiomyopathy has an arrhythmogenic potential, and may be the cause of sudden death in young age.

Carcinoid

Carcinoid often involves the tricuspid (and pulmonary) valve. Tricuspid valve and the tendons are thickened, fibrodysplastic, the valve is rigid, with a lack of coaptation of the leaflets, and often severely regurgitates. The origin of the leaflets is normal. In severe tricuspid regurgitation, the right ventricle as well as the right atrium is dilated and volume overloaded. Clinically, there is a flush in the face, upper part of the body and acral parts of the limbs, diarrhea and loss of weight. The gastrointestinal tumor carcinoid may be diagnosed by CT or MRI, and, if endocrinologically active, by increased serum level of serotonin and its metabolite 5-hydroxy-indol-acetic acid in urine or by production of other vasoactive substances.

References

1. Dearani JA, O'Leary PW, Danielson GK. Surgical treatment of Ebstein's malformation: State of the art in 2006. Cardiol Young 2006; 16(Suppl 3): 12–20.
2. Attenhofer Jost CH, Connolly HM, Edwards WD et al. Ebstein's anomaly – review of a multifaceted congenital cardiac condition. Swiss Med Wkly 2005; 135(19–20): 269–81.
3. Gussenhoven EJ, Stewart PA, Becker EA et al. 'Offsetting' of the septal tricuspid leaflet in normal hearts and in hearts with Ebstein's anomaly. Am J Cardiol 1984; 54: 172.
4. Oechslin E, Buchholz S, Jenni R. Ebstein's anomaly in adults: Doppler-echocardiographic evaluation. Thorac Cardiovasc Surg 2000; 48(4): 209–13.
5. Inai K, Nakanishi T, Mori Y, Tomimatsu H, Nakazawa M. Left ventricular diastolic dysfunction in Ebstein's anomaly. Am J Cardiol 2004; 93(2): 255–8.
6. Attenhofer Jost CH, Connolly HM, O'Leary PW et al. Left heart lesions in patients with Ebstein's anomaly. Mayo Clin Proc 2005; 80(3): 361–8.
7. Celemajer DS, Cullen S, Sullivan ID et al. Outcome in neonates with Ebstein's anomaly. J Am Coll Cardiol 1992; 19: 1041–6.

8. Furer SK, Gomes JA, Love B, Mehta D. Mechanism and therapy of cardiac arrhythmias in adults with congenital heart disease. Mt Sinai J Med 2005; 72(4): 263–9.

9. Danielson GK, Maloney JD, Devloo RAE. Surgical repair of Ebstein's anomaly. Mayo Clin Proc 1979; 54: 185–92.

10. Carpentier A, Chauvaud S, Macé L et al. A new reconstructive operation for Ebstein's anomaly of the tricuspid valve. J Thorac Cardiovasc Surg 1988; 96: 92–101.

11. Chauvaud S, Berrebi A, Attellis N et al. Ebstein's anomaly repair based on functional analysis. Eur J Cardiovasc Surg 2003; 23(4): 525–31.

12. Dearani JA, Danielson GK. Surgical management of Ebstein's anomaly in the adult. Semin Thorac Cardiovasc Surg 2005; 17: 148–54.

13. Augustin N, Schmidt-Habelmann P, Wottke M, Meisner H, Sebening F. Results after surgical repair of Ebstein's anomaly. Ann Thorac Surg 1997; 63: 1650–6.

14. Miyamura H, Kanazawa H, Takahashi Y et al. Long-term results of valve replacement in the right side of the heart in congenital heart disease – comparative study of bioprosthetic valve and mechanical valve. Nippon Kyobu geka Gakkai Zasshi 1990; 38(8): 1298–303.

15. Chauvaud S, Fuzellier JF, Berrebi A et al. Bi-directional cavopulmonary shunt associated with ventriculo and valvuloplasty in Ebstein's anomaly: Benefits in high risk patients. Eur J Cardiothorac Surg 1998; 13(5): 514–19.

16. Akaishi J, Yamauchi H, Ochi M et al. One and a half ventricle repair for Ebstein's anomaly. Jpn J Thorac Cardiovasc Surg 2003; 51(12): 665–8.

17. Chen JM, Mosca RS, Altmann K et al. Early and medium-term results for repair of Ebstein's anomaly. J Thorac Cardiovasc Surg 2004; 127(4): 990–8.

18. Chauvaud SM, Brancaccio G, Carpentier AF. Cardiac arrhythmia in patients undergoing surgical repair of Ebstein's anomaly. Ann Thorac Surg 2001; 71(5): 1547–52.

19. Kumar AE, Fyler DC, Miettinen OS et al. Ebstein's anomaly: Clinical profile and natural history. Am J Cardiol 1971; 28: 84–95.

20 Gentles TL, Calder AL, Clarkson PM et al. Predictors of long-term survival with Ebstein's anomaly of the tricuspid valve. Am J Cardiol 1992; 69: 377–81.

21. Attie F, Rosas M, Rijlaarsdam M et al. The adult with Ebstein's anomaly. Outcome in 72 unoperated patients. Medicine (Baltimore) 2000; 79(1): 27–36.

22. Uhl HSM. A previously undescribed congenital malformation of the heart: Almost total absence of the myocardium of the right ventricle. Bull Johns Hopkins Hosp 1952; 91: 197–205.

15

Functionally single ventricle, Fontan procedure – univentricular heart/circulation

The issue and diagnosis of complex congenital heart disease (CHD) is, given its complexity, outside the scope of this monograph. Therefore, individual complex CHD are discussed only briefly. Rather than on understanding the complex morphology, emphasis is placed on understanding the principle of Fontan procedure, Fontan physiology, and residual findings and complications following the procedure, which can also be encountered by adult cardiologists not specialized in the management of CHD.

Definition, anatomical notes and prevalence

Nomenclature and definition of the univentricular heart has remained controversial and a matter of debate for many years. The morphological heterogeneity contributes to this controversy, in particular the recognition that truly solitary ventricles are rare (a hypoplastic or rudimentary ventricle or outlet chamber is frequently present). The terms functionally single ventricle and univentricular heart are frequently used interchangeably, and describe the fact that there are not two well-developed ventricles. Thus, the group of congenital heart defects with univentricular heart includes heterogeneous, complex defects whose only common feature being that they cannot be repaired surgically to a circulation with two ventricles (biventricular repair). The situation is managed surgically by what is known as *univentricular circulation (Fontan procedure/circulation)*, or its modification total cavo-pulmonary connection (TCPC) (Figure 15.1). The systemic venous connection is detoured directly into the pulmonary artery, the intracardiac anatomy is left in situ, and the subaortic ventricle only acts as a pump for the systemic circulation. In the presence of complete cavo-pulmonary anastomosis, cyanosis is completely (or almost completely) eliminated, as all systemic venous blood travels directly into the pulmonary artery regardless of the intracardiac morphology.

Some patients with a functionally single ventricle may survive without surgery until adulthood, in the presence

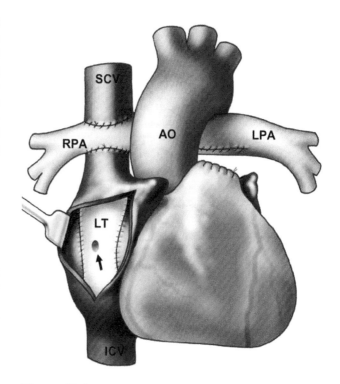

Figure 15.1
Total cavo-pulmonary connection with fenestration (arrow), type of Fontan operation. SCV, Superior caval vein; ICV, inferior caval vein; LT, lateral tunnel; AO, aorta; RPA, right pulmonary artery; LPA, left pulmonary artery.

of favorable hemodynamics and balanced pulmonary artery flow associated with significant pulmonary stenosis. Under certain circumstances, Fontan procedure or some of its modifications can be performed, even in adulthood. The main condition for Fontan procedure indication is normal pulmonary artery pressure. In adults with functionally single ventricle, this may be achieved by the existence of pulmonary stenosis, severe enough to prevent development of pulmonary hypertension and pulmonary vascular obstructive disease (Eisenmenger syndrome) (see Chapter 16).

The most common complex congenital heart diseases (CHD) with univentricular circulation, which may be surgically managed by Fontan circulation, usually TCPC, are discussed below.

Tricuspid atresia

Tricuspid atresia (TA) accounts for some 0.7% of all CHD. In TA, the tricuspid valve is absent, and there is no anatomic connection and direct communication between the right atrium and right ventricle; a fibrotic septum is usually present at the site of the tricuspid valve (Figures 15.2 and 15.3). In this defect, systemic venous blood runs from the right atrium, via the patent foramen ovale or secundum atrial septal defect, to the left atrium, where the blood blends with oxygenated blood from the pulmonary veins. The only functional ventricular chamber in this heart is the left ventricle. The right ventricle is rudimentary, there is no inlet and trabecular part, the infundibulum communicates with the left ventricle via the bulboventricular orifice. The pulmonary artery arises from the hypoplastic right ventricle. In 90% of patients, the great arteries are in a normal position and the bulboventricular orifice is restrictive (subpulmonary stenosis with protection of the pulmonary vascular bed against pulmonary vascular disease). The great arteries are transposed in 10% of the patients with tricuspid atresia, and the bulboventricular orifice is nonrestrictive. In addition to complications due to chronic hypoxemia, risks in the long run include progression of mitral regurgitation and failure of the left ventricle with volume overload.

Double-inlet left ventricle

This type of functionally single ventricle accounts for about 1.3% of all CHD. In double-inlet left ventricle (DILV), there are two atria; however, both atria empty into a single ventricle, which is a morphological left ventricle. The atrioventricular (AV) connection can be established by one single AV valve or by two (right and left) AV valves (Figures 15.4–15.6). The right- and left-sided AV valves are on the same plane, and these valves are neither morphological tricuspid nor mitral valves. The right AV valve orifice is overriding the ventricular septum and is predominantly (>50%) connected with the single left ventricle. The large left ventricle may communicate via the bulboventricular orifice with a hypoplastic infundibular right ventricle (Figure 15.7), which gives rise to the pulmonary artery (often hypoplastic or stenotic in adulthood). This arrangement protects the pulmonary vascular bed against excessive blood flow, allowing the patient to survive until adulthood without pulmonary hypertension. In patients with transposition of the great arteries, it is the aorta, which arises from the hypoplastic right ventricle.

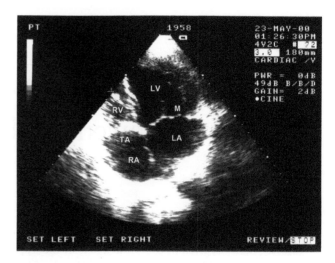

Figure 15.2
Tricuspid atresia (TA); transthoracic echo, apical four-chamber view. RA, Right atrium; RV, hypoplastic right ventricle; LV, left ventricle; M, mitral valve; LA, left atrium.

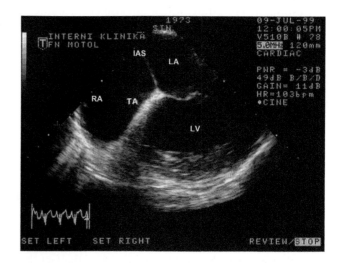

Figure 15.3
Tricuspid atresia (TA); transesophageal echo, transversal projection. RA, Right atrium; IAS, interatrial septum; M, mitral valve; LV, left ventricle with hypertrophic wall.

Double-outlet right ventricle

Double-outlet right ventricle (DORV) encompasses virtually the entire spectrum of congenital cardiac anatomy and physiology. Both great arteries arise predominantly (>50%) from the morphologically right ventricle (Figures 15.8 and 15.9). In adult survivors, subvalvular stenosis of the pulmonary artery is often present. The left ventricle often communicates with the right ventricle by a large ventricular septal defect, whose location in relation to the great arteries (subaortic, subpulmonary, doubly committed) determines the physiology. The left ventricle is usually hypoplastic with no great artery arising from it. Provided an adequately big left ventricle, *biventricular*

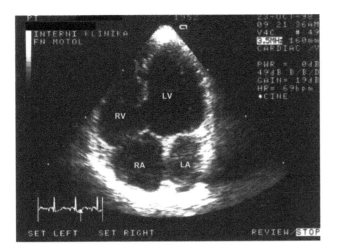

Figure 15.4
Double-inlet left ventricle, two atrioventricular valves, both on the same level. Transthoracic echo, apical four-chamber view. LV, Left ventricle, functionally common; LA, left atrium; RA, right atrium; RV, hypoplastic right ventricle.

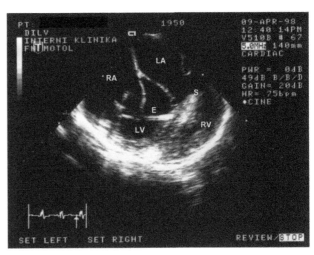

Figure 15.6
Double-inlet left ventricle; transesophageal echo, four-chamber transversal view. LV, Left ventricle; RV, hypoplastic right ventricle; E, electrode of the permanent pacemaker is fixed atypically to the rest of the interventricular septum (S); LA, left atrium; RA, right atrium.

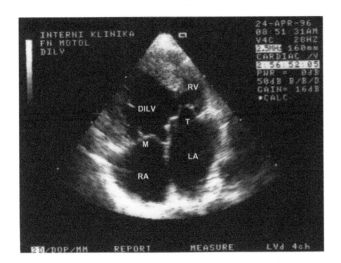

Figure 15.5
Double-inlet left ventricle (DILV); transthoracic echo, apical four-chamber view. Two atrioventricular (AV) valves, functionally common ventricle, functionally left (DILV) is on the right side; RV, hypoplastic right ventricle (on the left), the valve on the left side has tricuspid morphology (T), the AV valve on the right side has mitral morphology (M). RA, Right atrium; LA, left atrium.

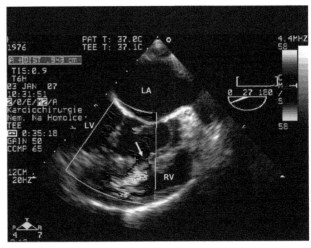

Figure 15.7
Double-inlet left ventricle (DILV) with restrictive ventricular septal defect and normal position of the great arteries. Transesophageal echo, 27 degrees. This patient was unoperated on until 31 years of age. Due to the restrictive muscular ventricular septal defect (arrow), which functionally served as subvalvular pulmonary stenosis, this patient did not have pulmonary hypertension and it was possible to perform total cavo-pulmonary connection in adulthood. LA, Left atrium; LV, left ventricle = DILV; RV, right ventricle.

repair can be considered. This type of DORV would not be classified as a functionally single ventricle.

A functionally single ventricle in the heterotaxy syndrome

The heterotaxy syndrome accounts for some 2% of all CHD (see Chapter 23 for more details). In this syndrome, the heart usually has a common atrium, a complete AV septal defect, a common AV valve, and often a common, morphologically right ventricle (Figures 15.10–15.12). The pulmonary artery usually has valvular and subvalvular stenosis. Patients with this syndrome usually have systemic and pulmonary vein anomalies, and the coronary sinus may be absent. Often a right and a left superior vena cava are

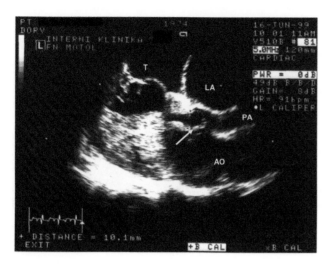

Figure 15.8
Double-outlet right ventricle; transesophageal echo, longitudinal view. T, Tricuspid valve; AO, dilated aorta in front due to the transposition of the great arteries; PA, hypoplastic pulmonary artery behind aorta with subvalvar obstruction due to the prolapsing fibrotic tissue (arrow).

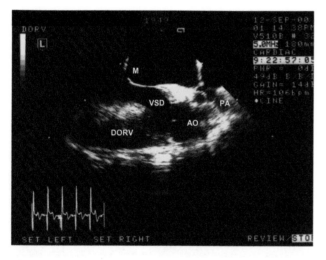

Figure 15.9
Double-outlet right ventricle (DORV); transesophageal echo, longitudinal view. AO, Broad aorta in front; PA, stenotic and hypoplastic pulmonary artery in the back; VSD, ventricular septal defect; M, mitral valve.

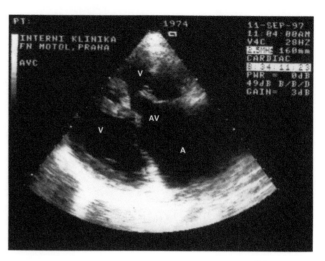

Figure 15.10
Heterotaxy syndrome; transthoracic echo, parasternal longitudinal view. AV, Functionally common atrioventricular valve; A, functionally common atrium; V, functionally common ventricle.

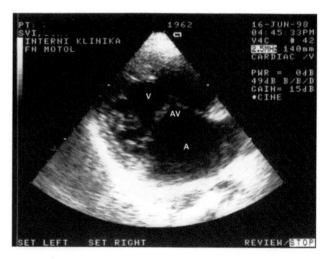

Figure 15.11
Functionally common ventricle in heterotaxy syndrome; transthoracic echo, apical view. A, Common atrium; V, common ventricle; AV, common atrioventricular valve.

Clinical notes

Patients with a functionally single ventricle, and reasonable degree of pulmonary stenosis and adequate pulmonary blood flow, may have a balanced physiology (pulmonary/systemic circulation) and survive without surgery until adulthood. Despite significant cyanosis and low oxygen saturation, their condition is not critical, enabling them to perform some physical activity (see Chapter 16). Their adaptation to hypoxemia (present ever since their birth), makes this possible. The diagnosis is established by echocardiography or, possibly, by transesophageal echocardiography.

present. The inferior vena cava is often absent, and it is drained via the venous azygos or hemiazygos systems to the superior vena cava. Hepatic veins empty into the common atrium directly and separately (Figure 15.13). Patients with interruption of the inferior vena cava may undergo Fontan procedure by connecting the vena cava superior with blood flowing from the azygos vein (or, alternatively, from both venae cavae superior) to the right branch of the pulmonary artery. The result is *cavo-pulmonary anastomosis according to Kawashima*.

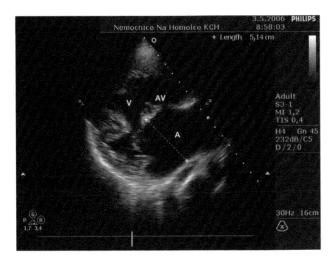

Figure 15.12
Functionally common ventricle in heterotaxy syndrome; transthoracic echo, parasternal view. A, Common atrium; V, common ventricle; AV, common atrioventricular valve. Patient was unoperated on until 44 years of age, when palliative bidirectional Glenn shunt was performed.

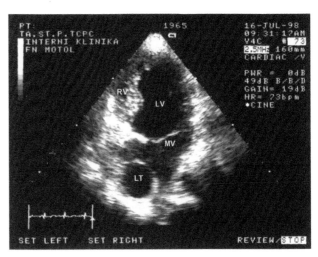

Figure 15.14
Tricuspid atresia after total cavo-pulmonary connection; transthoracic echo, apical view. LT, Lateral tunnel; LV, left ventricle; RV, severely hypoplastic right ventricle; MV, mitral valve.

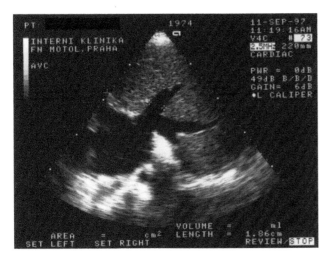

Figure 15.13
Transthoracic echo, subcostal view, heterotaxy syndrome with dextroisomerism. Dilated left-sided hepatic veins draining the common atrium in heterotaxy syndrome with the liver on both right and left sides.

Attention should be given to the course and connection of systemic and pulmonary veins. Patients considered for an intervention require catheterization to determine whether the capacity of the pulmonary vascular bed is adequately high and pulmonary vascular resistance adequately low, so that Fontan circulation would be functioning. However, preoperative determination of pulmonary vascular resistance in the presence of a low cardiac output may be inaccurate. Underestimation of increased pulmonary vascular resistance may be the cause of postoperative complications.

Surgical management

Palliative Fontan procedure consists of surgical connection of the systemic venous return directly into the pulmonary artery. Originally described by Fontan, it has undergone many modifications.[1-6] Fontan procedure eliminates the contractile function of the subpulmonary, right ventricle. While, initially, the procedure was intended by Fontan for patients with tricuspid atresia, it was later used for most types of functionally single ventricle which are not suitable for biventricular repair.

The procedure, as originally designed by Fontan in 1971, consisted of connecting the right atrium to the pulmonary artery by means of a conduit with a valve.[1] However, in the long run, this type of procedure resulted in extensive right atrial dilatation with the risk of atrial fibrillation and thrombus formation; therefore, a variety of surgical modifications have been devised. The technique used most often today is *TCPC* (total cavo-pulmonary connection), involving connection of the superior vena cava as well as inferior vena cava directly to the pulmonary artery according deLeval.[4] The inferior vena cava is connected using an intra-atrial tunnel (Figure 15.14) or, alternatively, an extracardiac prosthesis. In high-risk patients, the intra-atrial tunnel may be fenestrated (Figures 15.1, 15.15 and 15.16). This results in a small right-to-left shunt with usually insignificant cyanosis, but it helps in the case of high venous pressure. TCPC can be performed as a one-step or multistep procedure. If performed in several steps, the first procedure is a *bidirectional cavo-pulmonary anastomosis* (Figure 15.17), connecting the superior vena cava with the right pulmonary artery. Subsequent completion to Fontan circulation of total cavo-pulmonary connection consists of also connecting the

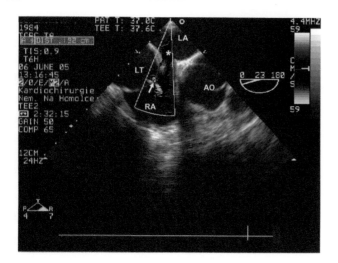

Figure 15.15
Tricuspid atresia after total cavo-pulmonary connection;
transesophageal echo, 23 degrees. The lateral tunnel (LT) with
small fenestration and small right-to-left shunt (arrow). LA, Left
atrium, *, atrial septal defect; AO, aorta; RA, right atrium.

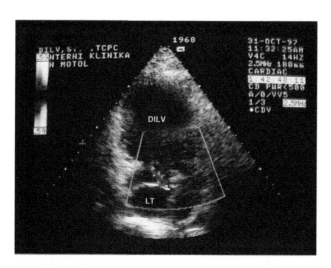

Figure 15.16
Double-inlet left ventricle (DILV) with total cavo-pulmonary
connection and small fenestration; transthoracic echo, apical
view. The small red jet indicates the small right-to-left shunt from
the lateral tunnel (LT) to the atrium.

inferior vena cava to the pulmonary artery, most often using
a lateral intra-atrial tunnel (Figures 15.1 and 15.14).

Risks and residual findings

Patients undergoing Fontan procedure are at permanent
risk of the following:[7–9]

- *Arrhythmias:* Atrial flutter or atrial fibrillation are frequent, and their incidence increases over time. It may

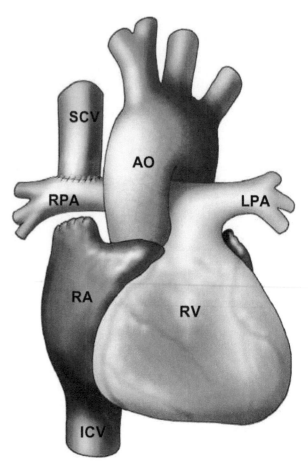

Figure 15.17
Bidirectional cavo-pulmonary anastomosis, bidirectional Glenn
procedure. SCV, Superior caval vein; IVC, inferior caval vein;
RPA, right pulmonary artery; LPA, left pulmonary artery;
AO, aorta; RA, right atrium; RV, right ventricle.

lead to significant deterioration of the hemodynamic
state. Late sequels may include AV block.

- *Thromboembolism:* May be systemic as well as pulmonary. Most often, it is caused by a thrombogenic state
and thrombus formation in the presence of slow, non-
pulsatile blood flow in systemic veins, intra-atrial tunnel
or in the severely enlarged right atrium in classical
Fontan procedure. A spontaneous echo-contrast is
invariably present in the intra-atrial tunnel in adults examined by transesophageal echocardiography. Development
of thrombosis in this conduit may result in direct
embolism into the pulmonary artery, which is dismal
(Figures 15.18–15.23). The subsequent rise in pulmonary artery pressure leads to severe venous hypertension in the cavo-pulmonary system and in systemic
veins, which is associated with edema and enteropathy
up to the collapse of Fontan circulation. Systemic
embolism may be associated with atrial fibrillation and
thrombophilic states (e.g. protein C, protein S and

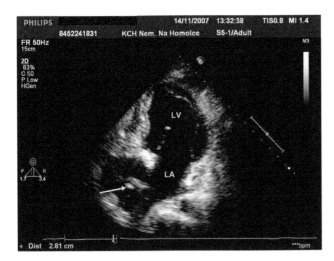

Figure 15.18
Tricuspid atresia with calcifications inside the lateral tunnel (arrow); transthoracic echo, apical view. This patient had thrombus in the lateral tunnel and protein-losing enteropathy. LV, Left ventricle; LA, left atrium.

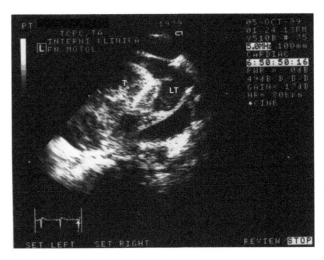

Figure 15.20
The same patient as in Figure 15.19. Transesophageal echo, longitudinal view. T, Partly calcified thrombus; LT, lateral tunnel.

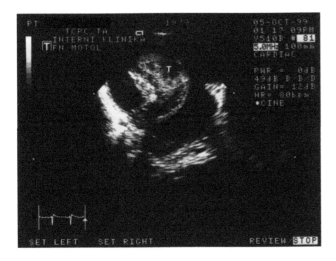

Figure 15.19
Tricuspid atresia with total cavo-pulmonary connection; transesophageal echo, transversal view. The lateral tunnel is obturated by thrombus (T), which is partly calcified. This patient had syncope and severe shortness of breath due to pulmonary embolism.

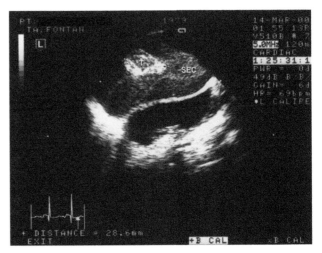

Figure 15.21
The same patient as in Figures 15.19 and 15.20. Tricuspid atresia with total cavo-pulmonary connection and thrombus (T) in the lateral tunnel, after 1 year of anticoagulation therapy. The thrombus is smaller, severe spontaneous echocontrast (SEC) in the lateral tunnel.

antithrombin III deficiencies, activated protein C resistance). Intracardiac thrombus was found in 12% of 235 adults with Fontan circulation, with an overall mortality of 18%; the mortality in hemodynamically unstable patients was 75%. Residual clots were seen after 1 year in 39% of survivors.[10]

- *Protein-losing enteropathy:* A high venous pressure and venous congestion in the splanchnic area lead to fluid and protein losses into the intestinal lumen. Impaired drainage and increased pressure in the superior vena cava result in an increased pressure in the thoracic duct and intestinal lymphangiectasia. This condition results in chronic diarrhea, and hypoproteinemia; it may be associated with ascites, peripheral edema, and pleural and pericardial effusions. Increased fecal levels of alpha-1-antitrypsin were demonstrated, as was hypalbuminemia in serum. Protein-losing enteropathy occurs after Fontan procedure in 3.7–10% of cases, even as long as 10 years postoperatively. Management is most difficult: high-protein diet, albumin infusion, diuretics, conduit

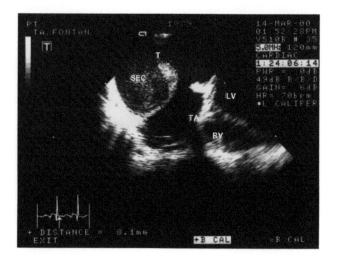

Figure 15.22
The same patient as in Figure 15.21. Transesophageal echo, transversal view. Severe spontaneous echocontrast (SEC) in the lateral tunnel with only small thrombus (T) at the medial wall. LV, Left ventricle; RV, right ventricle; TA, atretic tricuspid valve.

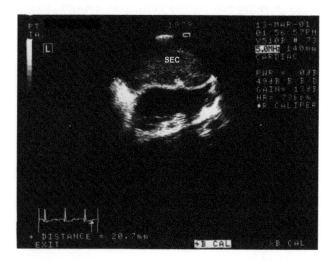

Figure 15.23
The same patient as in Figures 15.19–15.22. The thrombus disappeared after 2 years of anticoagulation therapy, spontaneous echocontrast (SEC) in the lateral tunnel remains.

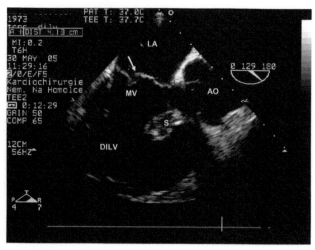

Figure 15.24
Double-inlet left ventricle (DILV) after total cavo-pulmonary connection; transesophageal echo, 129 degrees. Mitral valve (MV) has dilated annulus and prolapse of the anterior cusp (arrow). Severe mitral regurgitation caused pulmonary hypertension and required reoperation with mitral valve repair. AO, Aorta; S, rest of interventricular septum; LA, left atrium. Tricuspid valve (connected to the left ventricle) cannot be seen in this projection.

- *Residual cyanosis:* This may be due to residual shunts, e.g. from the hepatic veins, which were left entering the atrial space directly (so that hepatic venous blood bypasses the lungs), persistent left superior vena cava not detoured into the pulmonary artery, persistent fenestration. Other factors potentially contributing to cyanosis may include systemic venous to pulmonary venous collaterals, or formation of arteriovenous intrapulmonary collaterals (especially after conventional Glenn operation). Transcatheter treatment is feasible.[11]
- *Recurrent pleural and pericardial exudates* require frequent draining and long-term diuretic therapy.
- *Infectious endocarditis* may require reoperation.

Reoperation or reintervention of Fontan circulation

- In the presence of high venous pressure, with signs of systemic venous congestion and protein-losing enteropathy, fenestration between the intra-atrial tunnel and atria can be created surgically, a procedure which, while resulting in a right-to-left shunt, will reduce excess pressure in the systemic venous bed.
- In patients with stable hemodynamics following Fontan operation with fenestration related to excess desaturation, the fenestration can be closed by a transcatheter approach.

fenestration, reoperation, heart transplantation, corticosteroids, unfractionated heparin, somatostatin, etc.

- *Progressive failure of the subaortic single ventricle:* Worsening regurgitation of the AV valve(s), reduced myocardial compliance and systolic dysfunction, increase in pulmonary artery pressure and pulmonary vascular resistance result in congestive heart failure and failure of Fontan circulation (Figure 15.24).
- *Deterioration of hepatic function:* Congestive hepatopathy in the presence of increased venous pressure, hepatic fibrosis and cirrhosis.

- In the presence of atrial arrhythmias after conventional Fontan procedure, a TCPC conduit/extracardiac Fontan (conversion from a classic Fontan to an extracardiac Fontan) can be created, and the dilated right atrium reduced in size. These reoperations should be always preceded by a preoperative electrophysiology study, radiofrequency ablation and/or intraoperative antiarrhythmic surgery (isthmus ablation, modified right atrial maze or Cox-maze III). The arrhythmia recurrence after surgery was 12.8%.[12]
- Cyanosis due to venous–venous collaterals, or intrapulmonary AV malformations, can be occluded by catheter techniques.
- Failure of Fontan circulation with retractable protein-losing enteropathy, or failure of the common ventricle, may require heart transplantation.

Pregnancy

Pregnancy is possible in patients undergoing Fontan operation, yet it does pose a significant circulatory load. Pregnancy can only be considered in women without residual findings, with good functional exercise capacity and excellent function of the systemic ventricle and Fontan circulation. A multicenter study reported 33 pregnancies in 14 women after Fontan operation.[13,14] About one-third of women had a miscarriage in the first trimester; the percentage of live births was 45% of all pregnancies. There is a risk of arrhythmias, thromboembolic complications, and deterioration of hemodynamic state.

Follow-up

A specialized tertiary referral center, preferably the center where the patient was operated on, in cooperation with an adult cardiologist with expertise in CHD is required.

Prognosis

The procedure is not a corrective one; it is a palliative procedure with a completely nonphysiological circulation, which may fail, especially in cases where pulmonary artery pressure rises due to many reasons.[7,8] Fontan operation will eliminate cyanosis, and improve physical performance and prognosis of patients with a functionally single ventricle. After the procedure, most patients are in functional NYHA Class I or II. However, there is a discrepancy between the subjective report of the functional class and the objective assessment of the work capacity (e.g. oxygen uptake), as these patients have learned to adapt to a lower exercise capacity. Operative mortality in children is about 6%. The 10-year survival of patients after Fontan operation was some 60%; the figure is about 80–93% for TCPC, and in more recent studies the 20-year survival is 84–87%.[15–19] Total cavo-pulmonary connection failure in the late postoperative period occurred in 7.6% of cases; the risk factors of failure included subaortic obstruction and high pressure in the cavo-pulmonary connection system. Although contemporary techniques have improved long-term outcome, the Fontan circulation remains a palliation.[19]

Development of protein-losing enteropathy following Fontan operation implies a very grim prognosis. This complication occurs in 3.7–25% of patients undergoing Fontan operation, most often at 4 years postoperatively; still, it may occur even later. The incidence of protein-losing enteropathy also depends on the eligibility of patients scheduled for Fontan operation; the figure was a mere 1.3% in the series of Pediatric Heart Center of the Prague Motol University Hospital.[20] In an international multicenter study including more than 3000 patients after Fontan operation, protein-losing enteropathy was found in 3.7% of the survivors. The survival of patients developing protein-losing enteropathy was 59% at 5 years and <20% at 10 years.[21]

Reoperation after Fontan operation is associated with high mortality rates – as high as 75% in patients with existing protein-losing enteropathy.[15] Freedom from reoperation after Fontan procedure was 76% at 20 years.[18]

A cerebrovascular event was reported in a total of 17.8% of patients with a functionally single ventricle; about a half of these events were secondary to embolism, intracranial hemorrhage or ischemia following TCPC.[20]

References

1. Fontan F, Baudet E. Surgical repair of tricuspid atresia. Thorax 1971; 26: 240–8.
2. Kreutzer G, Galindez E, Bono H, De Palma C, Laura JP. An operation for the correction of tricuspid atresia. J Thorac Cardiovasc Surg 1973; 66(4): 613–21.
3. Björk VO, Olin CL, Bjarke BB, Thoren CA. Right atrial–right ventricular anastomosis for correction of tricuspid atresia. J Thorac Cardiovasc Surg 1979; 77(3): 452–8.
4. de Leval MR, Kilner P, Gewillig M, Bull C. Total cavo-pulmonary connection: A logical alternative to atriopulmonary connection for complex Fontan operations. Experimental studies and early clinical experience. J Thorac Cardiovasc Surg 1988; 96: 682–95.
5. Bridges ND, Lock JE, Castaneda AR. Baffle fenestration with subsequent transcatheter closure. Modification of the Fontan operation for patients at increased risk. Circulation 1990; 82(5): 1681–9.
6. Giannico S, Corno A, Marino B et al. Total extracardiac right heart bypass. Circulation 1992; 86 (5 Suppl): II110–II117.
7. Hager A, Kaemmerer H, Eicken A, Fratz S, Hess J. Long-term survival of patients with univentricular heart not treated surgically. J Thorac Cardiovasc Surg 2002; 123(6): 1214–17.
8. Gewillig M. Ventricular dysfunction of the functionally univentricular heart: Management and outcomes. Cardiol Young 2005; 15 (Suppl 3): 31–4.
9. Khairy P, Poirier N, Mercier LA. Univentricular heart. Circulation 2007; 115: 800–12.
10. Tsang W, Johansson B, Salehian O et al. Intracardiac thrombus in adults with the Fontan circulation. Cardiol Young 2007; 24: 1–6.

11. Suqiyama H, Yoo SJ, Williams W, Benson LN. Characterization and treatment of systemic venous to pulmonary venous collaterals seen after the Fontan operation. Cardiol Young 2003; 13(5): 424–30.

12. Deal BJ, Mavroudis C, Backer CL. Arrhythmia management in the Fontan patient. Pediatr Cardiol 2007; Epub Sep 8.

13. Canobbio MM, Mair DD. Pregnancy outcomes after the Fontan repair. J Am Coll Cardiol 1996; 28(3): 763–7.

14. Drenthen W, Pieper PG, Roos-Hesselink JW et al. Pregnancy and delivery in women after Fontan palliation. Heart 2006; 92(9): 1290–4.

15. Connelly MS, Webb GD, Somerville J et al. Canadian consensus conference on adult congenital heart disease 1996. Can J Cardiol 1998; 14(3): 395–452.

16. Giannico S, Hammand F, Amodeo A et al. Clinical outcome of 183 extracardiac Fontan patients: The first 15 years. J Am Coll Cardiol 2006; 47(10): 2065–73.

17. Mitchell ME, Ittenbach RF, Gaynor JW et al. Intermediate outcomes after the Fontan procedure in the current era. J Thorac Cardiovasc Surg 2006; 131(1): 172–80.

18. Ono M, Boething D, Goerler H et al. Clinical outcome of patients 20 years after Fontan operation – effect of fenestration on the late mortality. Eur J Cardiothorac Surg 2006; 30(6): 923–9.

19. d'Udekem Y, Iyengar AJ, Cochrane AD et al. The Fontan procedure: Contemporary techniques have improved long-term outcomes. Circulation 2007; 116 (11 Suppl): 1157–64.

20. Reich O, Chaloupecký V, Hučín B et al. Results of the treatment of congenital heart disease with one ventricle with the method of total cavo-pulmonary connection. Cor Vasa 2001; 43(4): 172–8.

21. Mertens L, Hagler D, Somerville J, Sauer U, Gewillig M. Protein losing enteropathy after the Fontan operation: An international multicenter evaluation. J Thorac Cardiovasc Surg 1998; 115: 1063–73.

16

Cyanotic congenital heart diseases in adulthood

Cyanotic congenital heart diseases (CHD) in adulthood include patients with pulmonary arterial hypertension (Eisenmenger syndrome is at the extreme end of the spectrum) and those without pulmonary arterial hypertension. Each group must be distinguished given the essential difference in pathophysiology and the potential for surgical repair in those without pulmonary arterial hypertension. Still, general risks and preventive measures are similar in either group.

Cyanotic congenital heart diseases without pulmonary hypertension

These conditions include shunt-related defects with restricted pulmonary blood flow in the presence of significant obstruction across the pulmonary outflow tract (i.e. subvalvular, valvular, and/or supravalvular pulmonary stenosis or atresia). These cases include tetralogy of Fallot, pulmonary atresia with ventricular septal defect (VSD), a functionally single ventricle with significant pulmonary stenosis or tricuspid atresia (see Chapter 15), Ebstein anomaly with atrial septal defect (ASD; see Chapter 14), significant subvalvular, valvular or supravalvular pulmonary stenosis with atrial and/or ventricular septal defect, etc. While most of these CHD have been managed by surgical repair in childhood, some children who have not had surgery may survive until adulthood. Some of these CHD can be managed by univentricular or biventricular repair even in adulthood.

The exact diagnosis, using transthoracic or transesophageal echocardiography and catheterization, must be established in a specialized center; and the decision on optimal treatment also has to be tailored individually. There has not been a consensus as to whether and when adults with cyanotic CHD and restricted pulmonary blood flow should undergo surgery if their defect is repairable, and if their clinical condition is stable. The decision is based on the nature of the defect, surgical risk, age, 'natural' history and comorbidities. The procedure can only be performed in a specialized center of congenital cardiac surgery with high-volume experience.

Patients on nonsurgical (medical) therapy have similar risks as those with cyanosis associated with pulmonary arterial hypertension, and require the measures specified below.

Cyanotic congenital heart disease with pulmonary arterial hypertension – Eisenmenger syndrome

Definition and anatomical notes

Eisenmenger syndrome is an extreme form of pulmonary vascular obstructive disease with irreversible pulmonary hypertension in the presence of high pulmonary vascular resistance associated with shunt-related CHD. The ratio of systolic pulmonary artery pressure to systolic arterial pressure in the systemic vascular bed is >0.9, while that of pulmonary to systemic blood flow (Qp/Qs) is <1.5.[1]

Eisenmenger syndrome occurs in unoperated, non-restrictive VSD, in a large patent ductus arteriosus. It can also occur in association with other CHD such as ASD, common arterial trunk, complete transposition of the great arteries (TGA) (atrioventricular concordance and ventriculo-arterial discordance) with a nonrestrictive VSD, functionally single ventricle without significant stenosis across the pulmonary outflow tract or in the presence of a big (surgically created) aortopulmonary shunt. Eisenmenger syndrome occurs only rarely in patients with ostium secundum defect (see Chapter 3).

The term Eisenmenger syndrome refers to the development of pulmonary vascular obstructive disease with a characteristic histologic pattern and remodeling of the pulmonary vascular bed (Figure 16.1). Heath and Edwards established a histopathologic classification (six-point scale) which is useful in assessing the potential for reversibility of pulmonary vascular disease:[2]

1. Hypertrophy of the media of small muscular arteries and arterioles.
2. Intimal cellular proliferation with migration of muscular cells into the intima.

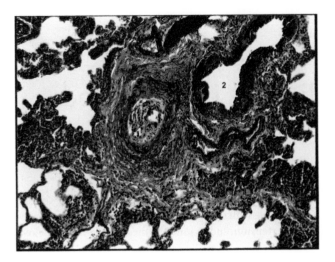

Figure 16.1
Eisenmenger syndrome – open lung biopsy, plexogenic pulmonary arteriopathy. Hematoxylin-eosin staining, elastic fibers, original magnification approx 160 times. 1, A small preacinary pulmonary artery with plexiform changes in the lumen, and with medial hypertrophy and muscularization. 2, Bronchiole. (Kindly provided by Associate Professor V Povýšilová, Institute of Pathology and Molecular Medicine, Charles University, School of Medicine 2 and Motol University Hospital, Prague.)

3. Intimal proliferation and concentric fibrosis with luminal narrowing and obliteration of small arteries and arterioles (transformation of intimal myofibroblasts with formation of muscle, collagen and elastin).
4. Development of plexiform lesions. Plexiform lesions are unorganized projections of pulmonary arteries made up of numerous channels and proliferating intimal cells; believed to develop as a result of intraluminal thrombosis, recanalization and proliferation with the formation of new anastomosing vessels.
5. Complex plexiform, angiomatous and cavernous lesions, and hyalinization of intimal fibrosis.
6. Necrotizing intimal and medial arteriitis with pulmonary artery occlusions.

These changes are assessed by histology of a specimen with pulmonary tissue, obtained by open (surgical) lung biopsy. While grades 1–3 are considered reversible, grades 4–6 are regarded as irreversible (Figure 16.1). Rabinovitch has introduced a morphometric approach to reflect and to classify histological changes.[3] Open lung biopsy can, and should only, be considered when the reversibility of the pulmonary hypertension is uncertain from the hemodynamic data. It is potentially hazardous and should be done only at centers with substantial relevant experience in CHD.[1] In addition, the pathologist must be very experienced to provide an accurate Heath-Edwards classification. Today, open lung biopsy is almost never considered.

Prevalence

Five to 10 per cent of patients with CHD develop pulmonary arterial hypertension of variable severity.[4] The development of Eisenmenger syndrome depends on timely detection and operation of a shunt-related CHD in childhood. Exact data on its incidence are not available, and its frequency is declining due to advances in the management of CHD. Eisenmenger syndrome is reported to account for about 4% among contemporary adult CHD patients at tertiary care centers.[4] Increased awareness and improved infrastructure, diagnostic and therapeutic options for the management of children with CHD will further decrease the number of patients with Eisenmenger syndrome due to simple defects. In contrast, there will be an increasing number of patients with complex CHD, with or without palliative surgery, who will develop pulmonary arterial hypertension.

Pathophysiology

High pulmonary vascular resistance develops as a result of high pulmonary flow rates and transmission of high systemic pressure to the pulmonary vascular bed in patients with a major left-to-right shunt at the levels of the ventricles and/or great arteries, most often soon after birth. In some cases, the high pulmonary vascular resistance from the fetal period may not have even declined (persistent pulmonary hypertension of the newborn). Pulmonary vascular obstructive disease is a dynamic, progressive, multifactorial process, and leads to pulmonary vascular bed remodeling, initially reversible to later become irreversible. Among others, activation of the nitric oxide pathway, prostacyclin pathway and endothelin system is the landmark for the remodeling of the pulmonary vascular bed and development of pulmonary arterial hypertension: imbalance of vasoconstriction and vasodilatation in favor of vasoconstriction, proliferation of endothelial cells, smooth muscle cells and fibroblasts, inflammatory process, release of cytokines and others.[4–6] Thrombus formation in the enlarged central pulmonary arteries, and thromboembolic complications, can occur in patients with advanced pulmonary arterial hypertension (Figures 16.2 and 16.3).

Pulmonary hypertension leads to pressure overload of the right ventricle with subsequent concentric hypertrophy. Patients with preserved systolic right ventricular function do not show signs of right-heart decompensation. This occurs in the presence of end-stage right ventricular systolic dysfunction and dilatation with secondary tricuspid regurgitation.

Victor Eisenmenger first described both the clinical and pathological features of irreversible pulmonary vascular disease in a 32-year-old man with a nonrestrictive VSD.[7] Sixty years later, Paul Wood elucidated the distinctive clinical and physiologic characteristics in 127 individuals with Eisenmenger physiology in his classic 1958 work on Eisenmenger syndrome.[8] Any large communication between

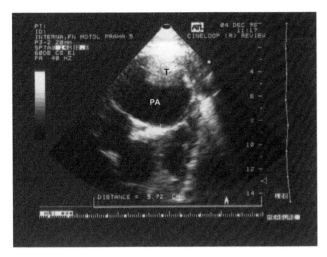

Figure 16.2
Transthoracic echo, short-axis projection on the level of great arteries. Severely dilated pulmonary artery (PA) with thrombus (T) in a patient with Eisenmenger syndrome, severe pulmonary hypertension. Pulmonary artery is dilated to 57mm.

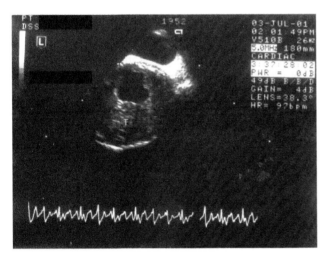

Figure 16.3
Eisenmenger's syndrome; transesophageal echo, longitudinal projection. Severely dilated pulmonary artery (78mm) with circular thrombus (T).

the systemic and pulmonary circulation may result in similar physiologic condition, when a markedly increased pulmonary vascular resistance occurs. Eisenmenger syndrome was defined as pulmonary hypertension with reversed (predominantly right to left) or bidirectional shunting at any level; 'it matters very little where the shunt happens to be'.[8]

The result is reduced arterial oxygen saturation (usually <90% at rest), and oxygen saturation tends to further decrease abruptly during exercise. Chronic hypoxemia leads to stimulation of juxtaglomerular cells in kidneys with increased erythropoietin production, and to secondary erythrocytosis. Secondary erythrocytosis is a physiologic response to chronic

hypoxemia and increases the capacity for oxygen transport and, consequently, oxygen delivery to the tissue. Increased red blood cell mass with an increase in hematocrit is, thus, a physiologic adaptive mechanism in the presence of a chronic right-to-left shunt.[9–12] There is an inverse relationship between the hemoglobin level and oxygen saturation. The hemoglobin reflects the severity of cyanosis: the lower the oxygen saturation, the higher the hemoglobin. Normal hemoglobin levels in these patients already signal 'anemia'.

Sideropenia, which may develop due to often inadequate phlebotomy or, alternatively, chronic infection, is associated with the development of microcytes with a reduced ability to deform and transit through the capillary bed. Tissue hypoxia predisposes to the development of infectious foci, both skin (furunculosis) and more serious brain abscesses. Increased heme degradation results in increased biliary levels of unconjugated bilirubin, and in the development of bilirubin cholecystolithiasis. Cyanotic CHD, especially when hematocrit >65%, is usually associated with thrombocytopenia, platelet dysfunction and abnormalities of the (intrinsic and extrinsic) coagulation pathways.

In patients with a right-to-left shunt, megakaryocytes do not pass from the systemic venous bed through the pulmonary circulation but enter, in a nonfragmented form, systemic arterioles and capillaries. Once there, platelet growth factors, i.e. platelet-derived growth factor (PDGF) and transforming growth factor beta (TGFB), start to release from their cytoplasm, which causes local proliferation of fibroblasts and smooth muscle, and protein synthesis.[13] This explains osteoarthropathy with drumstick fingers (clubbing) in cyanotic CHD, and also glomerular changes.[14]

In cyanotic CHD, the epicardial coronary arteries are widely dilated and tortuous (Figures 16.4 and 16.5), but they show a reduced ability of vasodilation and are atheroma-free because hypocholesterolemia acts in concert with the antiatherogenic properties of upregulated nitric oxide, hyperbilirubinemia, hypoxemia, and low platelet counts.[15–17] In addition, severe endothelial dysfunction of the systemic vascular bed is evident, and reflects the multisystem disorder of cyanotic CHD.[18]

Clinical findings and diagnosis

Symptoms

Patients with Eisenmenger syndrome are adapted to pulmonary hypertension and hypoxemia, so they may not have major complaints for some time and may lead a relatively normal life if they avoid strenuous physical exercise. When they reach middle age, usually their forties, these patients develop decompensation of their condition with progressive dyspnea, fatigability, exertional syncope and sudden death, or they show signs of heart failure.[18–21]

- Exertional dyspnea and fatigability are experienced by 84% of patients with Eisenmenger syndrome.[19]

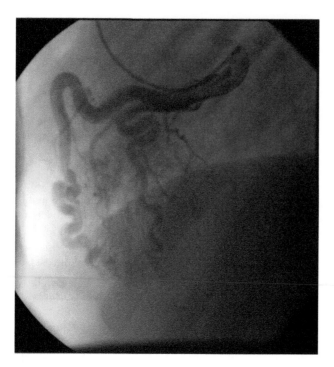

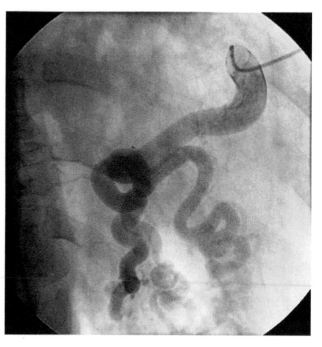

Figure 16.4
Selective coronarogram in a patient with untreated cyanotic congenital heart disease; 41-year-old female with, so far, unoperated d-transposition of the great arteries with ventricular septal defect, severe longstanding cyanosis. The coronary arteries are extremely ectatic and tortuous without signs of atherosclerosis, left coronary artery. This is the same patient as in Figures 11.20–11.22. Courtesy of Dr M Rubacek, Faculty Hospital Ostrava, Czech Republic.

Figure 16.5
Selective coronarogram in a patient with untreated cyanotic congenital heart disease, 41-year-old female with, so far, unoperated d-transposition of the great arteries with ventricular septal defect, severe longstanding cyanosis. The coronary arteries are extremely ectatic and tortuous without signs of atherosclerosis. This is the same patient as in Figure 16.4, and Figures 11.20–11.22. Courtesy of Dr M Rubacek, Faculty Hospital Ostrava, Czech Republic.

However, patients often disregard these problems and tend to adjust their lifestyle accordingly. The symptoms are due to a low cardiac output and progression of hypoxemia on exertion. Patients with Eisenmenger syndrome have the poorest exercise performance and maximum oxygen uptake among patients with CHD.[22]

- Palpitations occur in 21% of patients with Eisenmenger syndrome.
- Hemoptysis has been reported in 11% of patients; it does not develop until after 15 years of age. Coagulation disorders and mucosal bleeding are frequent.[10]
- Syncope occurs in 9% of cases.[19]
- Dehydration and hyperviscosity symptoms are associated with headache, visual disturbances, vertigo, tinnitus, myalgia, and paresthesia. However, similar symptoms may be caused by iron deficiency, particularly if hematocrit is <65%.[9,10]
- Neurological symptoms, headache and febrile spells lead one to consider brain abscess.

Clinical examination

- Central cyanosis may often be relatively inconspicuous at rest, and will increase during exercise. Helpful clues in

establishing the diagnosis may include conjunctival hyperemia and cyanosis of the tongue, lips and mucosa.
- Cyanotic CHD are associated with drumstick fingers (clubbing) and watch-crystal nails on the upper and lower limbs (Figures 16.6).
- There is usually increased jugular vein filling in the presence of tricuspid regurgitation with active pulsation.
- The second sound above the pulmonary artery is accentuated. Diastolic murmur above the pulmonary artery may be heard in the presence of pulmonary regurgitation. Because of balanced pressures in both ventricles and the great arteries, murmurs typical of VSD and patent ductus anteriosus are absent.
- Hepatomegaly, ascites, and lower limb edema are not present until the development of chronic right-heart decompensation, usually after the age of 40.
- Patients with cyanotic CHD may have varicose veins, and be at risk for skin ulcers and infection.

Laboratory investigations

The following parameters should be monitored regularly: blood count with special emphasis on hematocrit, erythrocyte count and indices, platelet counts, iron, ferritin, coagulation

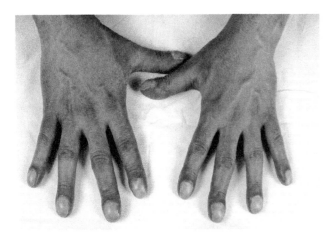

Figure 16.6
Fingers in 45-year-old patient with unoperated cyanotic congenital heart disease; drumstick fingers (clubbing) and watch-crystal nails.

parameters, uric acid, urinalysis, ureate, creatinine, aspartate aminotransferase (ASAT), alanine aminotransferase (ALAT), bilirubin, gamma glutamyltranspepsidase (GGT), alkaline phosphatase (ALP), total protein and albumin. Hyperbilirubinemia and increased GMT are early markers of congestive hepatopathy. Ferritin is an early and sensitive marker of reduced iron stores if its serum levels fall to <15µg/l. However, ferritin levels tend to rise in chronic infectious and inflammatory diseases irrespective of iron stores. Microcytosis develops in cases of chronic iron deficiency. Hyperhomocysteinemia due to folate or vitamin B12 deficiencies may mask iron deficiency.[10,23]

Laboratory precautions:

- *Coagulation parameters:* Caution is required for accurate measurement of the coagulation parameters because plasma volume is decreased due to secondary erythrocytosis. Adjustment of the amount of the liquid anticoagulants is essential for accurate measurement of the coagulation parameters.
- *Hematocrit:* Level of hematocrit must be determined by automated electronic particle counts because microhematocrit centrifugation results in plasma trapping and falsely elevated hematocrit.
- *Blood glucose:* In vitro glycolysis is increased and results from the greater than normal number of red blood cells. Thus, reduced blood glucose levels are common (artifical 'hypoglycemia'). Sodium fluoride added to the tube prevents red cell glycolysis.

Electrocardiogram (ECG)

The findings include P pulmonale and signs of right ventricular hypertrophy, consistent with right ventricular overload.

Echocardiography

- In the presence of balanced pressures in both ventricles, a VSD is not associated with the typical shunt-like flow, and the VSD must be visualized morphologically. Just as in Eisenmenger syndrome due to a nonrestrictive patent ductus arteriosus, there is no evidence of continuous flow through the ductus, which may make establishing the diagnosis difficult.
- An intracardiac right-to-left shunt will be documented by contrast echocardiography, whereby a contrast medium is administered into the venous bed to identify the site of the shunt. Agitated saline is the cheapest, and the contrast medium of choice to confirm or to exclude a shunt. Rarely, the procedure may be complicated by transient ischemic attack due to microembolism (air embolism) into the central nervous system.
- In Eisenmenger syndrome, the right ventricle shows a notably hypertrophic myocardium (concentric right ventricular hypertrophy); in many patients, the right ventricle may not initially be dilated in the presence of a nonrestrictive shunt at the ventricular or arterial level (Figure 16.7). It tends to dilate later, as does the right atrium, with the development of tricuspid regurgitation (with high velocity, usually >4 m/s) in the occurrence of pulmonary arterial hypertension. When right ventricular systolic hypertension is diagnosed, right ventricular outflow tract obstruction must be ruled out to avoid the misdiagnosis of pulmonary arterial hypertension (e.g. VSD with severe infundibular stenosis).
- Systolic and mean pulmonary artery pressure levels are derived from the gradient on the tricuspid valve, whereas end-diastolic pulmonary artery pressure can be calculated from the end-diastolic gradient on pulmonary regurgitation when adding estimated right ventricular end-diastolic pressure (right atrial pressure).
- A cursory examination of a compensated patient with trace tricuspid regurgitation, the presence of Eisenmenger syndrome may be overlooked (Figure 16.7). Patients with Eisenmenger syndrome due to a patent arterial ductus may be misdiagnosed as having idiopathic pulmonary arterial hypertension (Figures 16.8 and 16.9). A comprehensive examination, and the presence of differential cyanosis, will establish the correct diagnosis.
- Both right and left ventricular function must be assessed, as the function of both ventricles may be progressively deteriorating.
- Transesophageal echocardiography will thoroughly evaluate intracardiac morphology, as well as the morphology of the central segment of the pulmonary vascular bed; it may reveal patent arterial duct and vegetations in infectious endocarditis (IE). If sedation is used for transesophageal echocardiography, the risk of an increase in the right-to-left shunt should be considered because of subsequent hypotension. In addition, oxygen saturation

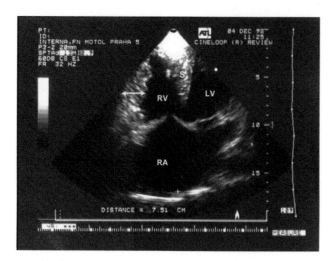

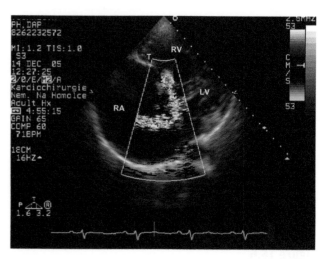

Figure 16.7

Eisenmenger syndrome; transthoracic echo, apical four-chamber view. Severe hypertrophy of the right ventricular lateral wall (arrow) and septum (S); the right ventricle chamber (RV) is not dilated, right atrium (RA) is dilated. However the tricuspid regurgitation is only trace and the diagnosis of Eisenmenger syndrome and severe pulmonary hypertension could be underestimated. LV: left ventricle.

Figure 16.9

Eisenmenger syndrome with patent ductus arteriosus and right-heart decompensation. Transthoracic echo, apical view. Severe dilatation of the tricuspid annulus; severe tricuspid regurgitation (color jet); extremely dilated right atrium (RA); RV, right ventricle; T, tricuspid valve; LV, small left ventricle.

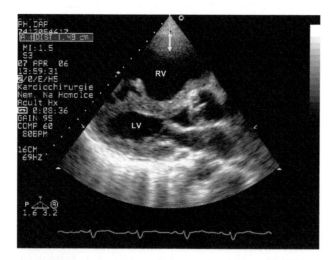

Figure 16.8

Eisenmenger syndrome; transthoracic echo, long-axis parasternal view. Thirty-two-year-old patient with severe pulmonary hypertension due to patent arterial duct. Severe hypertrophy of the right ventricular wall (arrow, 15mm), severe dilatation of the right ventricle (RV), small left ventricle (LV) with no intracardiac shunt. No murmur audible due to the systemic pressure in the duct.

can decrease to sedation and hypoventilation. In Prague, transesophageal echocardiography was employed to examine >100 patients with cyanotic CHD without sedation; the procedure was well tolerated by most patients. Important considerations include verbal contact with the patient, trust by the patient, explanation of the procedure to the patient, use of the technique of rapid probe insertion, and performance of the procedure by a very experienced and skilled physician. Another psychological boost for the patient may be inhalation of oxygen-enriched air while leaving the airways fully patent. Should nasal mucosa become congested, measures should be taken to eliminate it. Careful monitoring is crucial and surveillance by an anesthetist is highly recommended.

- Dilatation of the main pulmonary artery with or without thrombus formation is a frequent finding (Figures 16.2 and 16.3).[21,24,25]

Chest X-ray and spiral computerized tomography (CT) of the chest

In Eisenmenger syndrome, there is a massive dilatation of pulmonary trunk and dilatation of central pulmonary branches. There may even be aneurysmatic dilatation of the pulmonary artery (Figure 16.10). In the periphery, there is a distinct reduction of the lumen of pulmonary arteries, causing higher transparency of the lungs. The heart shadow is dilated due to the dilatation of the right ventricle, which may cause the elevation of the apex. There may be calcifications of the pulmonary artery or of hypertensive patent ductus arteriosus.

The distinctive radiologic findings were beautifully described recently.[26] The vascular lesions on chest radiographs and CT scans in Eisenmenger syndrome

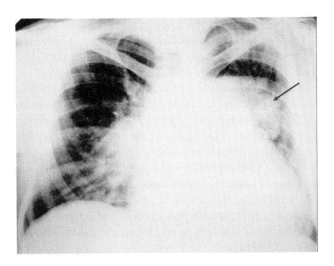

Figure 16.10
X-ray of a patient with Eisenmenger syndrome and aneurysmatic dilatation of pulmonary artery (arrow). The same patient as in Figure 16.3.

appear to be correlated histologically with collateral vessels that develop more extensively with post-tricuspid communications.

Should a chest X-ray show an infiltrate (e.g. in the occurrence of hemoptysis), spiral CT is the next diagnostic step to visualize intrapulmonary bleeding and to determine the extent of bleeding. It will also recognize thromboembolic disease in the differential diagnosis.[21,24,25] In these patients, bronchoscopy is associated with high risk and does not usually furnish therapeutically useful information.[13]

Catheterization

Catheterization is primarily indicated for full hemodynamic evaluation, and to determine pulmonary vascular resistance, including evaluation of its reversibility by use of vasodilators (O_2, NO, prostacyclines). Furthermore, it helps to specify the morphology of the underlying defect and the pulmonary vascular bed, or to perform coronary angiography. The epicardial coronary arteries are widely dilated and tortuous (Figures 16.4 and 16.5). However, pulmonary angiography in severe pulmonary hypertension is associated with high risk and may result in sudden death. Catherization of Eisenmenger patients is a high-risk procedure and should be performed only by skilled investigators with special expertise in CHD.

Magnetic resonance imaging (MRI)

This technique can be used to evaluate pulmonary vascular bed morphology, and to assess the presence of mural and obstructive thrombi.

Lung biopsy

In patients with Eisenmenger syndrome, this is a procedure associated with high risk, which can only be performed in centers with adequate experience. The procedure is indicated in cases whereby hemodynamic studies have not clearly established the reversibility of changes in the pulmonary vascular bed (Figure 16.1). Lung biopsy can be hazardous and is used only very rarely.[1]

CT of the brain

Headaches in patients with cyanotic CHD are not always caused by hyperviscosity symptoms. Brain abcess should be excluded, especially in the case of fever.

Management

- The generally accepted approach in Eisenmenger syndrome is conservative therapy and preventive measure. It is critical to strictly adhere to all safety measures – see below. Failure to observe these, or not paying adequate attention to them, is often the main cause of premature death of patients with Eisenmenger syndrome, rather than the disease per se.
- Vasodilators have become a cornerstone therapy for patients with idiopathic pulmonary arterial hypertension and pulmonary arterial hypertension associated with collagen disorders.[6,27] In contrast to 10 years ago, specific therapies are now available and approved for patients with Eisenmenger syndrome. The BREATHE-5 study and the BREATHE-5 open-label extension study have confirmed the efficacy and safety profile of Bosentan for patients with Eisenmenger syndrome secondary to VSD and ASD.[28–30]
- Surgical or catheter-based shunt closure is contraindicated in Eisenmenger syndrome, as it would result in right-heart failure. Surgery or catheter-based closure of patent ductus arteriosus can only be considered in patients with documented reversibility of pulmonary hypertension (see Chapter 12). Catheter-based closure after hemodynamic testing can be performed in patients with secundum atrial septum defects with some degree of pulmonary hypertension with or without pretreatment with vasodilators.[1] However, management of these cases is controversial and difficult.
- Lung or heart-lung transplantation is the last therapeutic resource and should be performed only in very experienced centers. The decision process (timing of listing), the procedure itself and post-transplant care require special expertise.
- Lung transplantation with surgical repair of the congenital heart defect is associated with 1- and 4-year survival rates of 70–80% and <50%, respectively.

- The 1- and 10-year survival rates of heart and lung transplantation have been reported to be 60–80% and <30%, respectively. Indications for transplantation include significant deterioration of the functional class, a history of syncope, and right-heart decompensation. Transplantation should be indicated in patients with a risk of death within 1 year in the presence of the natural course of the defect while not having common contraindications to transplantation.

Risks

The number of risk-related situations faced by cyanotic adults (with or without pulmonary hypertension) is incomparably higher than in CHD adults without cyanosis.

- General anesthesia and noncardiac surgery carry a risk of hypotension with augmented hypoxemia and high mortality.
- Dehydration, hypovolemia, use of diuretics, febrile states increase blood viscosity and exacerbate erythrocytosis.
- Vasodilators and hypotension can result in augmentation of the right-to-left shunt and augment hypoxemia.
- Bleeding occurs frequently because of blood coagulation disorders. The majority of bleedings are minor, but they can be dismal (e.g. hemoptysis). Hemoptysis is external and may not reflect the extent of intrapulmonary hemorrhage; it should be regarded as potentially life-threatening, and requires meticulous evaluation and expertise. Cyanotic patients with active bleeding should be referred to a tertiary care center with expertise in CHD, or managed in collaboration with such a care center.
- Repeat phlebotomies carry a risk for developing sideropenia and microcytosis, and the risk for ischemic events.[28]
- There is a high risk of infection in tissue hypoxia: lung and skin infection is frequent, prolonged vein cannulation may lead to the formation of brain abscesses, yet brain abscesses also occur in cyanotic CHD spontaneously.
- Paradoxical embolism may develop in deep vein thrombosis, from pacemaker electrode thrombosis, and paradoxical air embolism may result from venous cannulation.
- Increased bilirubin levels are associated with increased risk of gallstone and cholecystitis.

Measures taken in cyanotic adults with CHD:

- The administration of each new medication must be consulted with a cardiologist experienced in CHD.
- Prevention of dehydration and hypovolemia.
- Smoking cessation.
- Avoidance of strenuous physical activity.
- Avoidance of exposure to high altitudes, or only gradual ascent to high altitude (cable-car etc.).

- Air travel in a commercial aircraft is allowed only for patients with stable condition, and provisions made to ensure adequate fluid intake and to avoid inactivity to prevent deep vein thrombosis.[12]
- Careful consideration of indication for any noncardiac surgery because of the very high risk of fatal complications associated with general and epidural anesthesia, which must be induced and conducted by an experienced anesthesiologist; the surgeon must also be an experienced and fast-operating one.
- Prior to surgery, phlebotomy can be considered to decrease the hematocrit to approximately 65%; this strategy may increase platelet count and improve blood coagulation parameters, and reduce the risk of intraoperative bleeding; the blood so withdrawn should be reserved for autologous blood donation if required.
- Management of bleeding complications, including pulmonary hemorrhage, consists of discontinuation of aspirin, nonsteroidal anti-inflammatory drugs and oral anticoagulants immediately. Physical activity must be reduced (bedrest) and nonproductive cough should be suppressed. If bleeding persists, administration of fresh frozen plasma, cryoprecipitates and platelet concentrates in thrombocytopenia are recommended. In general, hemoptysis stops spontaneously and no specific therapeutic measures are required. *Precaution:* Bronchoscopy incurs risk and seldom provides useful information – it must be avoided.
- Cautious prevention of IE, exclusion of bacteremia, avoidance of infection. Annual flu shot and pneumovax (every 5 years) are recommended.
- Phlebotomy is only indicated in patients with moderate to severe hyperviscosity symptoms, usually with a hematocrit >65% *and* absence of iron deficiency and dehydration. Repeat phlebotomies should not be performed to maintain a predetermined hematocrit/hemoglobin to avoid ischemic complications. Phlebotomy is performed in symptomatic patients, not indiscriminately according to hematocrit levels. Over a period of 30–45 minutes, a total of 250–500ml of blood is withdrawn while the volume is replaced (e.g. 750–1000ml isotonic saline) before or during the procedure. ECG and pressure monitoring are appropriate before, during and after the procedure (up to 60 minutes after phlebotomy). Further fluid replacement may be necessary until the patient's blood pressure stabilizes. Frequent phlebotomy for no clearcut reasons result in iron deficiency, development of microcytosis, relative anemia, reduced oxygen carriers and tissue hypoxia, exacerbation of symptoms and reduced saturation. The symptoms of iron deficiency may resemble those of the hyperviscosity syndrome. Cautious iron supplementation is indicated in sideropenia, to be discontinued once hematocrit levels have increased; therefore, frequent (once every 1–2 weeks) blood count is to be performed.

- Prevention of iron deficiency: The bone marrow requires iron to produce red blood cells. Iron deficiency results in an inadequately low hemoglobin; it is hazardous for patients with cyanotic CHD and must be avoided using all means available. A low dose of ferrous sulfate (325mg once daily) is orally administered. However, parenteral iron therapy can be considered in patients who are intolerant of iron preparations, or in those with severe iron deficiency. Iron saccharose is a new preparation which is well tolerated intravenously and does not appear to have allergic side-effects.
- Prevention of bleeding: Chronic nonsteroid anti-inflammatory drugs should not be administered (or only with caution). Antithrombotic and anticoagulation therapy is associated with risks; it may be instituted in patients with chronic atrial fibrillation, with mechanical valvular prosthesis, those with documented thromboembolic complication, and solely under close clinical and laboratory monitoring. A target international normalized ratio (INR) between 2.0 and 2.5 is usually recommended; there are no evidence-based data.[10] The amount of sodium citrate must be adjusted to the hematocrit (see 'Laboratory investigations').
- Headache can be a symptom of a brain abscess; routine phlebotomy to improve headaches must be cautioned.
- Home oxygen therapy, while it may occasionally alleviate sensations of dyspnea, has not been shown to have an effect on survival or morbidity, and is not administered on a routine basis. Its prolonged use may result in psychological dependence, and the drying effect of the non-humidified oxygen may predispose the patient to epistaxis.[1,29]
- Drugs impairing renal function should be avoided, or administered with caution.
- Use of an airfilter to avoid systemic air embolism in the presence of an IV line.
- Maintenance of excellent oral hygiene. A toothbrush with soft bristles should be used to avoid bleeding; brushing should be gentle.

Pregnancy and delivery

In patients with significant cyanosis associated with pulmonary hypertension, pregnancy is contraindicated because of the high risk of maternal and fetal death. Systemic vasodilation in pregnancy results in augmentation of the right-to-left shunt and worsening of cyanosis; the risk of sudden death is increased.

The pathophysiology is different in cyanotic patients without pulmonary arterial hypertension. Fetal mortality was reported to be 100% at hemoglobin levels >180g/l. In more recent studies, there were only 8% of live births reported in women with *cyanotic CHD without pulmonary hypertension* and hemoglobin levels >200g/l, but 71% of live births at hemoglobin levels <160g/l. The rate of live births at

maternal saturation levels of >90% was 92%; however, women with oxygen saturation <85% had only 12% of live births. Cardiovascular complications occurred in 32% of cyanotic pregnant women without pulmonary hypertension. Hemoglobin and oxygen saturation were the most important predictors for successful pregnancy in patients without pulmonary hypertension.[30]

The risk associated with cyanotic *CHD and associated pulmonary hypertension* is incomparably higher. Mortality of pregnant women with Eisenmenger syndrome was reported to reach 52%.[31] Another study reported 35% mortality of pregnant women with Eisenmenger syndrome, and 39% infant mortality.[32]

Contraception

Intrauterine devices should not be used (risk of endocarditis and bleeding), nor should oral hormonal high-estrogen contraception. Advisable measures include condoms; combined products with low-dose estrogen (including three-stage combinations), or levonorgestrel-only contraceptives; alternatively, laparoscopic sterilization may be considered, but this procedure carries special risks related to general anesthesia and laparoscopy in this population. Anticonception counseling is crucial and must be performed in collaboration with both a cardiologist and a gynecologist with special expertise in CHD and high-risk pregnancy. Sterilization of the husband or male partner is not recommended as his longevity is much better: he will survive his female partner and may start a new relationship later in life.

Infectious endocarditis

All cyanotic CHD carry a high risk of IE; endocarditis prophylaxis is recommended.[33]

Follow-up

Follow-up should be overseen by a cardiologist in cooperation with a specialist center, or in a center specializing in CHD.

Prognosis

Most patients with Eisenmenger syndrome will survive to adulthood; heart failure does not usually occur before the age of 40. Patients with Eisenmenger syndrome have a more favorable natural prognosis compared with those with primary (idiopathic) pulmonary hypertension, as the pathophysiology and right ventricular remodeling is completely different.[34,35]

The most frequent causes of death of patients with Eisenmenger syndrome include sudden death (30%), congestive heart failure (25%), hemoptysis (15%), pregnancy and delivery, noncardiac intraoperative death, and infectious complications such as brain abscess and IE.[18–20] Independent predictors of mortality included supraventricular arrhythmia, higher NYHA classes, younger age at the time of diagnosis, and higher voltage in precordial leads in right ventricular hypertrophy (R in V1 and S in V5–V6 higher than 3mV).[19] Somerville[36] incriminated pregnancy, progression of resting hypoxemia and reduced exercise tolerance, right-heart failure, hemoptysis >100ml of blood, exertional syncope, surgery requiring general anesthesia, supraventricular arrhythmia and ventricular tachycardia runs, and the need for a permanent pacemaker as factors posing a risk of death over the next 1–2 years.

Transplantation as a therapeutic option is considered mainly in younger patients with Eisenmenger syndrome, below 35 years of age, in functional NYHA Class IV, at high risk of death. This is so because the outcome of heart and lung transplantation, or lung transplantation with cardiac surgical repair of CHD, is not very encouraging. The 5- and 10-year survival rates of patients with Eisenmenger syndrome undergoing heart and lung transplantation are 51.3 and 27.6%, respectively; however, these figures are not different from those reported for other transplant recipients.[37] In another study of adults with Eisenmenger syndrome, 44% of transplant recipients died during post-transplant hospitalization, while the figure was 33% for nontransplant patients; the mean age of both groups was 37.[19]

Patients with Eisenmenger syndrome and: ASD die at a mean age of 45 years; VSD die at a mean age of 43 years; patent ductus arteriosus die at a mean age of 42 years; atrioventricular septal defect and complex anatomy die at a mean age of 28 years.[19]

Erythrocytosis per se (formerly incorrectly referred to as polyglobulia or polycythemia), or the level of hematocrit, are not risk factors for the development of a completed stroke in patients with cyanotic CHD.[38] The most reliable predictors of cerebrovascular events are microcytosis (with erythrocyte volume <82fl), hypertension, and atrial fibrillation. Microcytosis, frequently caused by inadequate and repeat phlebotomies, remained the strongest risk factor after exclusion of patients with atrial fibrillation and systemic arterial hypertension.[28]

The improved survival of patients with Eisenmenger syndrome is currently attributed to improved preventive measures rather than to the potential of transplantation. Fewer therapeutic activities, with an emphasis on prevention of complications and education targeted at specialists in other branches of medicine, may be more beneficial for these patients than efforts to treat whatever the price.[36]

The new pulmonary vasodilating drugs (e.g. prostacycline and its analogues, bosentan, sildenafil) are under intensive research in patients with idiopathic (primary) pulmonary hypertension, or pulmonary arterial hypertension associated with collagen disorders. The safety profile and the efficacy by significant improvement in the 6-minute walk distance have been confirmed also in Eisenmenger patients.[39–41] However, the benefit on hard endpoints (e.g. quality of life, improved survival) for patients with Eisenmenger syndrome has to be determined.

References

1. Therrien J, Warnes C, Daliento L et al. Canadian Cardiovascular Society Consensus Conference 2001 update: Recommendations for the management of adults with congenital heart disease. Part III. Can J Cardiol 2001; 17(11): 1135–58.
2. Heath D, Edwards JE. The pathology of hypertensive pulmonary vascular disease: A description of six grades of structural changes in the pulmonary arteries with special reference to congenital cardiac septal defects. Circulation 1958; 18: 533–47.
3. Rabinovitch M, Haworth SG, Castaneda AR, Nadas AS, Reid LM. Lung biopsy in congenial heart disease: A morphometric approach to pulmonary vascular disease. Circulation 1978; 69: 655–67.
4. Diller GP, Gatzoulis MA. Pulmonary vascular disease in adults with congenital heart disease. Circulation 2007; 115: 1039–50.
5. Farber HW, Loscalzo J. Pulmonary arterial hypertension. N Engl J Med 2004; 351: 1655–65.
6. McLaughlin VV, McGoon MD. Pulmonary arterial hypertension. Circulation 2006; 114: 1417–31.
7. Eisenmenger V. Die angeborenen Defecte der Kammerscheidewand des Herzens. Z Klin Med 1897; 32 (Suppl): 1–28.
8. Wood P. The Eisenmenger syndrome or pulmonary hypertension with reversed central shunt. Br Med J 1958; II: 701–9, 755–62.
9. Perloff JK, Rosove MH, Child JS, Wright GB. Adults with cyanotic congenital heart disease: Hematologic management. Ann Intern Med 1988; 109: 406–13.
10. Oechslin E. Hematological management of the cyanotic adult with congenital heart disease. Int J Cardiol 2004; 97 (Suppl 1): 109–15.
11. Diller GP, Dimopoulos K, Broberg CS et al. Presentation, survival prospects, and predictors of death in Eisenmenger syndrome: A combined retrospective and case-control study. Eur Heart J 2006; 27: 1737–42.
12. Broberg CS, Bax BE, Okonko DO et al. Blood viscosity and its relationship to iron deficiency, symptoms, and exercise capacity in adults with cyanotic congenital heart disease. J Am Coll Cardiol 2006; 48: 356–65.
13. Perloff JK. Cyanotic congenital heart disease is a multisystem systemic disorder. Exp Clin Cardiol 1999; 4(2): 77–84.
14. Perloff JK, Latta H, Barsotti P. Pathogenesis of the glomerular abnormality in cyanotic congenital heart disease. Am J Cardiol 2000; 86: 1198–204.
15. Perloff JK. The coronary circulation in cyanotic congenital heart disease. Int J Cardiol 2004; 97 (Suppl 1): 79–86.
16. Chugh R, Perloff JK, Fishbein M, Child JS. Extramural coronary arteries in adults with cyanotic congenital heart disease. Am J Cardiol 2004; 94: 1355–7.
17. Fyfe A, Perloff JK, Niwa K, Child JS, Miner PD. Cyanotic congenital heart disease and coronary artery atherogenesis. Am J Cardiol 2005; 96: 283–90.
18a. Daliento L, Somerville J, Presbitero P et al. Eisenmenger syndrome. Factors relating to deterioration and death. Eur Heart J 1998; 19: 1845–55.
18. Oechslin E, Kiowski W, Schindler R et al. Systemic endothelial dysfunction in adults with cyanotic congenital heart disease. Circulation 2005; 112: 1106–12.
19. Cantor WJ, Harrison DA, Moussadji JS et al. Determinants of survival and length of survival in adults with Eisenmenger syndrome. Am J Cardiol 1999; 84(6): 677–81.

20. Oechslin EN, Harrison DA, Connelly MS, Webb GD, Siu SC. Mode of death in adults with congenital heart disease. Am J Cardiol 2000; 86: 1111–16.
21. Niwa K, Perloff JK, Kaplan S, Child JS, Miner PD. Eisenmenger syndrome in adults: Ventricular septal defect, truncus arteriosus, univentricular heart. J Am Coll Cardiol 1999; 34: 223–32.
22. Diller GP, Dimopoulos K, Okonko D et al. Exercise intolerance in adult congenital heart disease: Comparative severity, correlates, and prognostic implication. Circulation 2005; 112: 828–35.
23. Kaemmerer H, Fratz S, Braun SL et al. Erythrocyte indexes, iron metabolism, and hyperhomocysteinemia in adults with cyanotic congenital cardiac disease. Am J Cardiol 2004; 94: 825–8.
24. Silversides CK, Granton JT, Konen E et al. Pulmonary thrombosis in adults with Eisenmenger syndrome. J Am Coll Cardiol 2003; 42: 1982–7.
25. Perloff JK, Hart EM, Greaves SM, Miner PD, Child JS. Proximal pulmonary arterial and intrapulmonary radiologic features of Eisenmenger syndrome and primary pulmonary hypertension. Am J Cardiol 2003; 92: 182–7.
26. Sheehan R, Perloff JK, Fishbein MC, Gjertson D, Aberlee DR. Pulmonary neovascularity: A distinctive radiographic finding in Eisenmenger syndrome. Circulation 2005; 112: 2778–85.
27. Humbert M, Sitbon O, Simonneau G. Treatment of pulmonary arterial hypertension. N Engl J Med 2004; 351: 1425–36.
28. Ammash N, Warnes CA. Cerebrovascular events in adult patients with cyanotic congenital heart disease. J Am Coll Cardiol 1996; 28(3): 768–72.
29. Sandoval J, Aguirre JS, Pulido T et al. Nocturnal oxygen therapy in patients with the Eisenmenger syndrome. Am J Respir Crit Care Med 2001; 164: 1682–7.
30. Presbitero P, Somerville J, Stone S et al. Pregnancy in cyanotic congenital heart disease. Outcome of mother and fetus. Circulation 1994; 89: 2673–6.
31a. Broberg CS, Uebing A, Cuomo L et al. Adult patients with Eisenmenger syndrome report flying safely on commercial airlines. Heart 2006 Dec 12 (Epub ahead).
31b. Gleicher N, Midwall J, Hochberger D, Jaffin H. Eisenmengers's syndrome and pregnancy. Obstet Gynecol Surv 1975; 34: 721–41.
32. Vogel M, Bauer F, Abdul-Khaliq H, Lange PE. Outcome of pregnancy in patients with Eisenmenger reaction. Cor Vasa 1998; 40(5): K–210.
33. Wilson W, Taubert KA, Gewitz M et al. Prevention of infective endocarditis; guidelines from the American Heart Association. Circulation 2007; published ahead April 19, 2007.
34. Hopkins WE, Ochoa LL, Richardson GW, Trulock EP. Comparison of the hemodynamics and survival of adults with severe primary pulmonary hypertension or Eisenmenger syndrome. J Heart Lung Transplant 1996; 15: 100–5.
35. Hopkins WE. The remarkable right ventricle of patients with Eisenmenger syndrome. Coron Artery Dis 2005; 16: 19–25.
36. Somerville J. How to manage the Eisenmenger syndrome. Int J Cardiol 1998; 63: 1–8.
37. Stoica SC, Perreas K, Sharples LD. Heart-lung transplantation for Eisenmenger's syndrome: operative risks and late outcomes of 51 consecutive cases from a single institution. J heart Lung Transplant 2001; 20: 173.
38. Perloff JK, Marelli AJ, Miner PD. Risk of stroke in adults with cyanotic congenital heart disease. Circulation 1993; 87(6): 1954–9.
39. Schulze-Neick I, Gilbert N, Ewert R et al. Adult patients with congenital heart disease and pulmonary arterial hypertension: First open prospective multicenter study of bosentan therapy. Am Heart J 2005; 150: 716.
40. Galie N, Beghetti M, Gatzoulis MA et al; Bosentan Randomized Trial of Endothelin Antagonist Therapy-5 (BREATHE-5) Investigators. Bosentan therapy in patients with Eisenmenger syndrome: A multicenter, double-blind, randomized, placebo-controlled study. Circulation 2006; 114: 48–54.
41. Gatzoulis MA, Beghetti M, Galie N et al; on behalf of the BREATHE-5 Investigators. Longer-term bosentan therapy improves functional capacity in Eisenmenger syndrome: Results of the BREATHE-5 open-label extension study. Int J Cardiol 2007 Jul 19 (published ahead).

17

Pulmonary atresia with ventricular septal defect

Pulmonary atresia (PA) is rare and accounts for about 1% of all congenital heart diseases (CHD). This anomaly is a heterogeneous CHD and encompasses a broad range of anomalies, whose common feature is absence of continuity of blood flow from the right ventricle to the pulmonary vascular bed (PA at different anatomical levels), a subaortic ventricular septal defect (VSD) and a biventricular heart (Figure 17.1). PA with VSD may be considered as an extreme variant of tetralogy of Fallot. In echocardiography, PA may suggest unoperated tetralogy of Fallot, but one where the pulmonary artery will not be visualized even by transesophageal echocardiography, showing only a hypoplastic structure with no flow (Figure 17.2). PA may also develop secondary to unoperated tetralogy of Fallot with severe right ventricular outflow tract obstruction (RVOTO).

A critical factor regarding prognosis is the degree of development of pulmonary artery branches. The native pulmonary arteries can be normal, but they are frequently

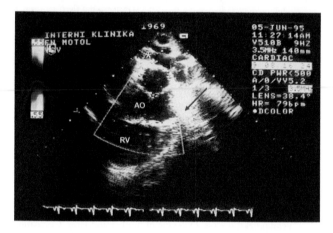

Figure 17.2
Pulmonary atresia; transesophageal echo, longitudinal view. There is fibrotic tissue in the region where pulmonary artery would be normally expected (arrow). In periphery, there are hypoplastic vascular structures (*) with reduced flow (in red) provided by collaterals. AO, Aorta; RV, right ventricle.

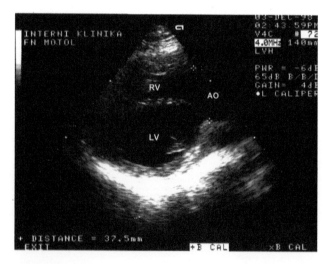

Figure 17.1
Pulmonary atresia; transthoracic echo, longitudinal parasternal view. Dilated aorta (AO) is overriding ventricular septal defect, two ventricles are present: LV, left ventricle; RV, right ventricle. This adult patient has pulmonary atresia; however, a similar picture could be seen in tetralogy of Fallot or double-outlet right ventricle. Differential diagnosis is achieved by visualization of pulmonary artery by transthoracic or transesophageal echo, or computerized tomography angiography.

hypoplastic and abnormal in structure. The right and left pulmonary artery may or may not communicate. Pulmonary blood supply is usually via a patent ductus arteriosus after birth in children with a well-developed pulmonary artery tree.

The pulmonary vascular bed, which can be hypoplastic, is assessed by angiography using the *McGoon index* – the ratio of the sum products of diameters of both pulmonary artery branches to the descending aorta diameter. An index >2 implies a nonrestrictive pulmonary vascular bed, whereas an index <0.8 is notably restrictive. The *Nakata index* gives the sum product of cross-sectional areas of the pulmonary artery branches divided by body surface area. A normal value is 330mm^2/m^2. Values <150mm^2/m^2 signal a hypoplastic pulmonary vascular bed. These indices are used in the decision-making of future therapy. In children with hypoplasia, or absence of the pulmonary arteries, pulmonary blood supply is provided by major aortopulmonary collateral arteries (MAPCA), which can arise from the descending aorta, aortic arch, subclavian arteries, or coronary arteries (Figures 17.3 and 17.4). There may be coronary fistulas between coronary and pulmonary arteries. Their

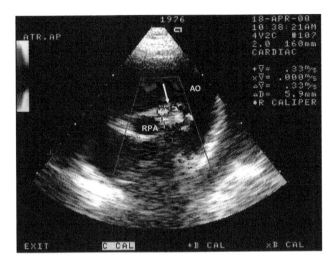

Figure 17.3
Pulmonary atresia, suprasternal view. Color flow Doppler shows systolic–diastolic flow from aortopulmonary collateral (arrow). AO, Aorta; RPA, right pulmonary artery.

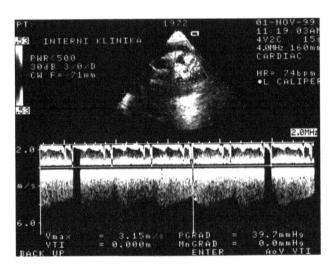

Figure 17.4
Pulmonary atresia, aortopulmonary collateral. Continuous Doppler examination from suprasternal view shows systolic–diastolic flow in aortopulmonary collateral.

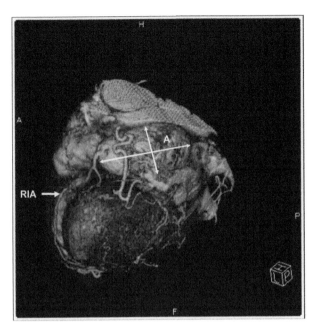

Figure 17.5
Computerized tomography angiogram with 3D reconstruction. Patient with pulmonary atresia after closure of left coronary-to-pulmonary artery fistula in childhood. Surprising giant aneurysm (A: 80 × 46mm) of the left coronary artery in adulthood. RIA, Ramus interventricularis anterior = LAD, left anterior descending coronary artery.

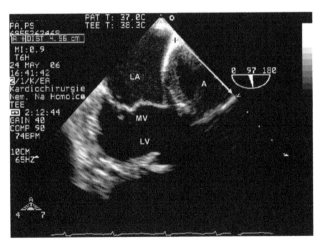

Figure 17.6
Pulmonary atresia; transesophageal echo, 97 degrees. The same patient as in Figures 17.5 and 17.6. The giant aneursym (A) of the left coronary artery is partly thrombotized and has diameter of 46mm. LA, Left atrium; LV, left ventricle; MV, mitral valve.

closure may result in late coronary artery aneurysm (Figures 17.5 and 17.6.).

Patients with well-developed pulmonary artery branches, supplied by a broad ductus arteriosus, are at the best end of the morphological spectrum and eligible for *reconstructive surgery* with perforation of the atretic pulmonary valve and/or implantation of a valved tube graft between the right ventricle and the pulmonary artery to establish luminal continuity between the right ventricle and the pulmonary artery (Figure 17.7). The VSD is closed with a patch. While the quality of life is good following successful reparative surgery, there is a risk of pulmonary conduit or homograft obstruction, hypertension of the right ventricle, residual shunts, arrhythmias, heart failure, aortic root and ascending aorta dilatation with aortic regurgitation, and infectious endocarditis (IE) in the long term.

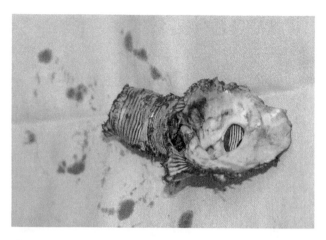

Figure 17.7
Explanted degenerated Hancock pulmonary conduit in 37-year-old patient with pulmonary atresia 21 years after intracardiac repair.

In the presence of hypoplastic or absent pulmonary artery branches, the pulmonary vascular bed is additionally supplied by MAPCA. It is a surgical challenge to create an independent pulmonary circulation in these patients with MAPCA-dependent pulmonary circulation. *Unifocalization* is a surgical technique to recruit pulmonary blood flow from MAPCA into a single, surgically accessible vessel: MAPCA are dissected, tied off and detached from the aorta, their proximal ends are rejoined to a single vessel, and anastomosed to the native pulmonary artery (if present) or to a tube graft (if a well-developed central pulmonary artery is absent). Unifocalization should be performed before the development of stenosis and pulmonary vascular disease in the MAPCA, but the child should be large enough to reduce surgical morbidity and mortality. There is a postoperative risk for thromboses in segmental branches, collaterals and conduit, as well as a risk of IE.

Prognosis

Estimated long-term survival rates in repaired patients are approximately 92% at 5 years, 86% at 10 years and 75% at 20 years.[1] The most common type of reintervention is pulmonary conduit replacement, being required in 36% of patients after 10 years of follow-up (Figure 17.7). Aortic valve replacement for hemodynamically significant aortic regurgitation is necessary in approximately 6% of cases 10 years after repair.[1]

In terms of prognosis, the least favorable condition is PA, whereby pulmonary artery branches are completely absent, with the pulmonary vascular bed supplied solely by *MAPCA*. These patients may not be candidates for reparative surgery (biventricular repair). In these cases, the pulmonary circulation is dependent exclusively on these MAPCA (Figures 17.3 and 17.4), or, alternatively, on *a surgically created aortopulmonary shunt*, e.g. *Blalock–Taussig shunt* (see Figures 7.22 and 7.23) or other *central systemic-to-pulmonary artery shunt*. However, high collateral pressure results, in pulmonary arterioles, in pulmonary vascular disease with plexiform changes and pulmonary hypertension. Progressive pulmonary vascular disease deteriorates further pulmonary perfusion and oxygen saturation. These patients may survive to young adult age. They present with chronic cyanosis, hemoptysis, occasionally even fatal, lung infection with a serious course, brain abscesses, cerebral vascular events (paradoxical emboli), IE, arrhythmias, and aortic root or ascending aorta dilatation. Their prognosis is poor. The only option would be heart and lung transplantation; however, this procedure is associated with poor long-term survival rates.

Follow-up

All patients with any type of PA are complex and must be followed-up by a cardiologist with special training and expertise in CHD. *PA with intact ventricular septum* is a duct-dependent defect incompatible with survival to adulthood without intervention/surgery.

Reference

1. Cho JM, Puga FJ, Danielson GK et al. Early and long-term results of the surgical treatment of tetralogy of Fallot with pulmonary atresia, with or without major aortopulmonary collaterals. Thorac Cardiovasc Surg 2002; 124: 70–81.

18

Congenital coronary artery anomalies

In adulthood, congenital coronary artery anomalies represent more often as an incidental finding rather than the cause of clinical complaints. However, in some cases, congenital coronary anomalies may cause atypical chest pains, anginal pain, arrhythmias, sudden death or heart failure, even in adulthood. But the majority of patients don't have a characteristic presentation and remain asymptomatic for a large portion of their lives. Normal coronary artery origins can be visualized in adults by transesophageal echocardiography (Figures 18.1 and 18.2). Coronary artery anomaly is defined as origin of a coronary artery from an ectopic position in the aorta.

Anomalous left coronary artery origin from the pulmonary artery

First to report this anomaly (ALCAPA) was Brooks, a pathologist, in 1885.[1] The clinical phenotype was first reported in 1933, and is named after the authors as Bland-White-Garland syndrome.[2]

Anatomical notes

In patients with this coronary anomaly, the left coronary artery usually arises from the left posterior sinus of the pulmonary artery, rarely as far as the pulmonary artery trunk or branch. Its branching pattern is usually normal into left anterior descending and left circumflex arteries. While not usually dilated in childhood, an anomalous left coronary artery is usually tortuous, dilated and thin-walled in adulthood, and resembles a vein (Figure 18.3). The right coronary artery is dilated and connected to the anomalous left coronary artery via abundant collaterals. Scars can be found on the left ventricular anterior wall as well as on the antero-lateral papillary muscle. The left ventricle may be dilated, and the mitral valve is regurgitant due to abnormal left ventricular geometry and/or mitral annular dilatation. Left ventricular endocardial fibroelastosis is a finding made in children more often than in adults.

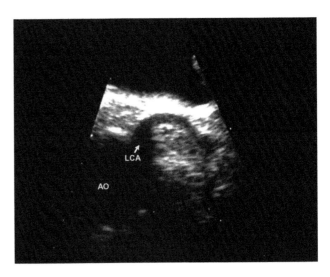

Figure 18.1
Transesophageal echo, short axis with aorta (AO) in 0 degrees and left main coronary artery (LCA) in the typical location.

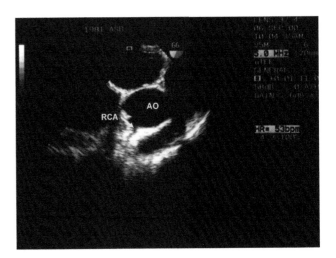

Figure 18.2
Transesophageal echo: aorta (AO) in 66 degrees and the origin of the right coronary artery (RCA) in typical location.

ALCAPA is usually an isolated anomaly; however, it may also be associated with other congenital heart diseases (CHD), such as patent ductus arteriosus, ventricular septal

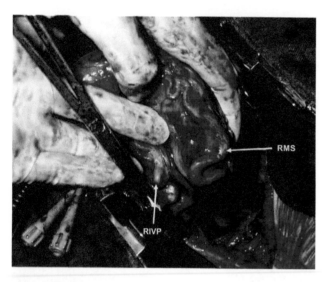

Figure 18.3
Anomalous left coronary artery (ALCAPA), a surgical view.
A meander-like course of the dilated left coronary artery arising
from the pulmonary artery. RMS, A dilated obtuse marginal
branch arising from the anomalous left coronary artery. RIVP, A
dilated posterior descending branch of the right coronary artery
supplying the anomalous left coronary artery by collaterals.
(Courtesy of Professor Jan Dominik, Clinic of Cardiac Surgery,
Hradec Králové University Hospital, Czech Republic.)

defect, tetralogy of Fallot, coarctation of the aorta, etc. In
rare cases, the right coronary artery may also arise from the
pulmonary artery.

Prevalence

The incidence of an anomalous origin of the left coronary
artery from the pulmonary artery is reported to be 0.22–
0.5% of all CHD.[3–5] ALCAPA accounts for 57% of all significant congenital coronary artery anomalies.[3]

Pathophysiology

There is a high pressure in the pulmonary artery of the fetal
circulation, the pulmonary artery blood is well oxygenated
and blood flows from the pulmonary artery to the anomalous
coronary artery. However, upon birth, the direction of flow
through the anomalous coronary artery is reversed, and
directed retrograde from the coronary artery to the pulmonary artery. The clinical course is determined by the extent
of the collateral vascular bed between the right coronary
artery and the anomalous left coronary artery. Poor collateral
vascular supply is associated with severe ischemia in the area
supplied by the left coronary artery,[6] with subsequent myocardial infarction, and/or endocardial fibroelastosis, left ventricular dysfunction, mitral regurgitation and heart failure. In the
presence of good collateral supply, the retrograde flow in the

left coronary artery causes the 'steal phenomenon' from the
capillary vascular bed with myocardial ischemia. The flow
from anomalous left coronary artery results in left-to-right
shunt, usually small in terms of the cardiac output but fairly
significant in terms of coronary circulation. Without surgery,
only patients with adequate collaterals will survive to adulthood. Natural survival is poor. Ninety per cent of the children
develop congestive heart failure due to myocardial ischemia
and die without surgical therapy.

Clinical findings and diagnosis

ALCAPA is usually surgically repaired in childhood; rarely the
coronary anomaly may remain undetected until adulthood.[7]

Symptoms

- Atypical chest pain.
- Dyspnea, particularly exertional dyspnea.
- Exertional angina pectoris.
- Arrhythmia.
- Signs of heart failure.
- Sudden death, especially during exercise.

Auscultatory findings

- Holosystolic murmur on the apex due to mitral
  regurgitation.
- Gallop in heart failure.
- Very quiet continuous murmur on the left upper sternal
  margin (similar to that heard in coronary arteriovenous
  fistula or small patent ductus arteriosus).

Electrocardiogram (ECG)

- Anterolateral Q wave myocardial infarction.
- Ischemic changes at rest or during exercise in the antero-
  lateral area.

Echocardiography

- Apical aneurysm and dilatation of the left ventricle may
  be present in adult survivors.
- Regional impaired left ventricular kinetics in the vascular bed supplied by the left coronary artery may be present at rest or during exercise echocardiography.
- The right coronary artery is usually significantly dilated.
- The origin of the left coronary artery arising from the
  left sinus of Valsalva in aorta cannot be identified.
- Color Doppler mapping will show an abnormal diastolic
  flow, directed retrograde from the anomalous left coronary artery to the pulmonary artery. To be examined by

transthoracic echo in patients easy to visualize and when using a high-quality echocardiographic device, or by transesophageal echocardiography in adulthood.

- Color Doppler mapping will visualize severely enlarged collateral vessels with a continuous flow pattern within the interventricular septum.
- There may be moderate to severe mitral regurgitation.
- Increased echogenity of the papillary muscles (papillary muscle fibrosis).
- Increased echogenity of the endocardium (endocardial fibrosis).

Catheterization and angiography

In children, catheterization and angiography are indicated in cases with unclear echocardiographic findings; in adults, the procedures should be performed as a rule. The left coronary artery may not be readily identified in selective coronary angiography. The right coronary artery is dilated and tortuous, collateral filling to the left coronary artery may be evident as well as late contrast-medium transit through pulmonary artery. Evidence of origin of an anomalous coronary artery may not be easy to obtain by pulmonary angiography; it can be obtained following partial pulmonary artery occlusion by the balloon.

Management

- The diagnosis of ALCAPA is an indication for surgical revascularization. Many surgical techniques have been applied during the last few decades.
- At present, left coronary artery reimplantation into the aorta with a patch in the pulmonary artery wall is performed. Alternatively, redirection of the anomalous left coronary artery can also be performed using an intrapulmonary conduit connection into the aorta (according to Takeushi).
- Previously, seriously ill children were scheduled for anomalous coronary artery ligation and coronary artery bypass grafting as a quick, simple, and palliative procedure. While it is no longer performed, some patients having undergone this procedure have survived to adulthood.
- Interventional closure (embolization) of the connection to the left pulmonary artery may be an option in selected patients (unpublished case reports). This therapeutic approach is reserved for selected patients and should be performed only by interventionalists highly experienced in CHD in high-volume centers. The patients are left with a coronary circulation depending on a single coronary artery.
- Modern heart failure management must be established in the presence of left ventricular dysfunction (ACE inhibitors, angiotensin II inhibitors, beta blockers, diuretics, etc.). Heart transplantation is a therapeutic option in selected patients with severe heart failure symptoms and poor quality of life.

Residual findings

- Late exertional ischemia requiring revascularization may occur in adulthood following anomalous left coronary artery ligation.
- Myocardial ischemia at rest or during exercise in patients with impaired patency of a reimplanted left coronary artery.
- Residual mitral regurgitation.
- Residual systolic left ventricular dysfunction.
- Residual shunt between the reimplanted anomalous coronary artery and the pulmonary artery.

Prognosis

The prognosis and outcome depend primarily on maintaining systolic and diastolic left ventricular function. Favorable factors in childhood include an adequate collateral vascular bed and a restrictive orifice of the anomalous left coronary artery into the pulmonary artery. Still, even asymptomatic adults not undergoing surgery are at risk of sudden death (especially so during exercise), angina, and heart failure. A surgical revascularization maintaining two coronary arteries is performed as the method of choice. The hospital mortality is approximately 14%.[8] Provided the coronary arteries are patent, and left ventricular and mitral valve function are not involved, the long-term prognosis is good. Survival of hospital survivors at 20 years was 94.8%.[8]

Follow-up

Regular follow-up visits are recommended in specialized CHD clinics.

Congenital coronary fistula
Definition and anatomical notes

The term coronary fistula refers to a communication between a coronary artery and cardiac chambers or great arteries without transit through the capillary vascular bed. The condition is a continuum of the embryonic state, whereby epicardiac coronary arteries are connected with intramyocardiac spaces via sinusoids. Coronary fistulas may arise from the right or left coronary artery while entering right-heart chambers in 90% of cases. Symptomatic coronary fistulas most often enter the right ventricle; less often the right atrium. Asymptomatic fistulas usually arise from

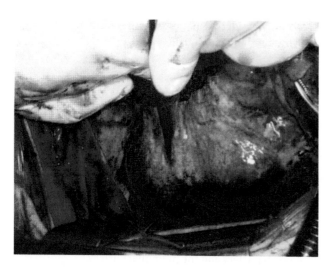

Figure 18.4

Giant coronary fistula. Surgical view of the giant aneurysm of the left circumflex coronary artery of diameter 10cm. This dilatation was caused by shunt flow in the coronary fistula between left circumflex coronary artery and right atrium. See also Figures 18.5–18.7. (Courtesy of M Semrad, 1st Clinic of Cardiac Surgery, 1st Medical School, Charles University, University Hospital, Prague.)

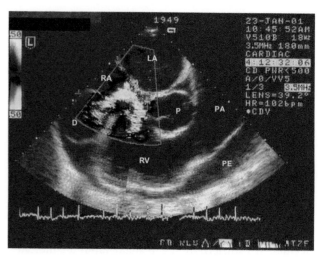

Figure 18.6

Transesophageal echo, longitudinal view; large coronary fistula. The same patient as in Figures 18.4 and 18.5. PA, Dilated pulmonary artery; RV, right ventricle; D, distal part of the large coronary fistula with the colored flow entering right atrium; P, proximal part of the coronary fistula; LA, left atrium; RA, right atrium; PE, pericardial effusion. The giant coronary artery causes significant left-to-right shunt with pulmonary to systemic flow Qp/Qs 2.7: 1.

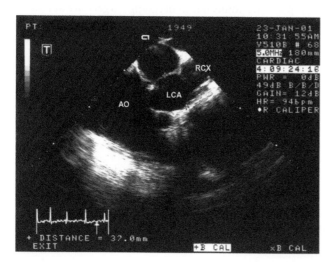

Figure 18.5

Transesophageal echo, transversal view; large coronary fistula. Dilated left main coronary artery, 37mm (LCA) from aorta (AO), dilated circumflex artery and coronary fistula from circumflex coronary artery (RCX) to right atrium.

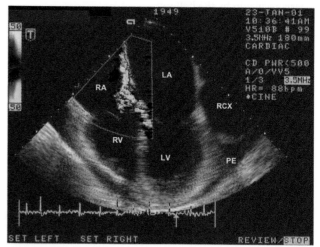

Figure 18.7

Transesophageal echo, transversal view; large coronary fistula. Color flow indicates left-to-right shunt via large coronary fistula to right atrium. All cardiac chambers are dilated. The same patient as in Figures 18.4–18.6. RCX, Large aneurysm of the circumflex artery with coronary fistula to right atrium; RA, right atrium; RV, right ventricle; LA, left atrium; LV, left ventricle; PE, large pericardial effusion.

Prevalence

Congenital coronary fistulas account for some 0.2–0.4% of all CHD, and 43% of all congenital coronary artery anomalies.[9,10] In large coronary angiography studies obtained

the left coronary artery and tend to enter the pulmonary artery.[9] More rarely, coronary fistulas may enter venae cavae, coronary sinus, left ventricle, aorta, or bronchial arteries. A coronary fistula may have multiple openings. At the site of fistula, the coronary artery will be dilated, elongated and tortuous; it may also be dilated in an aneurysm-like manner (Figures 18.4.–18.7).

from the general population, coronary fistulas were found incidentally in 0.13% of cases.[11,12] These incidentally identified fistulas were small and asymptomatic (Figures 18.8 and 18.9).[12]

Pathophysiology

A communication of a coronary artery with right-heart chambers creates a left-to-right shunt whose size is dependent on the fistula flow rate. In large fistulas, the shunt results in volume overload, right-heart chamber dilatation and increased pulmonary flow (Figures 18.4 and 18.6). In cases whereby the fistula empties into the left ventricle, blood flows through the fistula in diastole only, with the hemodynamic pattern resembling that in aortic regurgitation. A 'steal phenomenon' can be seen in the presence of blood flowing through a fistula at high rates and causing ischemia.

Clinical findings and diagnosis

The clinical relevance of a fistula depends on its size. Small fistulas are usually asymptomatic. Large fistulas may manifest themselves by heart failure in a major left-to-right shunt or ischemia: by angina, myocardial infarction, arrhythmias, heart failure or sudden death. A coronary fistula often does not become symptomatic until adulthood, most frequently not until the age of 40. Symptomatic coronary fistulas are associated with increased morbidity and mortality rates.

The physical finding is dependent on fistula size and location. Auscultation will detect continuous murmur in the precordium in cases where blood flow through the fistula is high enough, and the fistula enters low-pressure chambers. The murmur is only diastolic in cases where the fistula enters the left ventricle. The auscultatory maximum depends on fistula location.

The diagnosis is established by coronary angiography and echocardiography. Color Doppler mapping allows detection of the coronary fistulas in children using the transthoracic technique, while transesophageal echocardiography is sometimes more informative in adults. Echocardiography combined with color Doppler mapping is most useful to pinpoint the site of fistula opening (Figures 18.6–18.8). However, selective coronary angiography will clearly delineate the morphology, size and site of entry (Figure 18.9).

Management

- Small, asymptomatic, hemodynamically nonsignificant, coronary fistulas do not require any intervention; patients with these fistulas should only be on conservative follow-up without intervention.[9,12,13] Spontaneous coronary fistula closure has been reported in up to 23% of children.[9]

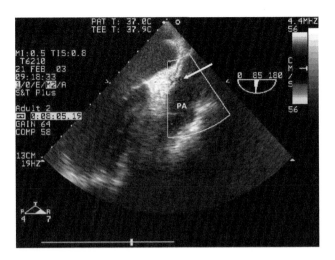

Figure 18.8
Transesophageal echo, longitudinal view. Small coronary fistula (2mm) from coronary artery to pulmonary artery in diastole (arrow). PA, Pulmonary artery.

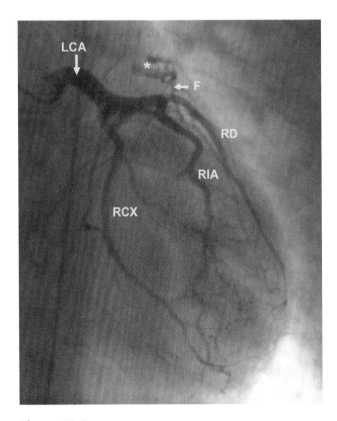

Figure 18.9
Small coronary fistula from left coronary artery to pulmonary artery. Selective coronarogram, anteroposterior projection. Accidental finding without hemodynamic significance. LCA, Left main coronary artery; RCX, ramus circumflexus; *, contrast agent from coronary fistula to pulmonary artery, small coronary fistula; RIA, ramus interventricularis anterior; RD, first diagonal branch.

- Moderate and large fistulas causing symptoms and/or complications require intervention, either surgical or percutaneous closure.[14]
- Morphologically suitable fistulas can be closed using a catheter. The most often used device is a detachable metallic spiral. Complete closure was obtained in 82% of cases. The procedure required special expertise in interventions in CHD.[15]
- Large, hemodynamically significant fistulas, refractory to catheter-based closure, are indicated for surgical management. The safest procedure involves complete closure of either end of the fistula using suture or a patch; in some cases, the procedure is complemented with coronary artery bypass grafting. Operative mortality with large and aneurysm-like dilated fistulas is some 6%.[16] Simple ligation of the origin of the fistula might result in thrombus formation with subsequent embolism in the dilated dead-end arm.

Risks

- Develompment of an aneurysm, accelerated atherosclerosis, fistula wall calcification, mural thrombosis, embolism.
- Myocardial infarction prior to or after surgical fistula closure (approx. 3%).
- Infectious endocarditis (approx. 4%).
- Fistula rupture.
- Fistula recanalization following its surgical closure (approx. 4%).

Congenital coronary aneurysm

Congenital coronary aneurysm without a fistula and a history of vasculitis has a poor prognosis with a risk of rupture, thrombosis or embolism. Surgical management is usually indicated.[17]

- *Acquired coronary artery aneurysms* may evolve in long-term outcome after coronary fistula ligation (Figure 18.10 and Figures 17.5 and 17.6).
- Another cause of acquired coronary aneurysms is *Kawasaki disease*, occurring predominantly in infants and young children. This acute systematic vasculitis involves small and medium-sized arteries, particularly the coronary arteries.[18,19] Those with persistent large (>8mm in diameter) or giant coronary artery aneurysms are known to be at risk of development of hemodynamically significant stenoses with myocardial ischemia or infarction (Figure 18.11). Calcification or thrombosis of these abnormal coronary arteries is frequent in long-term follow-up. Therapy with acetylosalicylic acid or surgery is recommended.[20]

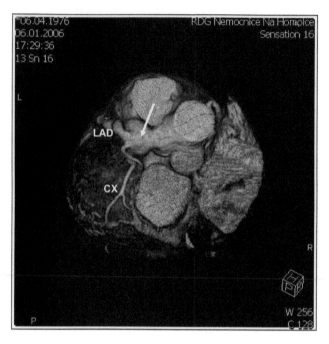

Figure 18.10
Computerized tomography angiogram with 3D reconstruction: large aneurysm of the left main coronary artery (arrow, diameter 22mm), dilation of the left anterior descending (LAD) coronary artery to 7mm; CX, circumflex artery. This patient has tetralogy of Fallot and had transcatheter closure of coronary fistula from LAD to right ventricle 7 years ago.

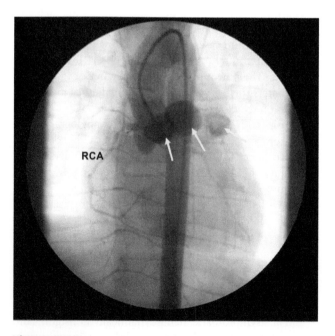

Figure 18.11
Kawasaki disease with three aneurysms on the left coronary artery (arrows), normal right coronary artery (RCA). (Courtesy of Petr Tax, Children Kardiocentrum, University Hospital Motol, Charles University, Prague, Czech Republic.)

Congenital variations of coronary artery origin

Congenital variations of coronary artery origin occur in 0.1–0.5% of coronary angiographic findings in the general population. However, the incidence was much higher (5.6%) in one of the few prospective analyses of a continuous series of 1950 consecutive patients studied by coronary angiography with strict diagnostic criteria.[6]

- The left coronary artery may arise from the right coronary sinus or from the right coronary artery. This anomaly occurs, for example, in some cases of tetralogy of Fallot. Coronary arteries with ectopic origin develop premature accelerated atherosclerosis; the coronary artery may be hypoplastic or absent. A coronary artery with an ectopic origin between the pulmonary artery and aorta (intramural course) may be compressed by the aorta in the presence of increased blood pressure or during exercise. Clinically, this condition may manifest itself for the first time in adulthood by anginal chest pain, arrhythmias, or by sudden death during exercise. In patients with an intramural course of the left coronary artery in front of the pulmonary artery, the left coronary artery may be injured during intracardiac repair of tetralogy of Fallot. A coronary artery with an ectopic origin and documented myocardial ischemia is indicated for revascularization, preferably by the use of the internal mammary artery for grafting.
- A single coronary artery is rarely present as an isolated anomaly.[21] It is more often associated with a bicuspid aortic valve and with conotruncal anomalies.
- In CHD, when the aorta is localized anteriorly and rightward to the pulmonary artery (e.g. transposition of the great arteries, double-outlet right ventricle with transposition of the great arteries), there are many variations of coronary arteries, which is beyond the focus of this book.

References

1. Brooks Jr HST. Two cases of an abnormal coronary artery of the heart arising from the pulmonary artery. J Anat Physiol 1885; 20: 26–9.
2. Bland EF, White PD, Garland J. Congenital anomalies of coronary arteries. Report of unusual case associated with cardiac hypertrophy. Am Heart J 1933; 8: 787–801.
3. Samanek M, Voriskova M. Congenital heart disease among 815,569 children born between 1980 and 1990 and their 15-year survival: a prospective bohemia survival study. Pediatr Cardiology 1999; 20: 411–17.
4. Valdes-Cruz LM, Cayre LO. Echocardiographic Diagnosis of Congenital Heart Disease. An Embryologic and Anatomic Approach, 1st edn. Philadelphia, PA: Lippicott-Raven Publishers, 1999.
5. Askenazi J, Nadas AS. Anomalous left coronary artery originating from the pulmonary artery: Report on 15 cases. Circulation 1975; 51: 976–87.
6. Angelini P. Coronary artery anomalies – an entity in search of an identity. Circulation 2007; 115: 1296–305.
7. Alexi-Meshkishvilli V, Berger F, Weng Y, Lange PE, Hetzer R. Anomalous origin of the left coronary artery from the pulmonary artery in adults. J Card Surg 1995; 10: 309–15.
8. Lange R, Vogt M, Horer J et al. Long-term results of repair of anomalous origin of the coronary artery from the pulmonary artery. Ann Thorac Surg 2007; 83(4): 1463–71.
9. Sherwood MC, Rockenmacher S, Colan SD, Geva T. Prognostic significance of clinically silent coronary artery fistulas. Am J Cardiol 1999; 83(3): 407–11.
10. Ogden JA. Congenital anomalies of the coronary arteries. Am J Cardiol 1970; 25: 474–9.
11. Yamanaka O, Hobbs RE. Coronary artery anomalies in 126,595 patients undergoing coronary arteriography. Cathet Cardiovasc Diagn 1990; 21: 28–40.
12. Gillebert C, Van Hoof R, Van De Werf F, Piessens J, De Geest H. Coronary artery fistulas in an adult population. Eur Heart J 1986; 7: 437–43.
13. Hobbs RE, Millit HD, Raghavan PV, Moodie DS, Sheldon WC. Coronary artery fistulae: A ten year review. Clev Clin Q 1982; 49: 191–7.
14. Collins N, Mehta R, Benson L, Horlick E. Percutaneous coronary artery fistula closure in adults: Technical and procedural aspects. Catheter Cardiovasc Interv 2007; 69: 872–80.
15. Armsby LR, Keane JF, Sherwood MC et al. Management of coronary artery fistulae. Patient selection and results of transcatheter closure. J Am Coll Cardiol 2002; 39: 1026–32.
16. Cheung DL, Au WK, Cheung HH, Chiu CS, Lee WT. Coronary artery fistulas: Long-term results of surgical correction. Ann Thorac Surg 2001; 71(1): 190–5.
17. Li D, Wu Q, Sun L et al. Surgical treatment of giant coronary artery aneurysm. J Thorac Cardiovasc Surg 2005; 130: 817–21.
18. Kawasaki T. Acute febrile mucocutaneous syndrome with lymphoid involvement with specific desquamation of the fingers and toes in children. Jpn J Allergy 1967; 116: 178–222.
19. Kato H. Cardiovascular involvement in Kawasaki disease: Evaluation and natural history. Prog Clin Biol Res 1987; 250: 277–86.
20. Niwa K, Tateno S. Kawasaki's disease. In: Gatzoulis MA, Webb GD, Daubeney PEF, eds. Adult Congenital Heart Disease. New York: Churchill Livingstone, 2003: 433–9.
21. Shirani J, Roberts WC. Solitary coronary ostium in the aorta in the absence of other major congenital cardiovascular anomalies. J Am Coll Cardiol 1993; 21(1): 137–43.

19

Persistent left superior vena cava

This is the most frequent anomaly of systemic veins, occurring in 0.3–0.5% of the general population, and in 1.5–10% of patients with congenital heart disease (CHD) (Figure 19.1). It usually empties via the coronary sinus into the right atrium, with the coronary sinus being dilated. While not causing a hemodynamic abnormality, its detection and differential diagnoses are important prior to any cardiac surgical procedure.[1]

If the persistent left superior vena cava is associated with a rare coronary sinus defect, it empties via this defect into the left atrium causing a right-to-left shunt (unroofed coronary sinus). Less often it may enter the left atrium directly. A persistent left superior vena cava is usually also present in the visceral heterotaxy syndrome (see Chapter 23).

A persistent left superior vena cava can be demonstrated by echocardiography, preferably by transesophageal echocardiography, visualizing it laterally to the left atrium in the transverse projection (Figures 19.2–19.4). The course

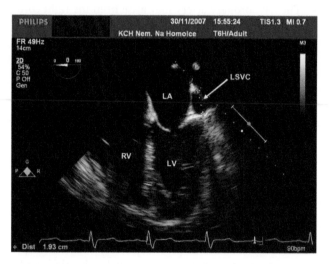

Figure 19.2
Transesophageal echo, 0 degrees. Persistent left superior vena cava (LSVC) is visualized laterally from the left atrium (LA). It is emptying into coronary sinus and right atrium. LV, Left ventricle; RV, right ventricle.

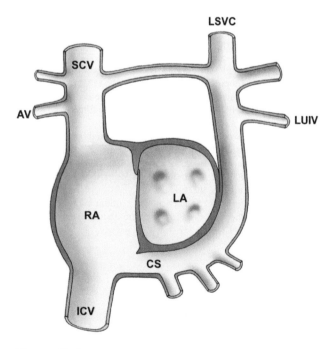

Figure 19.1
Persistent left superior vena cava (LSVC), usually empties into dilated coronary sinus (CS) and right atrium (RA). SCV, Right-sided superior caval vein; LUIV, left upper intercostal vein; ICV, inferior caval vein; AV, azygos vein; LA, left atrium with pulmonary veins ostia.

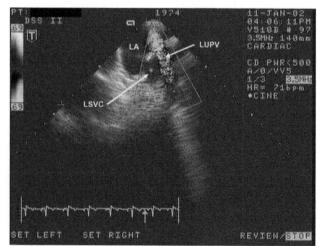

Figure 19.3
Transesophageal echo, transverse projection. Relation of the persistent left superior vena cava (LSVC) laterally from the left atrium (LA) and left upper pulmonary vein (LUPV). Incidental finding of LSVC in a patient with atrial septal defect type secundum, which is not visualized in this view.

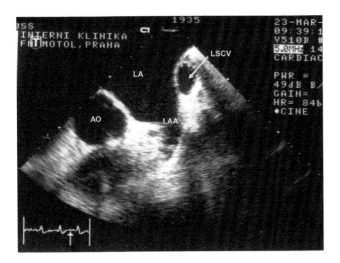

Figure 19.4
Transesophageal echo, transversal view. Relation between left superior vena cava (LSVC) and left atrial auricle (LAA). LA, Left atrium; AO, aorta. This patient has also atrial septal defect type secundum, which is not visualized.

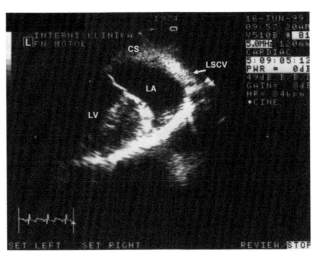

Figure 19.6
Transesophageal echo, longitudinal view. Persistent left superior vena cava (LSVC) enters dilated coronary sinus (CS), diagnosis confirmed by echo-contrast applied into left brachial vein. The contrast appears in the LSVC and CS, but it does not appear in the left atrium (LA) or the left ventricle (LV).

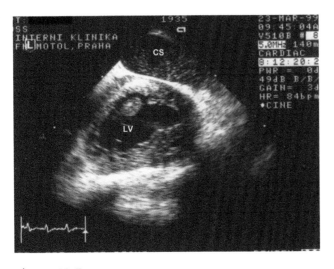

Figure 19.5
Transesophageal echo, longitudinal view. Persistent left superior vena cava enters dilated coronary sinus (CS), which empties into the right atrium. Confirmation was made by contrast echocardiography with application of the echo-contrast agent into the left brachial vein. Contrast can be seen in the dilated coronary sinus. LV, Left ventricle without contrast.

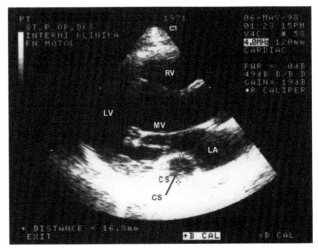

Figure 19.7
Transthoracic echo, long-axis parasternal view. Behind left atrium there is a dilated coronary sinus (CS), suspicious from persistent left superior vena cava entering the coronary sinus. It should not be mistaken for descending aorta, which can be differentiated by pulsed Doppler examination. LA, Left atrium; MV, mitral valve; LV, left ventricle; RV, right ventricle.

and entry of the persistent left-side superior vena cava is evident in the longitudinal projection (Figures 19.5 and 19.6). Suspicion of a persistent left superior vena cava is raised by the presence of an enlarged coronary sinus, dilated to >15mm in adults, which can also be well visualized by transthoracic echocardiography in the parasternal long-axis view (Figure 19.7). The diagnosis will be confirmed by contrast echocardiography with intravenous administration of agitated saline or an echo-contrast medium into the left brachial vein. The contrast medium will first appear in the left-side superior vena cava and in the dilated coronary sinus (Figures 19.5, 19.6, 19.8, and 19.9), and enters then the right atrium (Figure 19.10). The contrast medium applied to the left brachial vein does not appear in the right superior caval vein, unless there is a communicating vein between the right and left vena cava (Figure 19.11). In the presence of a

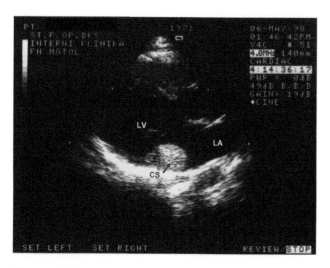

Figure 19.8
Transthoracic echo, longitudinal parasternal view; the same patient as in Figure 19.7. After application of contrast medium into left brachial vein, coronary sinus (CS) filled with contrast. LA, Left atrium; LV, left ventricle.

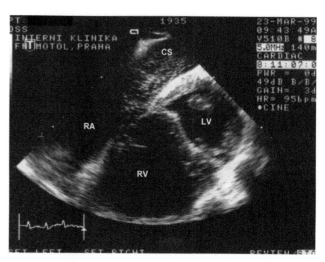

Figure 19.10
Contrast agent applied into the left brachial vein enters persistent left upper vena cava, coronary sinus (CS) and right atrium (RA). RV, Right ventricle; LV, left ventricle.

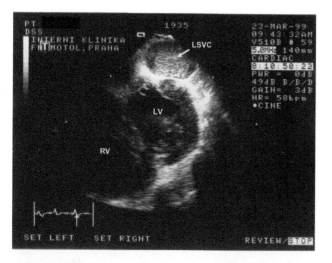

Figure 19.9
Transesophageal echo, transversal view. Shows dilated persistent left upper vena cava (LSVC) filled with contrast after the injection into the left brachial vein. LV, Left ventricle; RV, right ventricle.

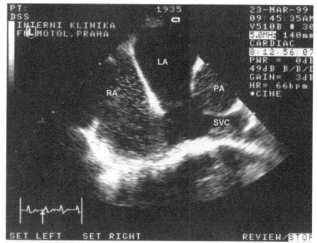

Figure 19.11
Transesophageal echo, longitudinal view, contrast echocardiography with application of the contrast to the left arm. Contrast agent is entering the right atrium (RA) via coronary sinus due to the presence of the persistent left superior vena cava, not via the right superior vena cava (SVC), which is without contrast. This patient has also atrial defect type sinus venosus superior (arrow). LA, Left atrium; PA, pulmonary artery.

coronary sinus defect, the contrast medium also appears in the left atrium (Figures 19.12 and 19.13).

Preoperative detection and description of a persistent left superior vena cava are crucial if a patient with either acquired or congenital heart disease is undergoing cardiovascular surgery (cannulation/heart-lung machine). In addition, the presence or absence of an innominate vein is important and must be described in this setting.

In the differential diagnosis, a dilated coronary sinus can also be seen in elevated right atrial pressure of any cause, e.g. significant tricuspid regurgitation. However, the dilatation is not as extensive as in the presence of a left superior vena cava emptying into the coronary sinus.

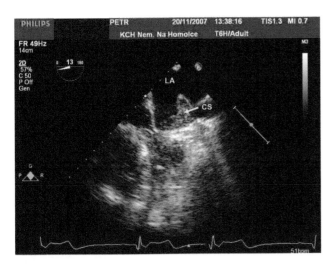

Figure 19.12
Transesophageal echo, 13 degrees. Patient with persistent left superior caval vein and coronary sinus defect. After application of the contrast medium into the left arm, the contrast enters left atrium (LA) via the defect in coronary sinus (CS).

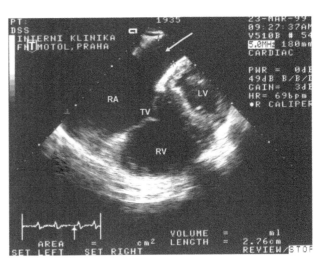

Figure 19.14
Transesophageal echo, transversal view. Dilated coronary sinus (27mm; arrow), could possibly be mistaken for atrial septal defect type primum by inexperienced echocardiographer. RA, Right atrium; RV, right ventricle; LV, left ventricle; TV, tricuspid valve.

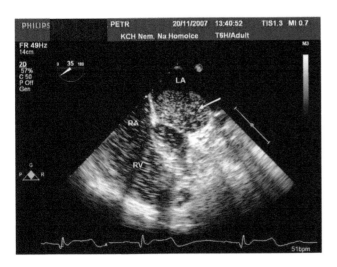

Figure 19.13
Transesophageal echo, 35 degrees; the same patient as in Figure 19.12. Contrast agent is filling the left atrium (LA) from the unroofed coronary sinus (arrow), rest of the contrast gets via coronary sinus into the atrium (RA) and right ventricle (RV).

Contrast echocardiography will reveal contrast medium regurgitating from the right atrium into the coronary sinus, but not contrast coming from inside the coronary sinus. A dilated coronary sinus may also be secondary to anomalous pulmonary venous connection (see Figure 20.14). However, in this case, the coronary sinus will not fill by agitated saline or the contrast medium administered intravenously into the left upper limb (see Figure 20.15). On cursory examination, a significantly dilated coronary sinus may be mistaken for ostium primum atrial septal defect (Figure 19.14).

There are other echogenic structures in the left atrio-ventricular groove to be considered, for example, aneurysm of the circumflex artery (see Figure 18.7), tumors, fat, etc.[1]

Reference

1. Zuber M, Oechslin E, Jenni R. Echogenic structures in the left atrio-ventricular groove: Diagnostic pitfalls. J Am Soc Echocardiogr 1998; 11: 381–6.

20

Anomalous pulmonary venous connection

Partial anomalous pulmonary venous connection

Partial anomalous pulmonary venous connection (PAPVC) describes abnormal connection of at least one, but not all, pulmonary veins to the right atrium or superior vena cava. It occurs in 0.3–0.6% of all congenital heart diseases (CHD). There is a wide anatomic spectrum of PAPVC. The most frequent anomaly is a connection of the right upper and middle lobe pulmonary veins to the right atrium or to the superior vena cava. This anomaly is associated in up to 95% of cases with a *superior sinus venous defect* (see Chapter 3). The diagnosis in adults is usually made by trans-esophageal echocardiography (Figures 20.1–20.5) or computerized tomography (CT) angiogram. Partial anomalous connection is reported to be associated also with 3–15% of cases of a secundum atrial septal defect.[1]

The so-called *scimitar syndrome* refers to cases whereby all right-sided pulmonary veins enter the inferior vena

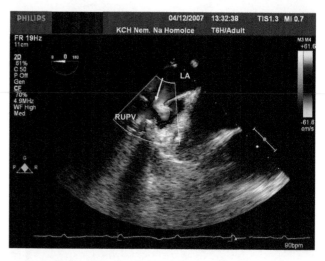

Figure 20.2
Transesophageal echo, 0 degrees, color Doppler; the same patient as in Figure 20.1. RUPV, Anomalous right upper pulmonary vein; arrow, atrial septal defect type sinus venosus superior; LA, left atrium.

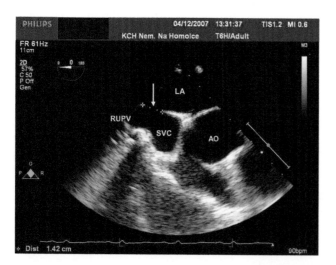

Figure 20.1
Transesophageal echo, 0 degrees, partial anomalous connection of the right upper pulmonary vein (RUPV) into the superior vena cava (SVC) just above the junction of superior vena cava with right atrium. An atrial septal defect type sinus venosus superior (arrow,14mm, between the two crosses) is almost always connected with partial anomalous pulmonary vein connection. LA, Left atrium; AO, aorta.

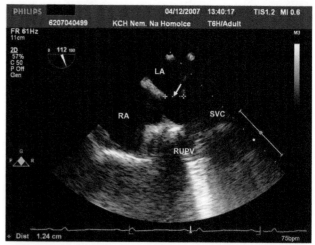

Figure 20.3
Transesophageal echo, 112 degrees, partial anomalous pulmonary venous connection of the right upper pulmonary vein (RUPV) into the superior vena cava (SVC) with sinus venosus superior defect (arrow, 12mm); the same patient as in Figures 20.1 and 20.2. RA, Right atrium; LA, left atrium.

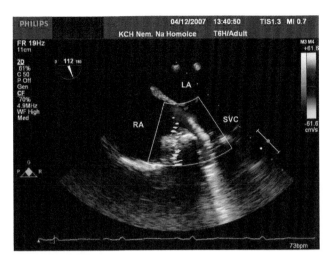

Figure 20.4
Transesophageal echo,112 degrees, color Doppler;
the same patient as in Figures 20.1–20.3. Partial
anomalous pulmonary venous return of the right upper
pulmonary vein (in red) into superior vena cava (SVC).
RA, Right atrium; LA, left atrium.

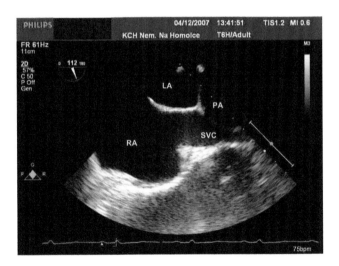

Figure 20.5
Transesophageal echo, 112 degrees; the same patient as in
Figures 20.1–20.4. The visualization of the partial anomalous
pulmonary venous return as well as the sinus venosus defect may
be difficult. RA, Right atrium; LA, left atrium; PA, pulmonary
artery; SVC, superior vena cava.

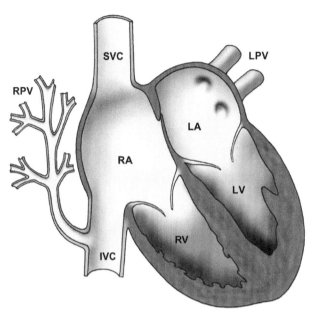

Figure 20.6
Partial anomalous pulmonary venous connection in scimitar
syndrome. Right pulmonary veins (RPV) are connected to inferior
vena cava (IVC). SVC, Superior vena cava; RA, right atrium;
LA, left atrium; LPV, left pulmonary veins; RV, right ventricle;
LV, left ventricle.

Abnormal connection of the left-sided pulmonary veins
from the left lung may enter, via the brachiocephalic vein,
into the superior caval vein (Figure 20.7) or to the coronary
sinus (Figure 20.8).

In terms of hemodynamics, a partially anomalous pulmonary venous connection causes a left-to-right shunt and
right ventricular volume overload. In contrast to a left-to-
right shunt in the setting of a defect at the atrial level (e.g.
secundum atrial septal defect, superior sinus venosus
defect), the shunt is fixed and does not vary according to the
diastolic function, or to filling pressures in the right- and
left-heart. The diagnosis is established by echocardiography
and/or angiography or CT angiogram or MRI. When using
transesophageal echocardiography, every effort should
always be made to check whether all four pulmonary veins
drain into the left atrium (Figures 20.9–20.11). Direct visualization of an anomalous pulmonary venous connection in
adulthood can be difficult (Figures 20.1–20.5).

Management

The degree of left-to-right shunt and the presence of symptoms direct the management. Surgical redirection of the pulmonary veins to the left atrium is the method of choice in the
presence of a hemodynamically relevant shunt and/or symptoms. In the presence of a superior sinus venous defect, the
anomalous pulmonary veins are redirected into the left atrium
using a patch closing the defect (Figures 20.12 and 20.13).

cava or the hepatic veins beneath the diaphragm (Figure
20.6). This syndrome is associated with various degrees of
right pulmonary artery branch hypoplasia and right lung
hypoplasia, anomalous blood supply from the systemic
arterial system to the right, and with or without pulmonary sequestration. Aortopulmonary collaterals to the
right lung may be present. The term was coined after the
name of the Turkish bent saber which CHD resembles on
the X-ray film.

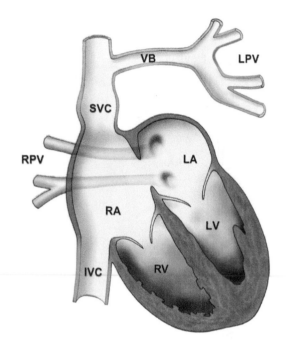

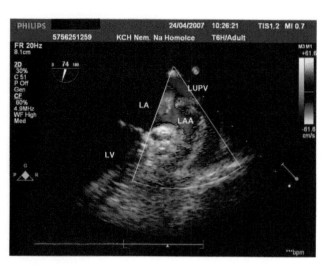

Figure 20.9
Transesophageal echo, 74 degrees, normal left upper pulmonary vein (LUPV) enters left atrium (LA). LAA, Left atrial auricle; LV, left ventricle.

Figure 20.7
Partial anomalous pulmonary venous connection, left pulmonary veins are connected via vena brachiocephalica (VB) with superior vena cava. Right pulmonary veins (RPV) are connected normally to left atrium (LA). RA, Right atrium; RV, right ventricle; LV, left ventricle; IVC, inferior vena cava.

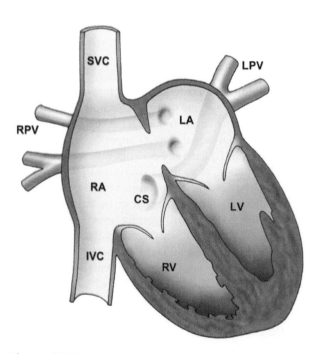

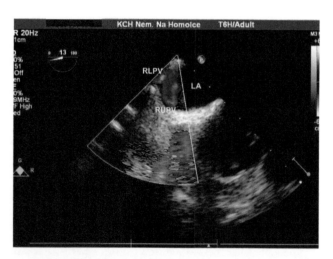

Figure 20.10
Transesophageal echo, 13 degrees, normal right upper (RUPV) and right lower pulmonary vein (RLPV) enter left atrium (LA).

Isolated partial anomalous connection of a single pulmonary vein without an atrial septal defect is usually not clinically relevant and can be left unoperated for follow-up. Natural history of patients with isolated PAPVC is usually excellent.

Total anomalous pulmonary venous connection

Total anomalous pulmonary venous connection (TAPVC) accounts for 0.8% of all CHD. The most frequently occurring

Figure 20.8
Partial anomalous pulmonary venous connection, left pulmonary veins (LPV) are connected to coronary sinus (CS), right pulmonary veins are connected normally to left atrium (LA). RA, Right atrium; RV, right ventricle; LV, left ventricle; SVC, superior vena cava; IVC, inferior vena cava.

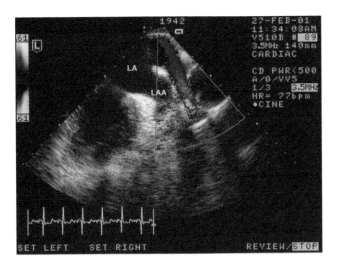

Figure 20.11
Normal left upper pulmonary vein (in red) entering left atrium (LA). LAA, Left atrial appendage.

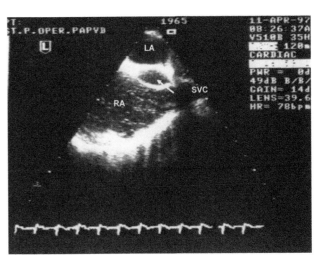

Figure 20.13
Transesophageal echo, longitudinal view, contrast echocardiography. Patient after operation of partial anomalous pulmonary venous connection; same patient as in Figure 20.12. After application of the contrast the left atrium (LA) as well as the tunnel derivation anomalous pulmonary vein (arrow) are without contrast. RA, Right atrium; SVC, superior vena cava.

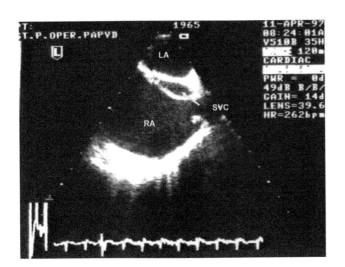

Figure 20.12
Transesophageal echo, longitudinal view. Patient after operation of partial anomalous pulmonary vein connection (PAPVC), redirection of PAPVC to the left atrium (LA) with pericardial tunnel (arrow) from superior vena cava (SVC). RA, Right atrium.

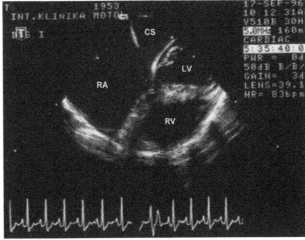

Figure 20.14
Transesophageal echo, transversal view. Adult patient with total anomalous pulmonary venous connection (mixed type), yet unoperated. Severely dilated coronary sinus (CS) with anomalous connection of the right pulmonary veins. The left pulmonary veins are connected to brachiocephalic vein and superior vena cava. RA, Dilated right atrium; RV, right ventricle; LV, left ventricle.

type is the supracardiac one (45% of TAPVC), whereby the pulmonary veins enter the ascending vertical vein draining into the brachiocephalic vein. With the cardiac type (25%), all pulmonary veins drain into the right atrium or the coronary sinus. With the infracardiac type (25%), the pulmonary veins enter jointly the hepatic veins, portal veins, or the inferior vena cava. The mixed type (5%) involves at least two of the above types.

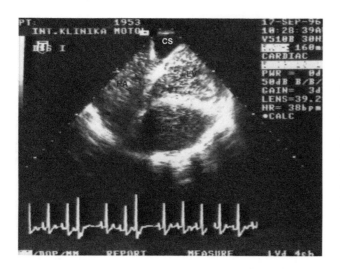

Figure 20.15

Transesophageal echo, transversal view. Adult patient with total anomalous pulmonary venous connection (mixed type), yet unoperated. Severely dilated coronary sinus (CS) with anomalous connection of the right pulmonary veins. The left pulmonary veins are connected to brachiocephalic vein and superior vena cava. After contrast injection into the left arm, the dilated right atrium (RA) and right ventricle (RV) are filled with contrast, as well as the left ventricle (LV). The left atrium and left ventricle are filled with contrast due to the existence of atrial septal defect. Only the dilated coronary sinus (CS) with the flow from right pulmonary veins stays without contrast.

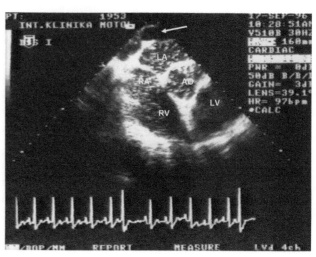

Figure 20.17

Transesophageal echo, transversal view; the same patient as in Figures 20.14–20.16, with unoperated total anomalous pulmonary venous connection. After application of the contrast agent, the left pulmonary veins, connected to brachiocephalic vein, stay without contrast (arrow). The other cardiac chambers are filled with contrast. LA, Left atrium; RA, right atrium; AO, aorta; RV, right ventricle; LV, left ventricle.

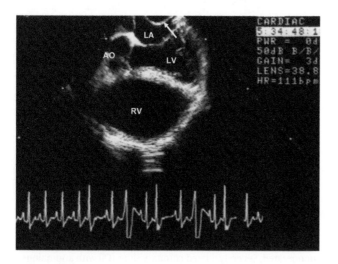

Figure 20.16

Transesophageal echo, transversal view; the same patient as in Figures 20.14 and 20.15. Adult patient with total anomalous pulmonary venous connection (mixed type), yet unoperated. Right pulmonary veins are connected to the coronary sinus, and left pulmonary veins are connected to brachiocephalic vein and superior vena cava. Arrow indicates the left pulmonary veins. LA, Left atrium; LV, left ventricle; RV, right ventricle; AO, aorta.

As a rule, TAPVC is associated with an atrial septal defect. Cyanosis, right ventricular dilatation and overload are present in these neonates who cannot survive in the absence of any additional shunt between the systemic and pulmonary circulation. The diagnosis is established using echocardiography and angiography. Adults with this CHD have been operated on in childhood. Rarely, we have seen patients with unoperated TAPVC surviving until adulthood (Figures 20.14–20.17). In this case, the defect must not be mistaken for a simple atrial septal defect, whose closure in TAPVC would entail circulatory collapse.

Patients with all the above defect types may develop pulmonary venous obstruction resulting in pulmonary edema. The defect is repaired surgically in the neonatal age. Operative mortality, presently <10%, was previously higher. Late postoperative complications include pulmonary venous restenoses.

Reference

1. Valdes-Cruz LM, Cayre LO. Echocardiographic Diagnosis of Congenital Heart Disease. An Embryologic and Anatomic Approach, 1st edn. Philadelphia, PA: Lippicott-Raven Publishers, 1999.

21

Psychosocial issues

Congenital heart disease (CHD) is one of the biggest success stories in medicine. However, health care givers have focused on medical, morphologic and hemodynamic problems, and have not adequately addressed psychosocial issues in patients with CHD. Indeed, health problems with limited exercise performance, recurrent hospital admission, interventions and operations, general anesthesia, cyanosis, absence from the family, friends and school, scar tissue, and other factors have an important impact on the psychosocial burden of adults with CHD.[1-3] Many children and adolescents were threatened by pain and even death during the excellent care provided by the pediatric health care givers. All stressors, including medical and psychological factors, act as a psychosocial injury or insult during childhood, and impact the psychosocial wellbeing and quality of life during adulthood.[4] Interestingly, the severity of the CHD seems to be marginally associated with patients' quality of life, and patients with CHD perceive their quality of life to be better than their peers.[5,6]

Adults with CHD have had the defect since childhood, so their mental state is often very vulnerable and different to that of cardiac patients who develop their defect in adulthood. Adults with CHD may feel unjustly ill-fated; occasionally, they may feel it is the physicians not helping them enough who are in fact responsible for their condition.

As adults with CHD have been physically affected since childhood, they are often faced with hyperprotective care on the part of their parents. As the adolescents mature, they must learn to take care of their heart and responsibility for their health. The periods of adolescence and early adulthood carry multiple risks:

- Inappropriate transition from the pediatric to the adult health care system.
- A change in the place of residence, loss of 'supervision' by their parents, and an effort not to be different from their peers may result in loss from regular follow-up by an adult cardiologist.
- A change in the place of residence and the general practitioner/family physician may involve loss of medical records including surgical reports.
- Children undergoing surgery in childhood are considered cured and the children or parents disregard the possibility of any residual findings, complications or even reoperation. Adults with CHD surgery during childhood are neither cured nor fixed, their hearts are only repaired.
- The patients do not get adequate information from their parents or pediatric cardiologists about future development and prognosis of their CHD, or of which situations carry a risk and, conversely, which activities and the extent of such activities they can practice without any worries.
- The level of risk of CHD or postoperative residual findings may be underrated, or even missed, by an adult cardiologist who does not have an adequate level of training and expertise, particularly in the presence of inconspicuous symptoms in young age.
- Conversely, the level of risk of CHD may be overrated by an adult cardiologist who may tend to advise their patients with nonsignificant CHD against practicing sports or becoming pregnant.
- An adult cardiologist may not have the necessary time and patience to take proper care of a patient with CHD.

Non-compliance may be a major problem in young adults with CHD during the transition from adolescence to adulthood. They can ignore the importance of regular follow-up visits, or even the importance of medications and meticulous surveillance of therapy (e.g. anticoagulants).

Social integration of adults with CHD is crucial. Partially or fully disabled patients who have retired because of serious CHD need to continue regular contact with their peers. As regards the prevention of depression and of social disintegration, it is critical to offer the patient an opportunity to perform work which is not physically vigorous, with adequate time for breaks and rest, and which does not require the patient to travel long distances from their home. The presence of depression was associated with unemployment in adults with CHD, and persisting cyanosis.[7]

Patients with CHD are successfully engaging in full adult responsibilities and roles, but they do experience specific psychosocial challenges that may impact emotional functioning, self-perception, and peer relationships. Lifestyle considerations in young adulthood are significant, and impinge on pregnancy considerations and exercise capabilities. Clinical management strategies include increased awareness and dialogue between patients with CHD and physicians regarding psychosocial concerns.[8] A clinical psychologist with a commitment to adults with CHD is a key pillar to provide comprehensive care.[9]

References

1. Van Rijen EH, Utens EM, Roos-Hesselink JW et al. Medical predictors for psychopathology in adults with operated congenital heart disease. Eur Heart J 2004; 25: 1605–13.
2. Van Rijen EH, Utens EM, Roos-Hesselink JW et al. Longitudinal development of psychopathology in an adult congenital heart disease cohort. Int J Cardiol 2005; 99: 315–23.
3. Van Rijen EH, Utens EM, Roos-Hesselink JW et al. Psychosocial functioning of the adult with congenital heart disease: A 20–33 years follow-up. Eur Heart J 2003; 24: 673–83.
4. Moons P, Van Deyk K, Marquet K, Raes E et al. Individual quality of life in adults with congenital heart disease: A paradigm shift. Eur Heart J 2005; 26: 298–307.
5. Moons P, Van Deyk K, De Geest S, Gewilling M, Budts W. Is the severity of congenital heart disease associated with the quality of life and perceived health of adult patients? Heart 2005; 91: 1193–8.
6. Moons P, Van Deyk K, De Bleser L et al. Quality of life and health status in adults with congenital heart disease: A direct comparison with healthy counterparts. Eur J Cardiovasc Prev Rehabil 2006; 13: 407–13.
7. Popelová J, Slavík Z, Škovránek J. Are cyanosed adults with congenital cardiac malformation depressed? Cardiol Young 2001; 11: 379–84.
8. Kovacs AH, Sears SF, Saidi AS. Biopsychosocial experiences of adults with congenital heart disease: Review of the literature. Am Heart J 2005; 150: 193–201.
9. Kovacs AH, Silversides C, Saidi A, Sears SF. The role of the psychologist in adult congenital heart disease. Cardiol Clin 2006; 24: 607–18.

22

Cardiac injury during surgery in childhood

Adults with congenital heart diseases (CHD) often underwent surgery while children, often decades previously. Surgical techniques, including myocardial protection, have a major impact on long-term residuae and sequelae. The surgical approach to treat the different types of CHD has been modified ever since. Surgical skills and techniques continue to improve, operative techniques and procedures change and evolve, and the body of experience with individual types of surgery grows. Therefore, on long-term follow-up of adults with CHD, the physician must bear in mind the period when the patient had surgery as well as the possibility of intraoperative injury to the heart. The latter may occasionally take some time to manifest itself.

- Surgery in childhood often results in *pericardial adhesions*. These may cause problems during reoperation, and may also contribute to diastolic ventricular dysfunction and render cardiac chamber dilatation impossible. The pericardium may become markedly thickened or, alternatively, calcified, and begin to show signs of constriction. The diagnosis is established by echocardiography and catheterization; with pericardial thickness potentially assessed by computerized tomography (CT) and magnetic resonance imaging (MRI).
- Operation of CHD may result in *conduction system injury* with subsequent development of bundle branch block (most often, right bundle branch block and/or left anterior hemiblock), or complete atrioventricular block. Because of anatomical arrangement, the risk of damage to the conduction system is highest with extensive ventricular septal defect, congenitally corrected transposition of the great arteries, and with atrioventricular septal defects.
- *Coronary arteries* may become damaged if featuring an atypical course or when they are poorly visible, e.g. during reoperation with pericardial adhesions. Iatrogenic dissection of a coronary artery will be shown by echocardiography as an akinesia or aneurysm in the region supplied by the artery in question and QS patterns on electrocardiogram (ECG). In bizarre ECG in CHD, the abnormal QS pattern may be mistaken for a conduction disturbance and not a sign of necrosis (Figure 22.1).
- *Right-heart ventriculotomy* involves the dissection of longitudinal myofibers of the right ventricle, which are important for the systolic right ventricular function. The

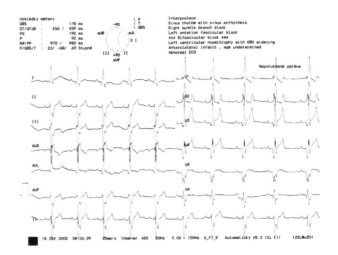

Figure 22.1
Electrocardiogram (ECG) in a patient after intracardiac repair of tetralogy of Fallot in childhood. Sinus rhythm, right bundle branch block, QRS waves of 178 ms, left anterior hemiblock, and right ventricular hypertrophy. Besides, there are pathological Q waves (QS) in the antero-lateral region (V4–V6) due to the operative injury of the left anterior descending coronary artery (ramus interventricularis anterior) with apical aneurysm of the left ventricle according echocardiography.

sequelae may take years to manifest themselves, especially during increased right ventricular workload.
- Areas with abnormal electrophysiological properties may form around the *scars and patches*, and, because of slow conduction, may result in the development of re-entry circuits and *tachydysrhythmias*. These areas tend to develop after extensive procedures involving the atria such as Mustard or Senning operation, Fontan procedure, or after repair of tetralogy of Fallot.
- *Myocardial injury* may also be due to inadequate cardioplegic protection of the myocardium, a prolonged surgical procedure and perioperative hypotension. In addition, many of our adults with CHD were cyanotic for many years during childhood, with subsequent ischemia/hypoxia of the myocardium, necrosis and fibrosis. These may be morphologic substrates for arrhythmias during adulthood.

23

Terminology remarks

Segmental analysis

A systematic approach to morphological description of congenital heart diseases (CHD), particularly complex CHD. The heart is considered in three segments: the atrial segment, the ventricular segment and the arterial segment. The philosophy of segmental analysis is founded on morphology. The chambers are recognized according to their morphology (leftness or rightness) rather than their position. Each chamber has its intrinsic morphologic features irrespective of location or distortion of malformation.

Rightness and leftness

Intrinsic morphologic features determine rightness or leftness.

Atria: Rightness and leftness of the atria are determined by the morphology of the atrial appendages. The morphological right atrial appendage has a broad base and a triangular shape; the morphological left atrial appendage has a narrow entrance and is hook-shaped. In addition, the right atrium has a terminal crest, which is an embryologic remnant of the right-sided sinus venosus valve; the left atrium has no terminal crest.

Lungs: The morphology of the lungs is determined by the position of the pulmonary arteries to their adjacent bronchi; the morphology of the lungs is *not* determined by the number of lobes. In the morphological right lung, the right pulmonary artery travels anteriorly to the adjacent (right upper) bronchus; in the morphological left lung, the left pulmonary artery travels posteriorly to the adjacent (left upper) bronchus. In general, a morphological right lung has three lobes and a morphological left lung has two lobes; a morphological right bronchus is shorter and more vertically oriented, and a morphological left bronchus is longer and more horizontally placed.

Situs solitus

Normal position of the viscera with the liver on the right. The cardiac situs is determined by the position of the morphological right atrium. In the presence of situs solitus, the morphological right atrium is on the right of the morphological left atrium, and the morphological right lung is on the right and the morphological left lung on the left. Usually, cardiac and abdominal situs are concordant.

Situs inversus

Inverse position of the viscera: the anatomical right atrium (right atrial appendage) is on the left to the left atrium, the morphological right lung and the liver are on the left side. This is a mirror-like image of situs solitus.

Situs ambiguus, visceral heterotaxy syndrome

The situs is indeterminate in the setting of isomerism (bilateral visceroatrial symmetry), there is either left isomerism or right isomerism. Isomerism describes a paired, mirror-image set of normally single or nonidentical organ systems (atria, lungs, viscera) and is frequently associated with other abnormalities. This condition occurs in about 2–4% of all CHD.

Right isomerism (asplenia syndrome)

Characterized by paired morphologically right structures: absence of the spleen (asplenia), symmetrical placement of the liver on the right and left sides (transverse liver), bilateral right (trilobed) lungs including bilateral right bronchi, and bilateral right atria. Complex CHD is usually present: common atrium, atrioventricular (AV) septal defects (complete AV septal defect, more than half of cases present with univentricular AV connection – double inlet ventricle); bilateral superior vena cava (left-sided superior vena cava may empty into the coronary sinus), if present; the inferior vena cava is usually not dissected and the hepatic veins drain directly into the atria. Total anomalous pulmonary venous connection to the systemic veins can be frequently seen; bilateral sinus node may be present.

Left isomerism (polysplenia syndrome)

Characterized by paired morphologically left structures: multiple spleens (polysplenia), whereby multiple accessory spleens are localized on the right and left sides; a symmetrical liver is placed in the midline (transverse liver), bilateral left bronchi and lung (the lungs and the tracheobronchial tree resemble the left lung with two lobes and morphologically left main bronchi on both sides), and two morphological left atria. Complex CHD is present: complete or partial AV septal defects, right ventricular outflow tract obstruction, etc. A typical feature of left isomerism is an interrupted inferior vena cava continuing via the azygos or hemiazygos venous system into the left- or right-sided superior vena cava. The hepatic veins may empty separately into the atria. The pulmonary veins empty into both atria. Sinus node may be absent.

Cardiac position

This term describes the position of the heart within the chest with regard to its location and the orientation of its apex. *Cardiac location* (e.g. levoposition, mesoposition, dextroposition): This describes the location of the heart within the chest, and is dependent of many factors including cardiac malformation, abnormalities of mediastinal and thoracic structures, tumors, kyphoscoliosis, etc. *Cardiac orientation*: This describes the axis between the base of the heart and the apex. Levocardia, apex directed to the left of the midline; dextrocardia, apex directed to the right of the midline; mesocardia, axis in the midline. Cardiac orientation (base to apex axis) is independent of the cardiac situs, position of the ventricles or great arteries.

Concordance

Appropriate connection between two structures (e.g. right atrium to right ventricle; right ventricle to pulmonary artery).

Discordance

Inappropriate connection between two structures. For example, AV discordance describes an inappropriate connection between the right atrium and left ventricle, while ventriculo-arterial discordance denotes that the pulmonary artery arises from a morphological left ventricle and that the aorta arises from a morphological right ventricle (synonym: double discordance or congenitally corrected transposition of the great arteries).

Morphological left or right ventricle

The term identifies the ventricle by its morphological features, not by its right- or leftward placement.

Erythrocytosis

A secondary increase in erythrocyte count in the presence of hypoxemia due to a right-to-left shunt in cyanotic CHD, or due to chronic pulmonary disease. This is a physiological adaptive mechanism, improperly also termed polyglobulia or polycythemia. It should be distinguished from polycythemia vera, which is a neoplastic transformation of all three blood cell lines associated with increased numbers of cells in the peripheral blood.

Atrioventricular valve 'straddling'

Straddling describes anomalous insertion of tendinous cords of papillary muscle to the contralateral ventricle (a ventricular septal defect is required). Of importance for surgical repair of defects.

Overriding

Overriding describes a malignment of the annulus of a semilunar or AV valve relative to the ventricular septum. Important for CHD nomenclature. For example, overriding of the aorta by <50%, tetralogy of Fallot; overriding by >50%, double-outlet right ventricle.

Restrictive defect

A small defect restricting free flow of blood from one ventricle to the other, which poses an obstruction to blood flow thus allowing the maintenance of a pressure gradient between the right and left ventricles.

Nonrestrictive defect

A defect allowing free mixing of blood without the maintenance of a pressure gradient between the ventricles, with balanced right and left ventricular pressure.

Note

For more definitions and terms (by Colman J, Oechslin E, Taylor D), visit http://www.achd-online.com/consensus/glossary.html

Index

Printed and bound by CPI Group (UK) Ltd, Croydon, CR0 4YY

23/10/2024

01778251-0019